ESSENTIALS OF EXERCISE PHYSIOLOGY

Larry G. Shaver

George Peabody College for Teachers
Vanderbilt University
Nashville, Tennessee

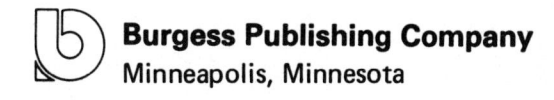

Burgess Publishing Company
Minneapolis, Minnesota

Artwork: Genesis 2 Inc. Nashville, Tennessee
Illustration and Cover Art: Genesis 2 Inc. Nashville, Tennessee
Cover Design: Priscilla Golz

Copyright © 1981 by Larry G. Shaver
Printed in the United States of America
Library of Congress Catalog Number 80-67145
ISBN 0-8087-4200-0

Burgess Publishing Company
7108 Ohms Lane
Minneapolis, Minnesota 55435

All rights reserved. No part of this book may be reproduced in any form whatsoever, by photograph or mimeograph or by any other means, by broadcasting or transmission, by translation into any kind of language, nor by recording electronically or otherwise, without permission in writing from the copyright holder, except by a reviewer, who may quote brief passages in critical articles and reviews.

J I H G F E D C

To my wife, JoAnn C. Shaver,
and children, Sherry Lynn and Laurie Ann

PREFACE

This book, *Essentials of Exercise Physiology,* is designed primarily for use as a basic text for undergraduate physical education students who are taking their first course in exercise physiology. The dominating purpose of this book is to provide the reader with the basic fundamentals necessary to the understanding of exercise physiology. A secondary purpose has been to approach this body of knowledge from a theoretical as well as a practical point of view by integrating and showing direct application to the concepts found in the research laboratory to the more practical problems that occur on the athletic field or in the gymnasia.

It is assumed that the student has some basic knowledge of anatomy and general physiology. At the same time, an attempt has been made to present the subject in terms that will not require an extensive background in physics, chemistry, or mathematics. Yet, the author has tried to maintain a completely scientific attitude throughout, hoping to leave the reader with as few vague generalizations as possible. Thus, those students who aspire to be athletic coaches will certainly find within the pages the scientific basis for their profession.

The book should be viewed as three related sections. Chapters 1 through 6 deal with the general effects of exercise on specific body systems and organs. Chapters 7 through 10 are directed at what are considered important problems in exercise and sport physiology today. Chapters 11 through 14 are intended as a synthesis. The purpose of these chapters is to apply the material of the foregoing chapters to specific topics. Chapters 11, 12, and 13 deal with the female, preadolescent, and elderly, respectively. Since the woman has played a leading role in recent years in all areas of sport, it was felt that a significant contribution in the field of exercise physiology would be to present the most recent physiological as well as anatomical findings concerning the female and compare these results with her male counterpart. In addition, since the number of participants taking part in competitive preadolescent sports (such as little league baseball, Pop Warner football, track and field, swimming, soccer, basketball, ice hockey, etc.) has grown tremendously in the past few years, and since much has been written (pros and cons) concerning their effects on the growth and development of the young participant, it was also felt that an important contribution would be to report on what is scientifically known concerning the effects of competitive sports on the normal growth and development of the preadolescent. And, with the population trend now moving toward one of older people, and with the popularity of recreation and age-group competition growing by leaps and bounds along with the fact that more and more senior citizens are now being used as subjects in research projects, it was felt that an important as well as significant contribution would be to present the latest physiological findings concerning the elderly in terms of the changes that accompany the aging process along with the specific training adaptations in the aged.

Finally, it is the writer's opinion that no exercise physiology textbook would be complete without a chapter on physical conditioning. Chapter 14 has been written primarily to provide sound information concerning the basic scientific principles and guidelines for constructing an effective general-type physical conditioning program. While it is beyond the scope of this book to get into discussion concerning specific training programs for specific sports, it is hoped that the information presented in this chapter can be of some benefit for the interested coach and player in developing an effective conditioning program for their particular sport or event.

In selection of the material for this book, an attempt has been made to meet the modern needs of the student in physical education. On the other hand, exercise physiology and more recently, sport physiology are such rapidly advancing sciences, that it is impossible to review all the current literature in a small book. The references cited at the end of each chapter include a sufficient number of recent papers to indicate important trends, and to suggest the sources of information that will enable the interested student to continue his education.

The author wishes to express his appreciation to the many students and colleagues who, in direct and indirect ways, have contributed to the writing of this book.

Larry G. Shaver

CONTENTS

1 **THE SKELETAL MUSCLE AND EXERCISE**   1
    Key Concepts to Be Gained from This Chapter   1
    Structure   2
    Muscle Fiber Types   4
    The Contractile Process: Sliding Filament Theory   8
    Energy for Contraction   11
    Summary   11
    Review References   12

2 **EXERCISE, ENERGY, AND METABOLISM**   13
    Key Concepts to Be Gained from This Chapter   13
    Definitions   14
    Sources of Energy   17
    Summary   45
    Review References   49

3 **THE RESPIRATORY SYSTEM AND EXERCISE**   50
    Key Concepts to Be Gained from This Chapter   50
    Structural Properties of the Lungs   51
    The Respiratory Muscles   52
    Regulation of Respiration   54
    Lung Ventilation Response to Exercise   58
    Gaseous Exchange   62
    Gaseous Transport   65
    Acids and Bases and Their Regulation   70
    Summary   71
    Review References   72

4 **THE HEART AND EXERCISE**   74
    Key Concepts to Be Gained from This Chapter   74
    Structural Properties of the Heart   74
    The Cardiac Cycle   79

Cardiac Output 81
Heart Rate 83
Stroke Volume 87
Cardiac Hypertrophy 90
The Electrocardiogram (ECG) 91
Summary 91
Review References 93

5 THE SYSTEMIC CIRCULATION AND EXERCISE 94
Key Concepts to Be Gained from This Chapter 94
Structural Properties of the Systemic Circulatory System 94
Hemodynamics: Physical Laws Governing Blood Flow 99
Regulation of Blood Flow During Rest and Exercise 101
Blood Pressure and Blood Flow Resistance Responses to Exercise 102
Summary 108
Review References 109

6 NEURAL CONTROL OF SKELETAL MUSCLE ACTIVITY 110
Key Concepts to Be Gained from This Chapter 110
Excitation of Contraction 112
The Synapse 113
Motor Units 115
The Chemical Transmitter 117
Voluntary Control of Muscular Activity 117
Involuntary Control of Muscular Activity 120
Reaction Time and Movement Time 126
Cross-Education 128
Summary 129
Review References 130

7 EXERCISE AND TEMPERATURE REGULATIONS IN HOT AND COLD CLIMATES 132
Key Concepts to Be Gained from This Chapter 132
Balance Between Heat Loss and Heat Production 133
Heat Gain 135
Regulation of Body Temperature 135
Temperature Measurement 136
Age 138
Sex 138
Diurnal Changes 138
Individual Differences 139
Exercise and Temperature Regulations in Hot Climates 139
Effects of Extreme Heat 143
Heat Acclimatization 144
Making Weight for Wrestlers 146
Exercise and Temperature Regulations in Cold Climates 148
Summary 151
Review References 153

8 EXERCISE AND ALTITUDE   155
Key Concepts to Be Gained from This Chapter   155
Effects of High Altitude on Physical Performance   156
Physiological Adaptations to Altitude   157
Altitude Training and Conditioning   161
Mountain (or Altitude) Sickness   164
Summary   165
Review References   166

9 NUTRITION, WEIGHT CONTROL AND PERFORMANCE   167
Key Concepts to Be Gained from This Chapter   167
General Nutrients of the Diet   168
Daily Food Requirements   174
The Essential Food Groups   176
Spacing and Number of Meals   177
Pre-Game Meal   177
Diet and Performance   178
Weight Control and Exercise   183
Body Composition   185
Methods for Assessing Body Composition   188
Determining Your Desired Weight   195
Summary   195
Review References   198

10 ERGOGENIC AIDS IN EXERCISE AND SPORTS   200
Key Concepts to Be Gained from This Chapter   200
Alcohol   201
Alkalies   201
Amphetamines   202
Anabolic Steroids   203
Aspartic Acid Salts   204
Blood Doping   205
Caffeine   205
Diet   206
Oxygen   206
Salt (Sodium Chloride)   207
Tobacco Smoking   208
Water   208
Summary   209
Review References   210

11 SEX DIFFERENCES IN EXERCISE   211
Key Concepts to Be Gained from This Chapter   211
Structural Characteristics   211
Physiological Characteristics   216
Gynecological Factors   222
Effects of Training and Athletic Competition on Pregnancy, Childbirth, and the Postpartum Period   223

Femininity 224
Female Injuries in Sports 225
Female Response to Stress 225
Trainability of the Female 226
Performance Comparisons in World Records (Male vs Female) 226
Summary 228
Review References 229

12 THE PREADOLESCENT AND COMPETITIVE SPORTS 230
Key Concepts to Be Gained from This Chapter 230
Growth and Development 231
Injury 236
Guidelines for Competitive Sports for the Preadolescent 238
Summary 239
Review References 240

13 AGING AND EXERCISE 242
Key Concepts to Be Gained from This Chapter 242
Physiological Changes Accompanying the Aging Process 243
Training Adaptation in the Aged 246
Basic Principles and Guidelines for Constructing an Individualized Cardiorespiratory Endurance Exercise Program for the Aged 247
Summary 251
Review References 252

14 PHYSICAL CONDITIONING 253
Key Concepts to Be Gained from This Chapter 253
General Principles of Physical Training 254
Development of Muscular Strength and Local Endurance 257
Factors Affecting Strength and Local Endurance 265
Retention of Muscular Strength and Local Endurance 266
Development of Aerobic and Anaerobic Endurance 267
Muscular Fatigue 281
Summary 283
Review References 285

APPENDIXES 287
A Units of Measure 287
B STPD 289
C BTPS 291

GLOSSARY 292

1
THE SKELETAL MUSCLE AND EXERCISE

KEY CONCEPTS TO BE GAINED FROM THIS CHAPTER

(1) The human body consists of three different types of muscles: skeletal (voluntary), cardiac (involuntary), and smooth (involuntary).

(2) Skeletal muscle fibers are identified according to their twitch contraction time.

(3) Fast-twitch muscle fibers are better suited for anaerobic work while slow-twitch fibers are better suited for aerobic work.

(4) Myofibrils are the contractile elements of sketetal muscle.

(5) The most immediate chemical source of energy for muscular contraction is ATP (adenosine triphosphate).

(6) The interaction of actin and myosin protein filaments by way of "cross bridges" plays an important role in the "sliding filament" theory of muscular contraction.

The primary physiological outcome in exercise is contraction of skeletal muscle. The human organism has over 600 muscles and a total of more than 6 billion muscle fibers dispensed among them. The main differnce in size between a small muscle in the foot and a larger muscle like the gastronemius of the lower leg is in the number of individual fibers in the muscle bundle. Although a muscle fiber is microscopically thin, it is very strong and can support one thousand times its own weight. During contraction, a muscle becomes shorter and thicker. In fact, some muscles can be contracted to approximately half their length as relaxed muscles.

There are three different types of muscles in the human body. When we talk about muscles used in weight lifting, swimming, jogging, etc., we mean *skeletal* muscles since they are attached to a part of the skeleton. Skeletal muscles are under almost complete voluntary control. The other types of muscle are *cardiac,* which is accountable for the pumping action of the heart, and *smooth,* which is concerned with movements of internal organs such as those of the stomach, intestines, visceral, and blood vessels. Both the smooth and cardiac muscle fall into the involuntry category of muscle over which there is no direct conscious control. Because the field of exercise physiology is primarily concerned with movement and external work, the remainder of this chapter will be devoted entirely to a discussion of the skeletal muscle, rather than smooth or cardiac muscle. The latter, however will receive special attention in Chapter 4.

I. STRUCTURE

A skeletal muscle consists of about 40% of the body weight. As the name implies, they are attached to the bony skeleton and are responsible for limb movement, etc. The units of skeletal muscle are long cylindrical muscle fibers which vary in length from 1 to 40 mm, and in diameter from 10 to 100 microns (1 micron is equal to 0.001 mm). Although the number of muscle fibers per muscle may vary somewhat depending upon the size and function of each muscle, it appears that by the time an embryo reaches a fetus stage of between 4 and 5 months of age, the actual number of muscle fibers per muscle is already established. Thus, the capability for an individual obtaining muscularity is apparently set genetically at the time of conception.

Each muscle fiber is composed of many smaller units called *myofibrils,* which lie parallel in the *sarcoplasm* muscle cell fluid similar to the intracellular fluid of other cells). Myofibrils are the contractile elements of the muscles, and they range from 1 to 2 microns in diameter (Fig. 1-1). Each muscle fiber is surrounded by a thin elastic noncellular membrane called the *sarcolemma.* The muscle fibers are contained in bundles by sheaths of connective tissue (*epimysium*) and groups of the bundles are again contained in yet tougher sheaths *(perimysium).* The various connective tissue sheaths spread throughout the whole muscle and they are structurally blended with the tendons, by which the muscle is connected to the bones of the particular joint it moves.

Under the electron microscope, the myofibrils appear as alternate light (I band) and dark (A band) areas (Fig. 1-1). Each myofibril consist of fine protein threads (myofilaments) called *actin* and *myosin*. The actin filament contains two important proteins called *troponin* and *tropomyosin,* while the myosin filament contains small protein projections called *cross bridges* (Fig. 1-1 and 1-4). Tropomyosin is a long, narrow molecule located on the surface of the actin filament with its ends fixed firmly in globular molecules of troponin. Along with the actin filaments, the cross bridges play an important part in the contraction mechanism, as will be seen subsequently. The light bands (I) arise where there is only one protein, whereas the dark bands (A) arise where both actin and myosin strands are found.

The area in the center of each A band is a less dense region called the H zone. Each I band is halved by a dark line called the Z line or Z membrane. The Z lines lend stability to the entire structure. They may also play a major part in the relaying of nerve impulses from the sarcolemma to the myofibrils. Thus, every myofibril is made up of units that encompass all elements between two Z lines. Each unit is called a *sarcomere* and is approximately 2 microns in length. The sarcomeres repeat themselves in a specific pattern in each myofibril. During relaxation, each A band is about 1.4 microns long, while the I band is approximately half this length.

The myofibrils are closely connected with an intracellular system referred to as the *sarcotubular system.* The system is composed of two distinct and separate types of tubules (both performing a somewhat separate function) called the *transverse* or *T-tubules* (T-system) and the *longitudinal* or *sarcoplasmic reticulum tubules* (Fig. 1-2). The system contains two sarcoplasmic reiticulum tubules which are fixed firmly in the A and I bands. These in turn surround the transverse or T-tubules which crosses into a myofibril alongside the Z line. The transverse tubule is a

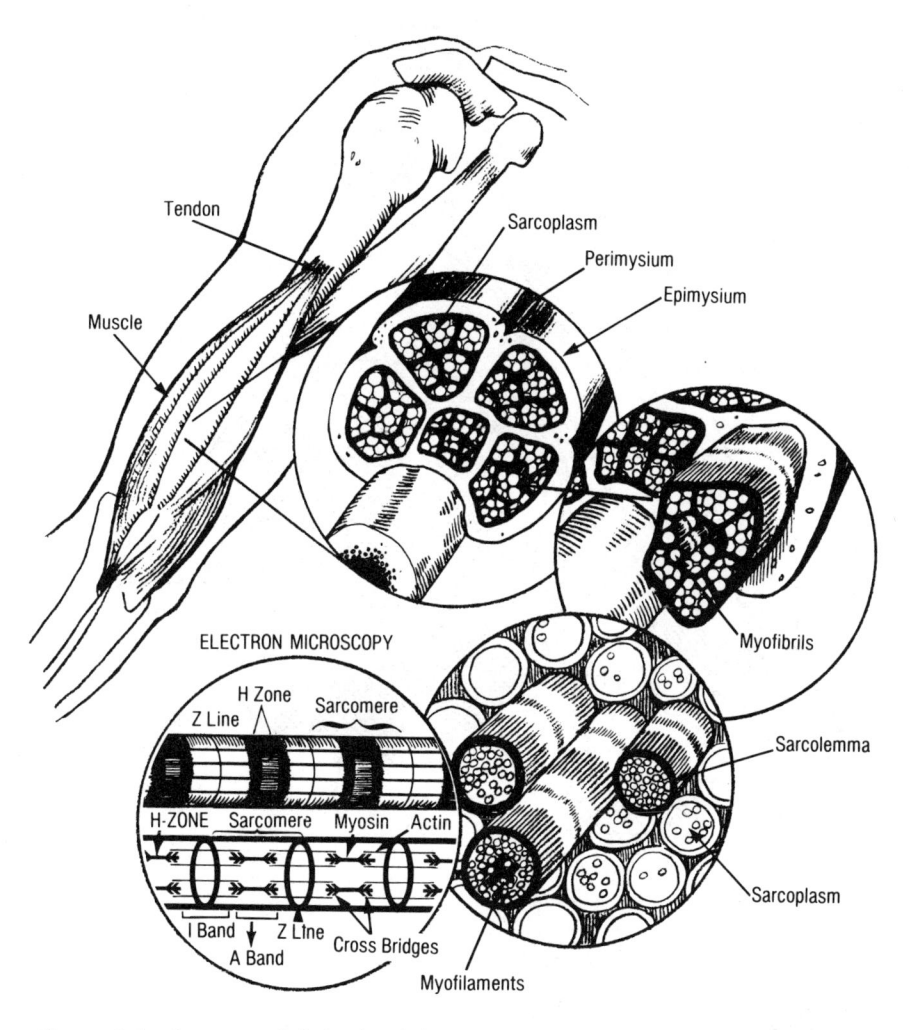

Figure 1-1 Structure of skeletal muscle.

small tubule that runs transversely through the muscle fiber between two layer channels referred to as *terminal cisternae*. At one point in the structure (the Z line area of the sarcomere), a transverse tubule comes together with two parts of the sarcoplasmic reticulum to form a *triad*. The ends of the transverse tubules open to the outside of the fiber and provides a pass by which the wave of electrical excitation can travel. The sarcoplasmic reticulum, on the other hand, does not come into contact with the cell membrane nor with the T-system. But instead, its terminal cisternae ends bind calcium (the muscle activating substance) where it can be readily discharged upon arrival of the wave of excitation. A more detailed discussion of the excitation of contraction may be found in a later chapter.

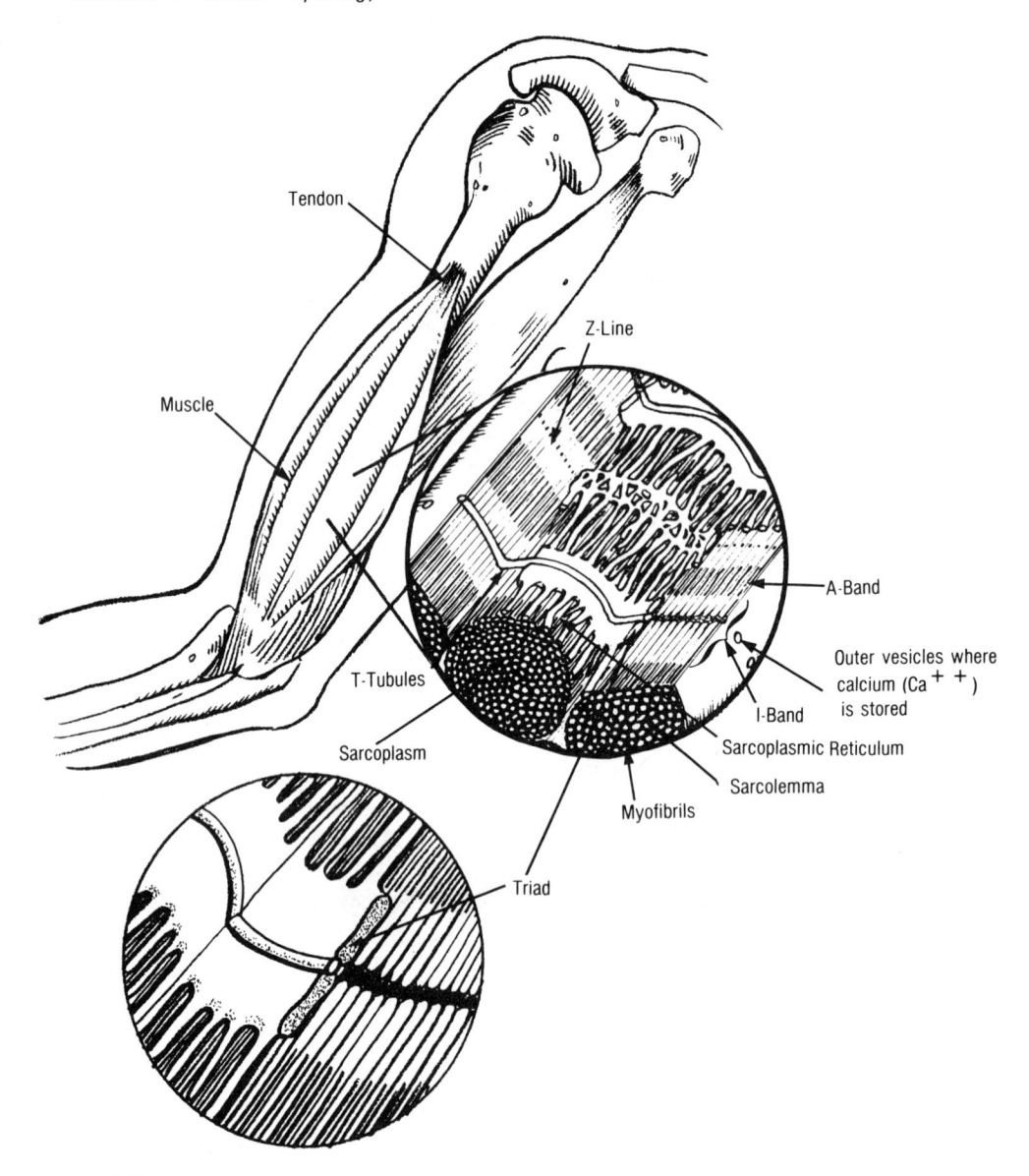

Figure 1-2 Structure of the sarcotubular system.

II. MUSCLE FIBER TYPES

A. SLOW (ST) AND FAST (FT) TWITCH MUSCLE FIBERS

All skeletal muscle fibers of humans and animals are not exactly the same. For instance, even though all fibers are able to carry out work under both anaerobic and aerobic situations, some are better prepared to perform anaerobically while others are better prepared to perform aerobically.

In humans, while the two main types of skeletal muscle fiber have been traditionally called *red* and *white*, researchers have recently insisted that it would be more relevant to identify the skeletal fibers according to their twitch contraction time. For example, if a muscle fiber finishes a contraction quickly, it is referred to as a *Type II* or *fast twitch (FT)* fiber as opposed to a *Type I* or *slow twitch (ST)* fiber who has a slow contraction time.

The ST fibers predominate in the postural, extensor muscles of the trunk and limbs, whereas the FT fibers predominate in flexor muscles which are better for making short, high-intensity contractions. Thus, ST fibers are better suited for submaximal endurance type activities that demand repetitive contractions over a long period of time such as long distance running and swimming, cross-country skiing, rowing, canoeing, and cycling. On the other hand, FT fibers are better adapted for explosive type exercises such as a weight-lifter lifting weights, a sprinter running a 100-meter dash, a high jumper and pole vaulter in the field events, or quick movements in team sports such as football, basketball, baseball, lacrosse, and soccer.

There are several reasons, as illustrated in Table 1-1, why ST fibers are better suited for long endurance type exercises (aerobic work) and FT fibers are used more for speed or power activities (anaerobic work). First of all, the FT fibers have high myosin ATPase activity and high glycolytic enzyme activity in comparison to the ST fibers. Since the splitting of *ATP (adenosine triphosphate* which is the most immediate chemical source of energy for muscular contraction) to release energy for muscular contraction is due to myosin ATPase activity, it is easy to understand how a higher level of myosin ATPase activity could bring about quicker contraction times. Because of the high glycolytic enzyme activity of *glycogen phosphorylase* and *phosphofructokinase* of the FT fibers, they are well equipped to handle rapid contractions where aerobic ATP production is unable to keep up with the ATP requirements of the working muscles such as during a 100-meter sprint. Note that glycogen phosphorylase and phosphofructokinase both have important functions in that they regulate the breakdown of glycogen and glucose to lactic acid, whereas the breakdown of glycogen and glucose are important for anaerobic ATP productions. More will be said about the splitting of ATP's in muscular contraction later in this chapter.

Table 1-1. Some Physiological Characteristics of Fast and Slow Twitch Muscle Fibers

	Fiber Type	
Physiological Characteristics	Fast(FT)	Slow(ST)
Short, Explosive-Type Exercises (Anaerobic)		
Myosin ATPase activity	High	Low
Glycolytic enzyme activity of glycogen phosphorylase and phosphofructokinase	High	Low
Long Endurance-Type Exercises (Aerobic)		
Mitochondrial enzyme activity of the Krebs cycle, the fatty acid oxidation cycle, and the electron transport system	Low	High
Myoglobin content	Low	High
Stores of intracellular fat	Low	High
Capillary density	Low	High

In addition, ST fibers are better suited for aerobic type work since they contain not only a greater sum of *mitochondrial* (aerobic ATP producing enzymes of the Krebs Cycle, the fatty acid oxidation cycle, and the electron transport system), but they also have a greater amount of *myoglobin*. Myoglobin is a red pigment which closely resembles hemoglobin both in its ability to combine with oxygen as well as in its chemical structure. Another advantage that ST fibers have for long duration exercise is that they tend to have larger stores of intracellular fat that can be summoned for energy when needed than is true for FT fibers. Finally, the density of the capillary network is more developed around the ST fibers which permits oxygen, glucose and fatty acids to be transported to these fibers quicker.

It is interesting to note that while the ST fibers are better adapted and are used preferentially in long, hard duration type exercise, as these fibers become tired and fatigued, the FT fibers may also be called into action to help out. In fact, with long extended work, both fiber types may actually become fatigued.

B. FIBER DISTRIBUTION AND PERFORMANCE

As indicated earlier, the human skeletal muscles have a mixture of slow (ST) and fast (FT) twitch fibers. While the range of fiber mixtures is relatively wide (ranging from 40 to 87 per cent for FT and 13 to 60 per cent for ST), biopsy* research has shown that there are specific muscles that are regarded as having predominantly either ST or FT fibers. For instance, the soleus, semitendinosus, vastus lateralis, rectus abdominis, and rectus femoris are just a few that contain a large percentage of ST fibers. At the same time, the biceps brachii, deltoid, gastrocnemius, and latissimus dorsi are a few that have high levels of FT fibers.

Investigations have also shown a rather interesting relationship between specific fiber types and certain athletic abilities. For example, world class sprinters are characterized by high percentages (up to around 74%) of FT fibers in their leg muscles, while at the same time, world class distance runners possess a much higher level of ST fibers (up to around 75%) in their leg muscles than normal proportion for untrained subjects. Biopsy studies also show that swimmers, bicyclists, and canoeists, when compared to untrained subjects, tend to possess a high percentage (between 60 and 70 per cent) of ST fibers in their shoulder muscles (see Fig. 1-3). The average proportion of ST fibers in the thigh and shoulder muscles for untrained subjects is around 35 and 45 per cent, respectively.

While it would appear that muscle fiber composition may play an important part in determining championship performance, an important question that needs to be answered is what effect does training have on an individuals inherited muscle fiber population. Is an individual's percentage composition of fibers in a certain muscle genetically limited or can training alter the fiber composition? Studies have shown that only the capacities and size of the fibers increase as the result of training and not the number or twitch contraction times. In other words, with endurance training, both fiber types become better suited for producing ATP for aerobic work, while at the same time, fiber types can still be clearly identified and separated on the basis of twitch contraction times since FT fibers remain FT fibers and are not changed into ST fibers. While training may cause an increase in size and capacities, in short, it does not bring about changes in the proportion of ST and FT fibers in a muscle. The only way that a ST fiber can be functionally

---

*Technique used for determining fiber types. This procedure requires that a small area of muscle be removed by way of a large biopsy needle, quickly frozen, thinly cut, and then examined under a laboratory microscope.

The Skeletal Muscle and Exercise 7

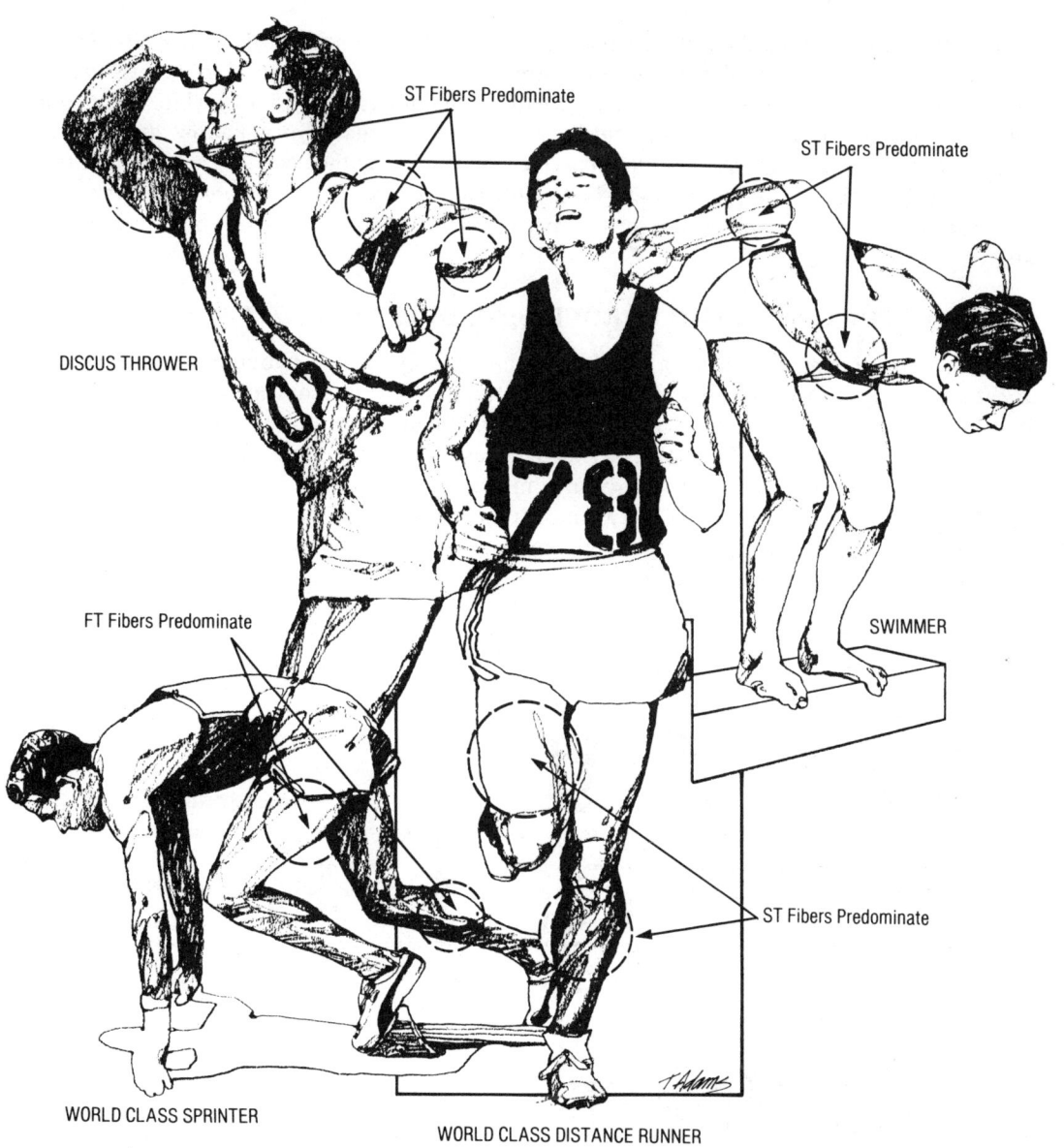

Figure 1-3 Specific fiber types of certain skeletal muscles in athletes with specific athletic abilities.

changed to a FT fiber or vice versa would be to actually remove the original motor nerve from one fiber type and transplant it to the other fiber or vice versa.

Do the considerations of heredity and muscle fiber populations mentioned in the previous discussion mean that someone who is born with a high proportion of ST muscle fibers in his legs is likely to be an outstanding distance runner? Will an individual who has a high percentage of FT fibers in the leg muscles be a world class sprinter? Maybe, but not necessarily. While muscle fiber composition is apparently important, there are many other factors that enter into making championship performances. Factors such as dedication, motivation, training, skill, body build, coaching, and in some cases, plain old luck that may actually overshadow an apparent physiological advantge such as fiber type. This is especially true at the lower levels of competition, whereas at the national and international levels, inheritance of fiber types probably plays a more important role in determining championship performance. More will be said about training in a later chapter.

III. THE CONTRACTILE PROCESS: SLIDING FILAMENT THEORY

Research utilizing the electron microscope has led scientist to hypothesize the currently accepted "sliding filament" theory of muscular contraction. During contraction the actin or thin filament is believed to slide over the myosin or thick filament toward the center of the sarcomere, thus shortening the muscle (Fig. 1-4). The exact elements involved in causing the sliding action of the filament during contraction has not been completely elucidated. It has been postulated that there is an interaction or "hook-up" between the two by way of "cross bridges" which allows the actin filaments to slide over the myosin filaments. This "hook-up" between actin and myosin forms a protein complex called *actomyosin* (A + M → AM).

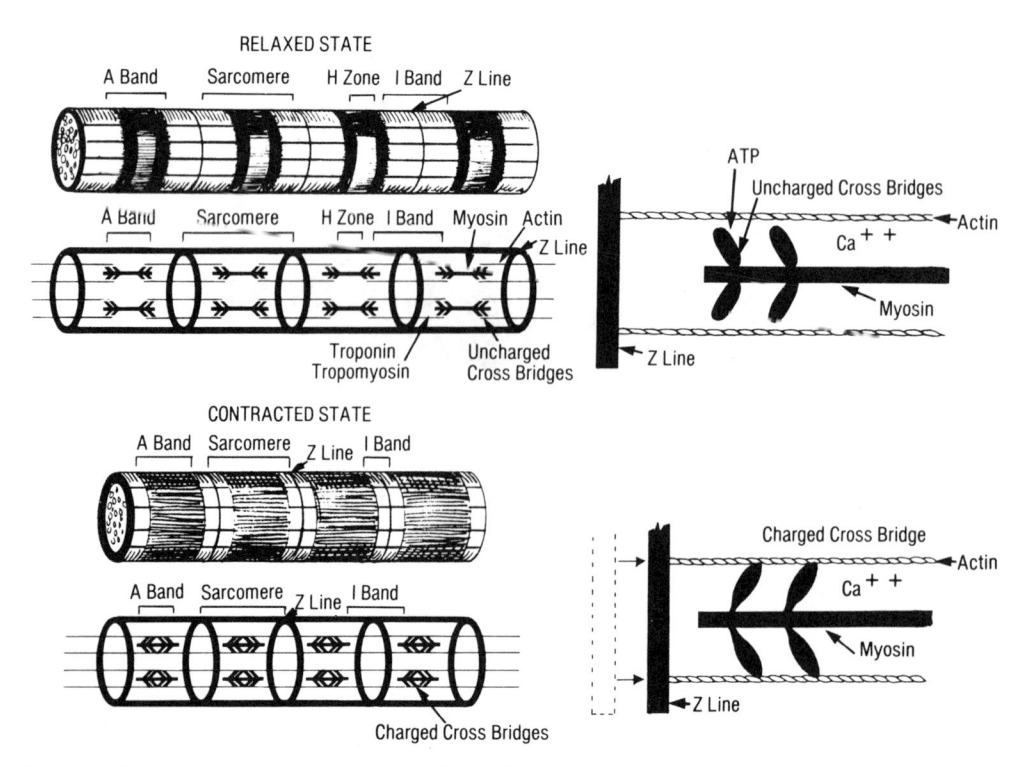

Figure 1-4 Illustration of the proposed sliding filament theory of muscular contraction during rest, contraction, and relaxation conditions.

A. REST

During rest, it is believed that the myosin cross bridges remain extended as a result of the electrostatic forces that exist at both ends of the bridges (Fig. 1-4). In other words, because both charges are negative (the high-energy ionized compound molecule called adenosine triphosphate—ATP which is present at the end of the cross bridge with a negative charge along with a fixed negative charge at the base of the cross bridge), the two ends repel each other, thus allowing the bridges to stay extended. Because the active sites on the actin protein filaments also possess a negative charge, the cross bridges do not hook-up to them during rest. During this period, this arrangement is referred to as an uncharged ATP cross bridge complex. It is generally believed that during rest, in the absence of calcium (Ca^{++}), these electrostatic charges in all of the aforementioned examples are due to the specific structure of actin, tropomyosin, and troponin which, in turn, prevents the myosin cross bridge from interacting with actin.

B. CONTRACTION

The following steps appear to be the normal process by which the bridges connect to the actin filaments so that contraction may occur. When the action potential (or stimulus delivered by a motor nerve fiber or electric shock) signal passes through the T system, Ca^{++} is released from the sarcoplasmic reticulum near the transverse tubules in the form of free Ca^{++}. The Ca^{++} diffuses to the active sites on the actin and myosin filaments and by some reaction involving tropomyosin, the Ca^{++} is quickly taken up by the troponin molecules on the actin filaments. It is believed that the chemical reactions involved in this process create electrostatic forces between the myosin ATP cross bridges and the actin protein filaments which cause them to attract each other and form actomyosin and thereby promote the sliding process. In other words, because Ca^{++}, with two positive charges, are attracted to the negative charges of the myosin ATP cross bridges and the active sites on the actin protein filaments, an electrostatic bond between actin and myosin is developed (thus, the uncharged ATP cross bridge complex is transformed into a charged ATP cross bridge complex) and is thus responsible for the formation of actomyosin (Fig. 1-4).

At the same time, the two positive charges of the Ca^{++} neutralize the two negative charges of the myosin ATP cross bridges and the actin filament. At this point, the cross bridges, which are now "hooked" up to the actin or thin filament, collapse and pulls the actin filament toward the middle of the sarcomere, thus causing the muscle to shorten (Fig. 1-4). It has been postulated that a single bridge hooks onto an active site, pulls the thin filament a short distance toward the center of the sarcomere, releases it, and then hooks onto the next active site. Thus, the actin filament slides along over the myosin filament by a "ratchet" mechanism, the actin molecule first locking with one cross bridge, then with the next, etc. Obviously, tension is developed during this movement since each actin filament is connectd to the Z line. It should be pointed out that any one myosin cross bridge may "hook-up" and "break" with the actin filaments a hundred or more times during a period of one second. At the same time, however, within any one sarcomere, the amount of tension build up and the shortening that takes place is generally somewhat small. On the other hand, it should be remembered that a high level of tension and shortening of intact muscle is due to several hundred sarcomeres contracting simultaneously.

Although the provision of energy for muscular contraction is a complex process (and for which it will be dealt with in more detail later), it would appear that at each cross bridge site where the protein of the two filaments are in contact, myosin acts as an enzyme (called myosin ATPase) to split a phosphate group from ATP and ADP and thus provide the energy for contraction. Once

Table 1-2. Basic Steps of the Muscular Contraction Process According to the Sliding Filament Theory

I. *Rest*
   (a) No nerve impulse
   (b) Myosin uncharged ATP cross bridges remain extended
   (c) Ca^{++} remains stored in sarcoplasmic reticulum
   (d) Specific structure of actin, tropomyosin, and troponin prevents myosin and actin from interacting

II. *Contraction*
   (a) Nerve impulse to muscle results in an action potential
   (b) Action potential causes Ca^{++} to be released from sarcoplasmic reticulum
   (c) Ca^{++} diffuses to active sites on actin and myosin where it is taken up by troponin
   (d) Myosin ATP cross bridges becomes charged
   (e) Actin and myosin interact to form actomyosin (A + M → AM)
   (f) Myosin ATPase splits a phosphate group from ATP and ADP
   (g) Energy for muscle contraction is provided from the splitting of phosphate from ATP and ADP (ATP → ADP + P + Energy) → Myosin ATPase
   (h) Muscle contracts by the actin sliding over the myosin

III. *Relaxation*
   (a) Nerve impulse stops
   (b) Sarcoplasmic reticulum removes Ca^{++} from troponin
   (c) Myosin ATP cross-bridge becomes uncharged
   (d) Actomyosin dissociates into actin and myosin
   (e) ATP is resynthesized
   (f) Muscle is now back to its resting state

ATP is replenished (see next section for this discussion) and the negative charges are restored. Figure 1-4 shows that the cross bridges are reextended and the whole process is repeated with new active sites on the thin protein filaments. Apparently, muscle contraction cannot take place (such as during rest) without this chemical bond between actin and myosin. That is, neither protein by itself is contractile. Figure 1-4 illustrates that neither the myosin nor the actin filaments decrease in length during normal contraction.

C. RELAXATION

Following the cessation of nervous impulses over the motor nerve innervating the muscle, the sarcoplasmic reticulum removes Ca^{++} from the troponin molecules on the actin filaments and stores it in the outer vesicles (Fig. 1-2). Once Ca^{++} has been withdrawn from the troponin, the actin filament is now no longer active. In addition, the myosin ATP cross bridge complexes are also now no longer able to form an electrostatic bond with the active sites of the actin filament. Since the myosin ATPase activity is now turned off, no more molecules of ATP can be split for energy. Thus, by way of elastic recoil, the muscle filaments return to and remain in a relaxed state (Fig. 1-4). Table 1-2 contains a summary of events that occur during rest, contraction, and relaxation as proposed by the sliding-filament theory.

IV. ENERGY FOR CONTRACTION

The energy for muscular contraction is provided by the splitting of ATP (adenosine triphosphate) to ADP (adenosine diphosphate) and phosphoric acid (ATP $\rightleftarrows$ ADP + Pi + energy for contraction). Thus, when one molecule of ATP splits to form one molecule of ADP and a molecule of phosphoric acid, approximately 8,000 calories of energy are released. It appears that it is this energy that creates the forces between the myosin and actin filaments that cause muscle contraction.

After ATP has been broken down into ADP and phosphoric acid, it is essential that these substances be reconverted into ATP for reuse at a later period. Hence, this is done by the metabolism of carbohydrates, fats, and proteins. For example, the metabolism of one molecule of glucose with oxygen to form carbon dioxide and water releases 680,000 calories of energy. The energy from this reaction is used to synthesize 38 molecules of ATP from ADP. Following contraction, the increased metabolism in a given muscle fiber restocks the chemical stores that are consumed during the contractile process. A more thorough discussion of energy metabolism is found in the next chapter.

V. SUMMARY

(1) There are three types of muscle tissue found in the human body. They are: (a) skeletal (voluntary) which provides the force for movement of the skeletal system: (b) cardiac (involuntary) which accounts for the pumping action of the heart: and (c) smooth (involuntary) which is concerned with the movements of internal organs such as those of the stomach, intestines, visceral, and blood vessels.

(2) There are two types of skeletal muscle fibers found in the human body: (a) slow twitch (ST) which have low myosin ATPase activity and low glycolytic enzyme activity, and (b) fast twitch (FT) which have high glycolytic and myosin ATPase activity.

(3) ST fibers predominate in the postural, extensor muscles and are better suited for long endurance type activities.

(4) FT fibers predominate in flexor muscles and are needed for explosive type exercises such as in sprinting or high jumping.

(5) At the national and international level of competition, inheritance of fiber types probably plays an important role in determining championship performances, whereas at the lower, less competitive level, factors such as motivation, training, skill, dedication, and coaching may overshadow an apparent physiological advantage such as fiber type.

(6) Each skeletal muscle fiber is composed of many myofibrils and within each myofibril is a series of sarcomeres (contractile elements of muscle).

(7) Each myofibril consist of two types of protein filaments: (a) actin which represents the light (I band) area under a microscope, and (b) myosin which represents the dark (A band) area. The actin filament contains two important proteins called troponin and tropomyosin, whereas the myosin filament contains small protein projections called cross bridges.

(8) The sliding filament theory of muscle contraction indicates that during contration, there is a "hook-up" between the myosin and actin filaments by way of the cross bridges which permit an electrostatic bond to be formed between the two filaments. This allows the actin to slide over the myosin filaments during muscle contraction. Ca^{++} is needed in order for this bond to take place. Following cessation of nervous impulses over the motor nerves innervating the muscle, the

sarcoplasmic reticulum removes the Ca^{++} from the troponin molecules on the actin filaments and stores it in the outer vesicles, thus restoring the muscle to its resting state.

(9) The immediate source of energy at the actomyosin filament level is the splitting of the high-energy phosphate bonds of ATP to ADP and phosphoric acid. The chemical breakdown of carbohydrates, fats, and proteins allow ADP and phosphoric acid to be reconverted into ATP for reuse at a later period.

VI. REVIEW REFERENCES

(1) Bergh, U., Thorstensson, A., Sjodin, B., Hulten, B., Piehl, K., and Karlsson, J. "Maximal Oxygen Uptake and Muscle Fiber Types in Trained and Untrained Humans," *Medicine and Science in Sports,* 10:151-54, 1978.
(2) Costill, D. L., Daniels, J., Evans, W., Fink, W., Krahenbuhl, G., and Saltin, B. "Skeletal Muscle Enzymes and Fiber Composition in Male and Female Track Athletes," *Journal of Applied Physiology,* 40:149-54, 1976.
(3) Costill, D. L., Fink, W., and Pollock, M. L. "Muscle Fiber Composition and Enzyme Activities of Elite Distance Runners," *Medicine and Science in Sports,* 8:96-100, 1975.
(4) Coyle, E. F., Bell, S., Costill, D. L., and Fink, W. "Skeletal Muscle Fiber Characteristics of World Class Shot-Putters," *Research Quarterly,* 49:278-84, 1978.
(5) Coyle, E. F., Costill, D. L., and Lesmes, G. R. "Leg Extension Power and Muscle Fiber Composition," *Medicine and Science in Sports,* 11:12-15, 1979.
(6) Edstrom, L. and Ekblom, B. "Differences in Sizes of Red and White Muscle Fibers in Vastus Lateralis of Musculus Quadriceps Femoris of Normal Individuals and Athletes: Relation to Physical Performance," *Scandinavian Journal of Clinical and Laboratory Investigation,* 30:175-81, 1972.
(7) Gollnick, P. D., Armstrong, R. B., Saubert, C. W. IV, Piehl, K., and Saltin, B. "Enzyme Activity and Fiber Composition in Skeletal Muscle of Untrained and Trained Men," *Journal of Applied Physiology,* 33:312-19, 1972.
(8) Huxley, H. E. "Review Lecture: Muscular Contraction," *Journal of Physiology* (London), 243:1-43, 1974.
(9) Huxley, H. E. "The Mechanism of Muscular Contraction," *Scientific American,* 213:18-27, 1965.
(10) Huxley, H. E. "The Structural Basis of Muscular Contraction," *Proceedings of the Royal Society of Medicine,* 178:131-49, 1971.
(11) Komi, P. V., Rusko, H., Vos, J., and Vihko, V. "Anaerobic Performance Capacity in Athletes," *Acta Physiologica Scandinavica,* 100:107-14, 1977.
(12) Prince, F. P., Hikida, R. S., and Hagerman, F. C. "Human Muscle Fiber Types in Power Lifters, Distance Runners and Untrained Subjects," *Pfugers Archives (Eur. J. Phys.),* 363:19-26, 1976.
(13) Thorstensson, A., Grimby, G., and Karlsson, J. "Force-Velocity Relations and Fiber Composition in Human Knee Extensor Muscles," *Journal of Applied Physiology;* 40:12-16, 1976.
(14) Thorstensson, A., Karlsson, J., Vitasalo, J. H., Luhtanen, P., and Komi, P. V. "Effect of Strength Training on EMG of Human Skeletal Muscle," *Acta Physiologica Scandinavica,* 98:232-36, 1976.
(15) Thorstensson, A., Larsson, L., Tesch, P., and Karlsson, J. "Muscle Strength and Fiber Composition in Athletes and Sedentary men," *Medicine and Science in Sports,* 9:26-30, 1977.

2

EXERCISE, ENERGY, AND METABOLISM

KEY CONCEPTS TO BE GAINED FROM THIS CHAPTER

(1) ATP (adenosine triphosphate) is the immediate source of energy for a muscle cell.

(2) CP (creatine phosphate) is the source of energy for ATP while the breakdown of food and glycolysis—the breakdown of glycogen resulting in the formation of lactic acid—is the ultimate source of energy for the regeneration of CP.

(3) There are two chemical or metabolic pathways by which ATP is formed. They are: (a) The anaerobic pathway (commonly referred to as glycolysis) which does not require oxygen and uses only carbohydrates in its production of ATP. This pathway results in an incomplete breakdown of glucose to pyruvate and eventually to lactic acid. (b) The aerobic pathway (Krebs, tricarboxylic acid, or citric acid cycle, and the electron transport enzyme system) requires the presence of oxygen and it can use all three foodstuffs such as carbohydrates, fats, and proteins in its production of ATP. This pathway involves a complete breakdown to carbon dioxide and water.

(4) Specific types of exercises call for specific metabolic pathways for its energy needs.

(5) During rest or steady-state exercise, the respiratory quotient (R.Q.) accurately indicates the metabolic foodstuff being oxidized for energy.

(6) Following exercise, the oxygen consumed above the normal rest conditions is called the oxygen debt. The debt has two parts: (a) the alactacid component and (b) the lactacid component.

(7) Under submaximal workloads, heart rate is linearly related to the workload and the oxygen consumption values.

(8) The indirect calorimetry procedure for measuring energy cost is the most practical for exercise physiologists and physical educators, and it is based upon knowing the sums of oxygen consumed and carbon dioxide produced.

(9) Negative work is somewhat more economical in terms of energy cost than positive work.

(10) Basal metabolic rate is based upon age, sex, and body surface area

---

Metabolism is the method by which foods are broken down and converted into energy and the energy is kept in reserve of the body. It includes all chemical reactions occurring within the body. By virtue of metabolism, cells are provided with the capacity to contract, conduct, secrete, absorb, grow, and reproduce. Hence, metabolism is the backbone for all physiological phenomena that one can see or measure.

Understanding energy expenditure and how it is measured during rest, exercise, and recovery is basic as well as essential for the exercise physiologist, physical educator, or coach. Thus, the purpose of this chapter will be to discuss energy metabolism and how it is determined during both rest and exercise as well as during recovery.

I. DEFINITIONS

In order to understand and fully appreciate the measurements of the metabolic processes during activity and recovery, we need to know the meaning of and relationships among (a) energy, (b) work, (c) power, (d) efficiency—gross and net, and (e) METS.

A. ENERGY

Energy is usually defined as the capacity to perform work. Normally, there are six forms of energy: mechanical, heat, light, chemical, electrical, and nuclear. Each can readily be converted from one form to another. This is done in accordance with the doctrine of the conservation of energy which implies that although it is possible to transform energies, one can neither create nor destroy energy. For example, our bodies are capable of converting chemical into electrical energy such as the stimulus for muscular contraction. In addition, a person exercising or playing basketball is converting chemical (foodstuffs) to heat and mechanical energy. Thus, it can be seen that in every human movement, whether it be contraction of the viscera within the body or the throwing of a baseball, the energy required to perform it is originated from food.

Since energy can be neither created nor destroyed, the total amount taken in by the body must be accounted for by the output by the body. This energy balance may be expressed in the following equation:

Energy input = energy output
(Chemical energy of food) = (heart energy + work energy ± stored chemical energy)

The energy of food as well as the work resulting from the energy can both be described in terms of calories. One Calorie (spelled with a capital C) or kilocalorie represents the heat (energy) required to raise the temperature of one kilogram of water by one degree Centigrade. Depending upon age, size, and sex, the average Calorie intake needed for maintaining body weight for most people during a normal day varies between 1,500-3,000 kilocalories (kcal) per day. During training (and depending on the type of training and competition), athletes need somewhere around 500-2,000 kcal per day extra to maintain body weight.

B. WORK

The physicist defines work rigidly as a product of force times the distance through which this force acts. This may be expressed in the following equation:

$$\text{Work} = \text{force} \times \text{distance}$$

Thus, lifting 5 pounds to a height of 5 feet will constitute 25 foot-pounds of work. Pushing an object horizontally for a distance of 5 feet and applying 5 pounds of constant pushing force throughout this distance will also result in 25 foot-pounds of work. In the case of the metric system, if an individual weighed 80 kilograms and climbed up to stand on a 3-meter diving board, he would have performed 80 kilograms times 3 meters, or 240 kilogram-meters of work

The physicist's definition of work is often unsatisfactory and unfair from the standpoint of physiology. For instance, if a man holds 5 pounds in his hand while his arm remains motionless in the horizontal position, he is not doing any work, since the distance is zero, yet he quickly gets fatigued. While it is common to express static or isometric work as the product of load and time, there are a number of other different terms by which work may be stated. These, along with various other energy units may be found in Appendix A.

C. POWER

The term power is used to represent work in a unit of time. It consists of strength and speed and may be stated as:

$$\text{Power} = \frac{\text{work}}{\text{time}}, \text{ or Power} = \frac{\text{force} \times \text{distance}}{\text{time}}$$

In the above example, if the 5-pound weight was raised 5 feet in 1 second, power would be expressed as:

$$\text{Power} = \frac{5 \text{ lb} \times 5 \text{ ft}}{1 \text{ sec}} = 25 \text{ ft-lb/sec}$$

Power may also be defined in terms of horsepower. For example:

$$1 \text{ hp} = 33,000 \text{ ft-lb per min} = 550 \text{ ft-lb per sec}$$

As an illustrative example of the calculations of horsepower, let us consider the above power illustration with the 5-pound weight. In terms of horsepower, the individual has worked at:

$$\frac{25 \text{ ft-lb/sec}}{550 \text{ ft-lb/sec}} = 0.045 \text{ hp}$$

Power may also be expressed in various other units. These may be found in Appendix A.

D. EFFICIENCY

While efficiency is written as a percent of total energy used, researchers have generally utilized two distinct methods for computing it. The first and simplest is *gross efficiency*, in which the total energy used is divided into the total measurable work. It is written as:

$$\text{Gross efficiency (percent)} = \frac{\text{external work output}}{\text{total energy used for work}} \times 100$$

"Work output" is generally expressed in terms of foot-pounds or kilocalories (1 kcal = 3,087 foot-pounds). For instance, if a man weighing 160 pounds climbs stairs to a height of 30 feet, he performs 30 × 160 = 4,800 ft-lb of work. The "total energy used" in performing muscular work is usually measured by the sum of the oxygen consumption (in liters) during work and recovery or it may be expressed in terms of the equivalent value in kilocalories of heat energy (1 liter of oxygen is equivalent to 4.83 kilocalories). In the above example, if the 160-pound man uses 10 kilocalories of energy for his 30-foot climb, his energy cost is 10 × 3,087 = 30,870 ft-lb, and the gross efficiency of his performance is as follows:

$$\text{Gross efficiency (percent)} = \frac{4,800 \text{ ft-lb}}{30,870 \text{ ft-lb}} \times 100 = 15.6\%$$

Note that work and energy should always be expressed in the same units of measure, such as foot-pounds, kilocalories, or horsepower.

The second method is called *net efficiency*. Since at any given time of the day a certain amount of the energy used up by the body is being used merely to maintain life (basal requirements), the calculated gross efficiency does not fairly represent the efficiency of the working muscles that are being appraised. In order to determine the net efficiency of the working body, the basal requirements should be subtracted from the total energy cost. Thus, the net efficiency is calculated with the following equation:

$$\text{Net efficiency (percent)} = \frac{\text{external work output}}{\text{total energy used} - \text{basal requirements}} \times 100$$

Net efficiency calculated in this manner yields a value higher than gross efficiency. The total energy used is generally measured by the sum of the oxygen consumption during work and recovery, whereas the net energy used is measured by the sum of the oxygen consumption during work and recovery corrected for the basal metabolic oxygen consumption.

As an illustrative example of the calculation of net efficiency, let us consider the above gross efficiency example. If the man's basal requirement is .25 liters of oxygen or 1.2075 kilocalories (1 liter of oxygen is equivalent to 4.83 kilocalories), then his total energy cost is 30,870 foot-pounds minus 1.2075 × 3,087 = 3,728 foot-pounds. Thus, net efficiency of his performance is as follows:

$$\text{Net efficiency (percent)} = \frac{4,800 \text{ ft-lb}}{30,870 \text{ ft-lb} - 3,728 \text{ ft-lb}} \times 100 = 17.6\%$$

Usually the performance of large muscle activities of men results in a net efficiency of 20 to 25 percent. There are, of course, individual differences, which include body size, fitness, and skill in performing a given task. Efficiency is also dependent upon the speed with which a task is performed. It should be realized that the other energy which does not appear as work appears

E. METS

In addition to those expressions found in Appendix A, the term "metabolic equivalents" or METS has also been employed recently in metabolic studies for purposes of expressing the energy cost of work. One MET represents the net energy cost during rest (approximately .25 liters of oxygen or 1.25 kcal); two METS corresponds to two times the resting value; three METS is three times the resting value, etc. In some situations where work and/or power is difficult to measure (such as in isometric work) and where direct measurement of the metabolic energy cost is not only time consuming, but requires rather expensive equipment, the MET concept undoubtedly has some practical value and will more than likely be used extensively in future metabolic investigations.

II. SOURCES OF ENERGY

A. ATP-CP

The energy set free during the breakdown of food is not utilized directly by the muscle cells. Instead, it is used by the body to build another, more complex powerhouse chemical compound known as *ATP (adenosine triphosphate)*. ATP is found in the cytoplasm of cells and it consists of a adenosine component and three "high-energy" phosphate groups. During the breakdown of ATP, one of these phosphate bonds is split or removed from the rest of the molecule, and approximately 8,000 calories (8 kcal) of energy are set free and free *phosphate (Pi)* plus *adenosine diphosphate (ADP)* are formed. This reaction is illustrated in Figure 2.1. Recall from Chapter 1 that the breakdown of ATP represents the immediate source of energy for the contractile process of the actin and myosin protein filaments of the myofibril.

In addition to ATP, *creatine phosphate (CP* or *phosphoryl creatine)* is another important chemical which provides stored energy. Although CP also contains the high-energy phosphate

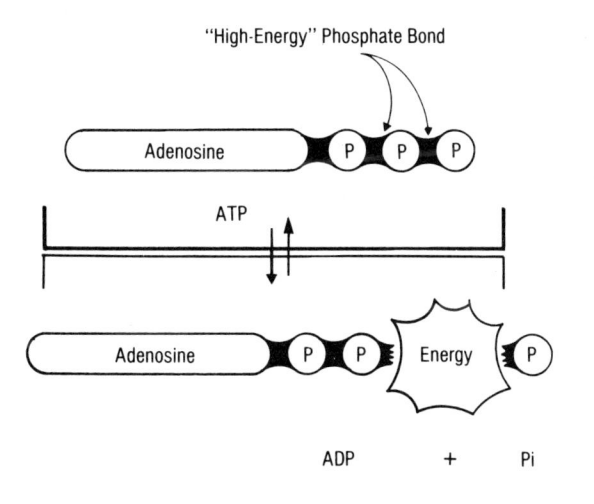

Figure 2-1 Schematic diagram of ATP along with its three "high-energy" phosphate groups. The diagram illustrates the breakdown of ATP to ADP and free phosphate (Pi).

bond, it cannot be used directly by the cells as a source of energy. Instead, it is used to resynthesize ATP from ADP. For instance, Figure 2-2 illustrates that during the breakdown of CP when its phosphate group is removed, a large amount of energy is set free and creatine plus free phosphate are formed. This energy is immediately available to re-form ATP. For example, when ATP is broken down during heavy work, it is continuously regenerated from ADP and Pi by the energy set free during the breakdown of the stored CP. CP, like ATP, is in short supply in the muscle and must be resynthesized continuously.

It is interesting to note that the only means by which CP can be regenerated from Pi and creatine is from the energy set free by the breakdown of ATP. Thus, there are two ultimate sources of energy for the resynthesis of the phosphagens (ATP and CP): (1) breakdown of food, and (2) glycolysis, the breakdown of glycogen resulting in the formation of lactic acid. The second of these processes is reversible: with an input of energy from food combustion, lactic acid is reconstituted to glycogen. These sources will be discussed in more detail later.

ATP and CP are not dependent on oxygen nor on a series of reactions and for this reason, they are extremely important not only during muscular work involving powerful quick starts of football players, high jumpers, sprinters, and basketball players, but also in events that require only a few seconds to complete such as sprinting up a flight of stairs.

B. AEROBIC AND ANAEROBIC METABOLISM (CARBOHYDRATE BREAKDOWN)

The major purpose of aerobic and anaerobic metabolism is to provide energy for the body's cells. Figure 2-3 illustrates a schematic drawing of both anaerobic and aerobic metabolic pathways for glycogen degradation in skeletal muscle. It can be seen that anaerobic metabolism uses carboyhydrates (glucose and glycogen) exclusively for the manufacture of ATP, whereas aerobic metabolism can use all three foodstuffs (carbohydrates, fats, and proteins) for its fuel. Since fat and protein are not used as anaerobic energy sources, they will be discussed separately later in this chapter.

Anaerobic Metabolism

From Figure 2-3, it can be seen that carbohydrates are broken down into glucose where it is transported by the blood and stored in the muscles and liver in the form of glycogen. It is generally believed that somewhere between 350 to 450 grams of glycogen are stored in the human body.

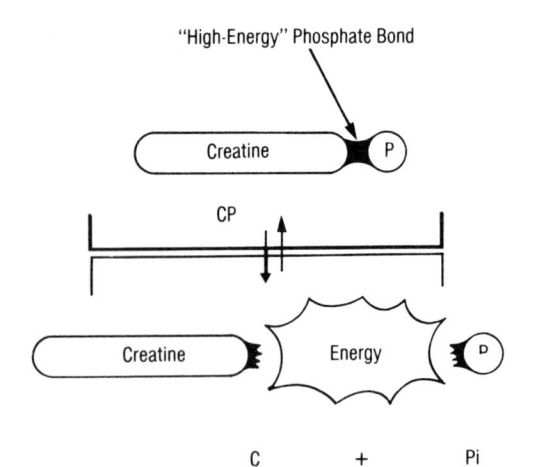

Figure 2-2 Schematic diagram of CP along with its "high-energy" phosphate bond. The diagram illustrates the breakdown of CP to creatine (C) and free phosphate (Pi) with energy being released.

Exercise, Energy, and Metabolism   19

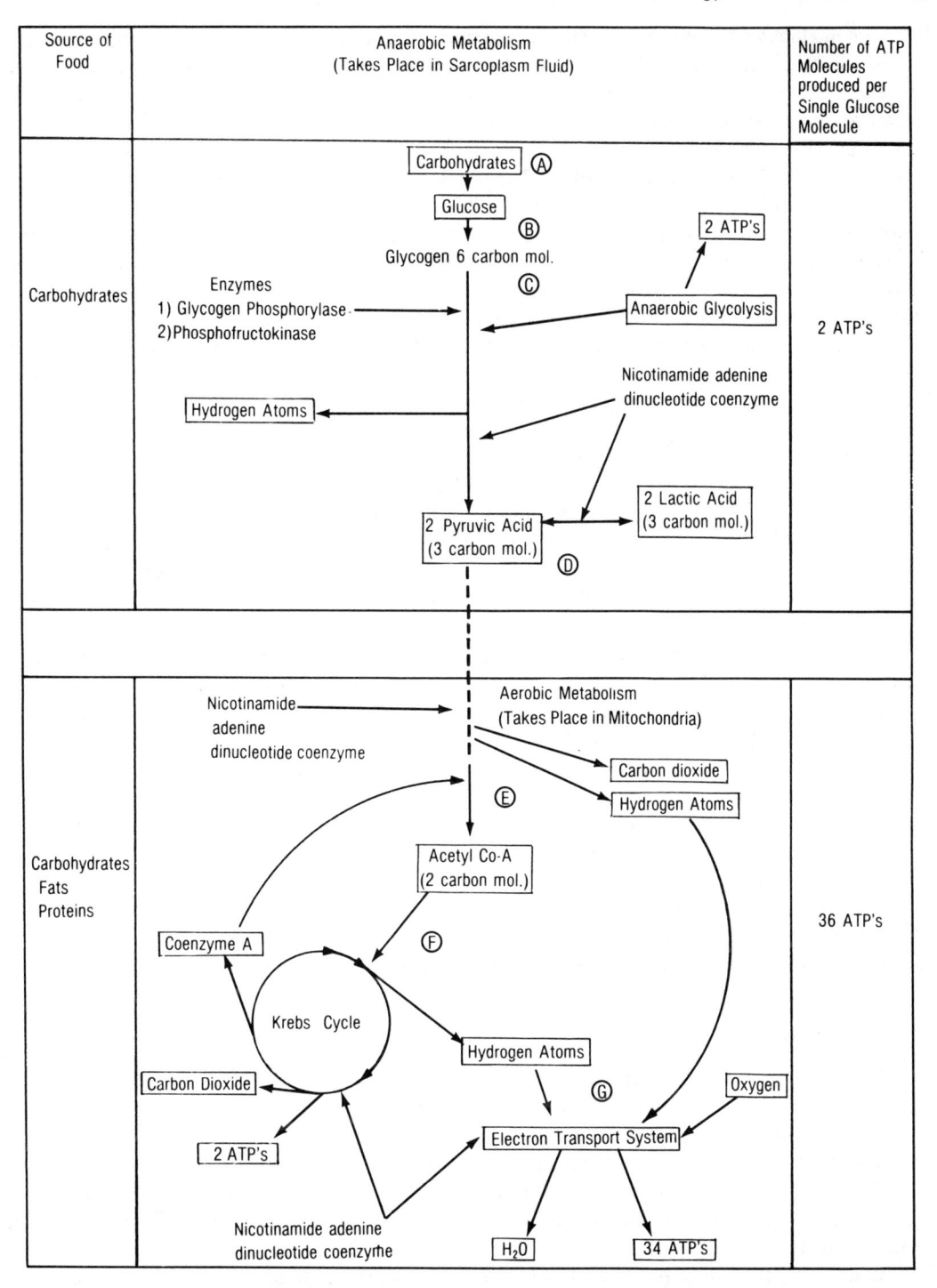

Figure 2-3 Schematic illustration of anaerobic and aerobic metabolic pathways for glycogen degradation in skeletal muscle.

While each glucose molecule is made up of 6 carbon atoms, glycogen molecules are merely clusters of glucose sugar molecules that are linked to each other in chain-like structures. The actual process of breaking down glycogen involves the removal of a glucose molecule from the chain-like structure one at a time (process called *glycogenolysis*).

Anaerobic metabolism (in the absence of oxygen) involves a series of chemical reactions starting with the 6-carbon glucose molecule being broken down partially from glycogen into two 3-carbon molecules of pyruvic or lactic acid. This process is referred to as *anaerobic glycolysis*. Anaerobic glycolysis takes place entirely in the sarcoplasm of the cell since all the enzymes that catalyze these reactions are located in this area. Note that it is generally believed that *glycogen phosphorylase* and *phosphofructokinase* are the two major enzymes that actually determine the rate of glycogen breakdown during the early stages of anaerobic metabolism. It is also commonly believed that in order for certain reactions in anaerobic metabolism to be able to take place such as reactions C and D, a coenzyme called *nicotinamide adenine dinucleotide* (NAD) must be present. Briefly, a coenzyme is classified as a nonprotein molecule that is required for the activity of an enzyme.

As stated earlier, the primary purpose of anaerobic metabolism is to provide energy for the body's cells and that glucose is used exclusively for the production of ATP. An important question at this point is exactly how much usable energy in the form of ATP molecules can be produced by way of anaerobic glycolysis? Figure 2-3 illustrates that for every single glucose molecule that undergoes glycolysis results in a net production of 2 ATP molecules. While this represents only approximately 5 percent of the total number of ATP molecules that can be produced when the same amount of glucose is completely broken down to carbon dioxide and water such as in aerobic metabolism, anaerobic metabolism is tremendously important to us, especially during high-intensity type work. For example, when the body is unable to supply oxygen to the cell in sufficient quantity such as in underwater swimming (breath holding) or as in sprinting a 220-yd run, anaerobic metabolism is able to furnish energy for muscular contraction. At the same time, however, it shoud be pointed out that while anaerobic metabolism may function in the total absence of oxygen, this process is inefficient when compared to aerobic metabolism since it results in the accumulation of lactic acid. Because there is a finite limit as to the amount of lactic acid that can be tolerated in the human body, this process can continue for only a short period of time before muscular fatigue sets in.

At this point, it should be mentioned that most of the reactions in Figure 2-3 are reversible. This means that when oxygen supply is sufficient, lactic acid can be changed back to pyruvic acid, which in turn, can then be broken down to carbon dioxide and water through aerobic metabolism.

Aerobic Metabolism

When oxygen is available in sufficient quantities, aerobic metabolism provides energy for the body's cells. While the breakdown of glucose from glycogen starts in the same manner as illustrated in Figure 2-3 for anaerobic glycolysis, the pyruvic acid molecules (under aerobic conditions) are not converted to lactic acid, but instead, they diffuse from the sarcoplasm fluid across the mitochondria membrane to the inside of the mitochondria where a series of chemical reactions take place to form carbon dioxide and water with the production of ATP's taking place simultaneously.

When oxygen supply is plentiful and the muscles are not under heavy stress (such as in exhaustive-type anaerobic work), a glucose molecule is completely broken down to carbon dioxide and water with 36 molecules of ATP being produced in addition to those found in the anaerobic glycolysis. This means that a sum total of 38 ATP molecules per glucose molecule is produced aerobically.

There are two important series of chemical reactions that play a vital part in aerobic metabolism: namely, the *Krebs cycle* and the *electron transport system*. Because of their importance, they will be mentioned separately.

The Krebs Cycle. From Figure 2-3, it can be seen that if sufficent oxygen is available to meet muscular demands, the 3-carbon pyruvic acid molecule is degraded to carbon dioxide and *hydrogen atoms* (which contains two *hydrogen ions* and two *electrons*). Following the removal of carbon dioxide, hydrogen ions, and electrons, the 2-carbon molecule that is left is called an *acetyl molecule*. The acetyl molecule then combines with a molecule commonly called *coenzyme A* (CoA) to form acetyl CoA. As illustrated in Figure 2-3, the acetyl CoA molecule then enters the Krebs cycle (also known as the *tricarboxylic acid (TCA) cycle* or the *citric acid cycle*). After entering the Krebs cycle, the 2-carbon acetyl CoA molecule undergoes a series of chemical reactions where two additional carbon dioxide molecules and four additional hydrogen ions and electrons are removed while producing two molecules of ATP. Thus, for each acetyl CoA molecule that passes through the Krebs cycle, two molecules of ATP is actually produced. While the carbon dioxide molecules are eliminated from the body by way of the respiratory system, in order to produce greater numbers of ATP from aerobic metabolism of pyruvic acid, the electrons and hydrogen ions that were released in the Krebs cycle must be transported to oxygen (to form the remaining end product of aerobic metabolism, water) via the *electron transport system* which will be discussed below.

The Electron Transport System. Located in the mitochondria, the electron transport system (also known as the *respiratory chain*) is where a chain of oxidative enzymes and coenzymes take place to combine oxygen that we breathe with the electronss and hydrogen ions that are released in the Krebs cycle to form water and ATP. It is generally believed that the key to aerobic metabolism is the ability of *flavoprotein* and *cytochromes* to receive the electrons and hydrogen ions from the Krebs cycle and then to pass them along the electron transport system to combine eventually with the oxygen that we breathe. In so doing, the majority of the energy is produced in this system. In fact, for each molecule of glucose entering the metabolic system, 34 molecules of ATP are produced via the electron transport system, 2 ATP molecules from both the Krebs cycle, and the anaerobic glycolysis for a net gain of 38 molecules.

From the previous discussion, it should be obvious that energy production is much more efficient when glucose is broken down through aerobic metabolism than by way of the anaerobic system. In fact, 19 times more ATP is produced per glucose molecule aerobically than by anaerobic glycolysis (38 ATP = aerobic; 2 ATP = anaerobic). This helps to explain partially why a marathoner or a laborer can run or work so much longer (and at higher efficiency levels) at submaximal or steady-state speed than at maximum speed.

C. FAT METABOLISM

It has been previously thought that carbohydrates (glucose and glycogen) were the main sources of producing ATP during exercise. However, it is becoming increasingly evident that the oxidation of fats can account for most of the ATP production during certain types of exercise.

The majority of fat (lipid) that is consumed by man is stored in the body as *triglycerides;* a 4-part molecule made up of three molecules of fatty-acids and one molecule of glycerol. It should be pointed out that this discussion will be restricted to the fatty-acid molecule since most of ATP production from fats come from the fatty-acid molecules that are split off (by an enzyme called *lipase*) from the triglyceride molecules of the adipose tissue. Note that each fatty-acid molecule is composed of 16 or 18 long chains of carbon atoms with hydrogen atoms attached to them.

Once the fatty-acid molecule splits off from the triglyceride molecule of the adipose tissue, it diffuses over into the blood where it is transported to the muscles and eventually undergoes a chemical transformation called *beta oxidation* in which the fatty-acid molecule is degraded to acetyl coenzyme A. As can be seen in Figure 2-3, the acetyl coenzyme A enters the Krebs cycle in the mitochondria cell in the same way to produce ATP as the carbohydrates.

The total ATP production from an 18-carbon fatty-acid molecule is 147 ATP molecules. When compared to the 38 ATP molecules per 6-carbon glucose molecule, it is quite obvious that fat comes out ahead. For the normal person, since approximately 35 to 40 percent of the calories in the diet come from fats, it is apparent that fats play an extremely important role as an energy source. This statement becomes even more apparent when it is realized that between approximately 30 and 50 percent of carbohydrates consumed are converted to triglycerides in the body.

Fat also appears to have the advantage over carbohydrates in terms of energy stored per unit of weight. For example, a gram of fat produces more than twice as much energy (9.5 kcal/gm) as a gram of carbohydrate (4.3 kcal/gm). Another advantage in which fats have over carbohydrates is that the human body is able to store in the cells of adipose tissue large quantities of fat, whereas body tissue, including muscle, is not able to store carbohydrates (glycogen) in very large quantities. This is a definite advantage for stored fat in the sense that it can be called upon for later use, especially during a long duration type of exercise or physical labor, whereas the body reserves of carbohydrates are too small to continue work for extended periods of time. Note that while carbohydrates have the ability to be converted to fat and stored in fat cells, fat does not have the ability to convert into carbohydrates and thus become a source of glucose.

Finally, in comparing fat to carbohydrate as a source of energy, carbohydrate is a more efficient food fuel in regards to ATP produced per molecule of oxygen consumed. For example, fats require 2.01 liters of oxygen for their oxidation while carbohydrates need only .75 liters. For producing 38 ATP molecules during aerobic metabolism of a 6-carbon glucose molecule, this turns out to be 6 oxygen molecules needed, whereas for producing 147 ATP molecules during the breakdown of an 18-carbon fatty acid molecule, 26 oxygen molecules are required.

From the previous discussion, it is rather clear that while both carbohydrates and fats are important food fuels, carbohydrates are the preferred source for short, maximal bouts of exercise and work, whereas fats are used mainly for longer endurance type activities. In addition, because carbohydrate is a more efficient food fuel, it is clear that even in long extended work (such as in long physical labor or marathon running) where performance is not only somewhat limited by the oxygen supply, but where it is also depended upon fat as a source of fuel, it is to the performers advantage to oxidize carbohydrates (glycogen) as long as possible.

It is interesting to note that research has shown that if a high carbohydrate diet is given during the first 2 or 3 days following exhaustive exercise (at which time the glycogen stores are depleted), the glycogen stores of the muscles depleted will increase to approximately 2 to 3 times the normal levels. In addition, if the individual fasts or consumes a low carbohydrate diet several days before beginning the high carbohydrate diet, further increases in glycogen stores can be stimulated. This information should be of interest to athletes and coaches since such a diet definitely increases muscle glycogen stores and thus increases muscular performance. More detail information on this topic can be found in Chapter 9 of this text.

D. PROTEIN METABOLISM

Contrary to popular opinion, protein makes only slight contributions to ATP production during exercise. In fact, it has been widely recognized that the breakdown of protein supplies only about 5 to 15 percent of the body's total energy. Thus, consuming a large amount of protein prior to an event or contest from the viewpoint of energy metabolism is not supported. While proteins are not a common source of fuel, they are, however, an important part of the diet. They are used primarily for construction of new body tissue cells.

Each protein molecule contains complex chains of carbon, oxygen, hydrogen, and nitrogen atoms with *amino acids* being the basic unit. In fact, 20 different amino acids have been determined to be present in proteins. Several of these amino acids such as *alanine, serine,* and *cysteine* can be broken down to pyruvic acid and thus enter the metabolic pathway at the Krebs cycle for oxidation and subsequent production of ATP. In addition, within the Krebs cycle, other amino acids can be converted into molecules for final oxidation and production of ATP. While it is obvious that proteins do have the potential for ATP production, they, unlike carbohydrates and fats, are not considered to be a primary source of energy. As a source of fuel, they are used only under extreme circumstances with their major contribution being that of building and repairing body tissue.

E. ENERGY METABOLISM DURING REST, EXERCISE, AND RECOVERY

Rest

Because oxygen consumption (approximately 0.25 liters/min) during rest remains relatively constant and is adequate to supply the required ATP, and because blood lactic acid level remains within the normal range (10 mg/100 ml), it is apparent that metabolism under resting conditions is aerobic. In fact, the aerobic breakdown of fats and glucose supplies all the ATP required by the body under resting conditions. Approximately two-thirds of the food source is contributed by fats, and the remaining one-third by glucose.

Exercise

Although Figure 2-4 illustrates quite clearly that both metabolic pathways (aerobic and anaerobic) contribute a certain amount of energy during maximal exercise of various durations, it is also clear that it is somewhat difficult to determine the major energy source in activities lasting

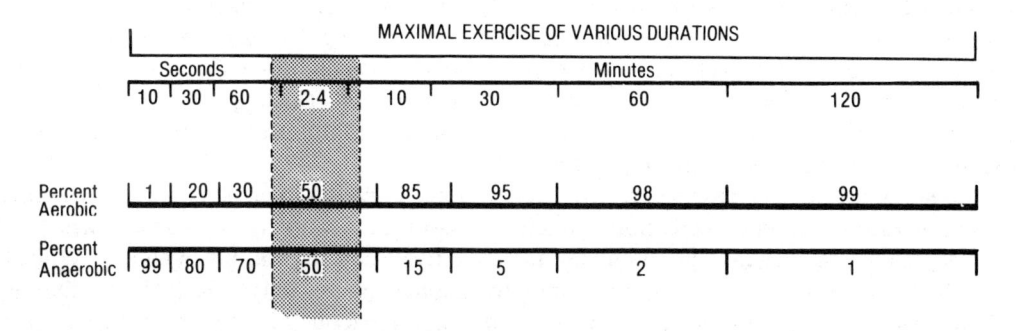

Figure 2-4 Illustration of aerobic and anaerobic energy contributions during maximal exercise of various durations.

from 2 to 4 minutes such as middle-distance events. During this time, the anaerobic and aerobic energy sources are of equal importance. In Figure 2-4, it can also be seen that at one extreme, maximal exercises of short duration are supplied via anaerobic metabolism, whereas exercises that can be performed for relatively long periods of time such as marathon running are supplied primarily by aerobic metabolism. For sake of simplicity, our discussion in this section will be divided into three categories: (1) short-duration, high-intensity exercises, (2) high intensity exercises lasting several minutes, and (3) long duration exercises.

Short-Duration, High-Intensity Exercises. Generally included in this category are activities which can be kept up for no more than one or two minutes. These include swimming events up to 200 meters or track events up to 800 meters. Also included are jumping, throwing, and vaulting in track, cycling sprints, weightlifting, fast-breaks in basketball games, the golf swing, and some gymnastic activities including apparatus routines.

The primary food fuel is the stored ATP and glycogen. If the maximal, all-out exercises are repeated many times with intervening rest periods (such as in football, basketball, and baseball games), then fatty-acids from the blood may play a minor role as an energy source. Apparently, ATP and CP are replenished during the intervening rest periods at the expense of not only glycogen, but perhaps blood glucose and fatty-acids as well. The predominant metabolic pathway is anaerobic with the aerobic cycle playing only a minor part.

According to Mathews and Fox, there are a couple of reasons why aerobic metabolism is not (and cannot be) the main source of energy for maximal work of short duration. First of all, every human being has a maximum rate and capacity for which he or she can take in oxygen and use it. For athletes, this capacity is around 4.5 (females) to 6.0 (males) liters per minute, whereas for untrained subjects, the capacity is around 3.0 (females) to 3.5 (males) liters per minute. Because a race such as the 100-yd dash is so fast and short and may require an oxygen consumption of somewhere around 45 to 60 liters per minute, it is obvious that the above oxgen consumption capacities for both the athlete and the nonathlete are not nearly adequate to furnish all the ATP molecules needed for this type of event.

Another important point is that even if it were possible to take in enough oxygen that would alone meet the energy or ATP requirement, it still takes the human body two or three minutes in which to adjust biochemically and physiologically to the new level of oxygen consumption requirement that is brought about by the exercise. By this time, the 100-yd race is over. This delay or adjustment period is needed when going from rest to exercise or from a low level of exercise to a high level.

High-Intensity Exercises Lasting Several Minutes. Any strenuous exercise lasting from 5 to 10 minutes such as middle-distance running, swimming, cycling, lacrosse, soccer, or basketball should be included in this section. Performances under these conditions require a blend of both anaerobic and aerobic energy sources with lactic acid formation. The major food fuels are stored ATP, creatine phosphate and muscle glycogen. Oxidation of fatty-acids contribute less than 10 percent of the energy cost of this type of activity.

Long Duration Exercises. Performances of long duration such as channel swimming, cycling, marathon running, recreational jogging, long-distance walking, or a laborer who works at a machine in a factory for eight hours require a relatively constant supply of energy. While the anaerobic breakdown of glycogen, ATP, and creatine phosphate contribute at the beginning of the exercise, the energy provided for this type of work is provided nearly exclusively from the aerobic breakdown of fat, glycogen and glucose with little or no lactic acid production. As the work is prolonged, and the glucose supply is nearly depleted, a greater contribution of the energy fuel comes from the stored fat as well as from the fatty-acids in the blood. This would seem to indicate that as exercise is prolonged, there is an increase activity of enzymes involved in the breakdown of fatty-acids.

It should be emphasized that in long duration activities of low intensity such as leisure walking, golf, etc., lactic acid levels do not go much above the resting levels. This is due to the fact that the stored ATP and creatine phosphate is sufficient to meet the demand until a steady state of oxygen consumption or aerobic metabolism is reached.

One rather interesting bit of information concerning lactic acid levels during and following long duration exercises is that blood lactate has been found to reach a high of 140 mg/100 ml blood when a final sprint was preceded by 35 minutes of hard work. On the other hand, when a final sprint was not permitted following 31 to 32 minutes of exhaustive running, lactate values were found to be around 38 to 47 mg/100 ml blood. In fact, at the end of marathon races (26.2 miles in about 2.5 hours) blood lactic acid levels have been found to be only about three times those found at rest (normal rest values are around 10 mg/100 ml blood). Fatigue brought on by this type of long duration activity is apparently not due to high blood lactic acid levels, but instead to factors such as low blood glucose levels and high body temperatures (which is brought on by the loss of water and electrolytes). Boredom and the overall physical beating that the body takes may also add to the fatigue. A more detail discussion of muscular fatigue may be found in Chapter 14 of this text.

Recovery

The primary purpose of the metabolic pathways during the recovery period following exercise is to repay the energy stores that were used up during the exercise period. This is accomplished solely by the aerobic (oxygen system) pathway.

The Oxygen Debt. The oxygen debt notion has been of interest to exercise physiologists for a number of years. The term was coined many years ago by A. V. Hill, an English physiologist. An oxygen debt is defined as all postexercise oxygen consumption above the basal oxygen consumption level. This means that the oxygen taken in during recovery over and above that which would have normally been consumed for the same period of time during rest is used to provide energy for repaying the energy stores that were used up during exercise. This is illustrated schematically in Figure 2-5.

Since there is generally a lag in the circulatory-respiratory systems during the transitional period of rest and exercise, a small oxygen debt can occur even in light exercise for which a *steady state* (when the rate of work is such that the metabolic demand can be met aerobically) can be attained (Fig. 2-5A). Ordinarily, this oxygen debt is paid off quickly during the recovery period. During high-intensity work (anaerobic) in which a steady state cannot be achieved, the oxygen debt will continue to rise until work ceases (Fig. 2-5B). The duration of the exercise is generally limited by the individual's ability to tolerate a large oxygen debt. Research has illustrated that in maximal, all out work where anaerobic metabolism furnishes most of the energy needs, the length of work is restricted to approximately 30 seconds while recovery may last as long as 90 minutes. The untrained sedentary person will usually stop work when an oxygen debt of about 10 liters has been reached, wheres with endurance training the debt capacity may be increased to somewhere around 17 to 18 liters. Apparently, the highly trained athlete is able to tolerate a much larger oxygen debt than the untrained.

In determining the oxygen debt, two measurements are required: (1) the resting oxygen consumption, and (2) the oxygen consumed during the recovery period. For example, let us

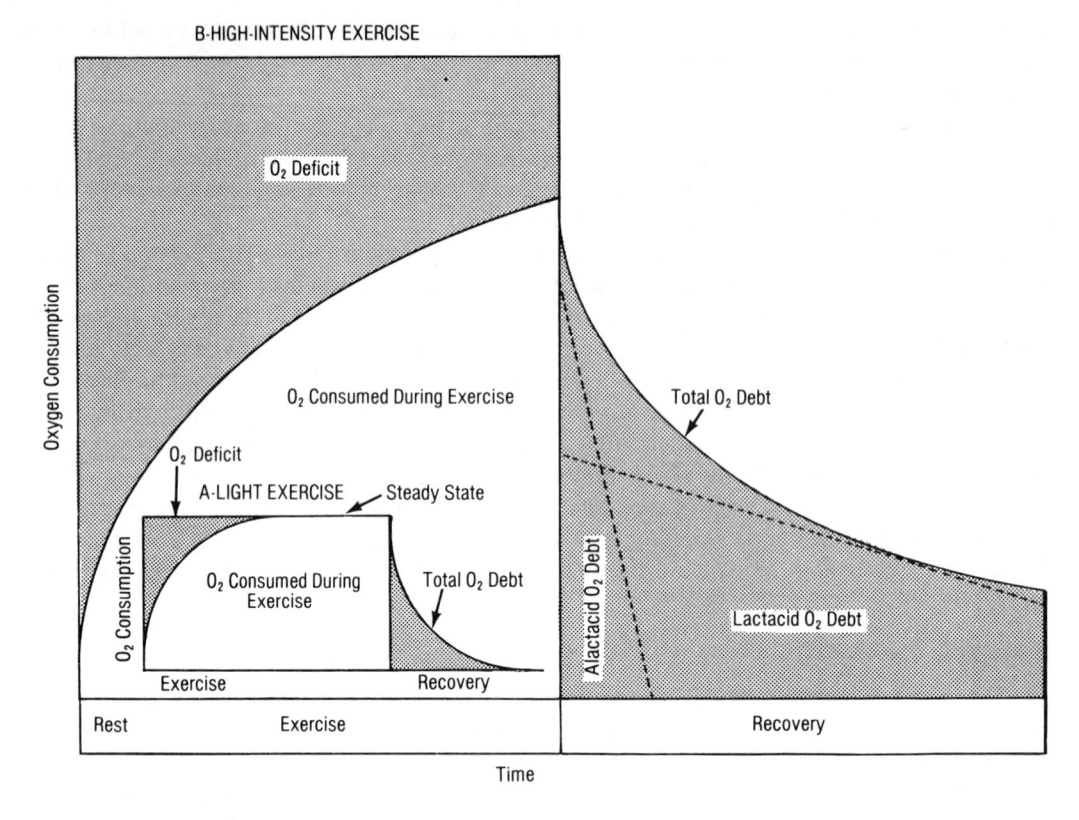

Figure 2-5 Schematic diagram of oxygen debt. *A,* Oxygen debt occurred during light exercise. *B,* Oxygen debt occurred during high-intensity work.

assume that we found during a 5-minute rest period the subject consumed 2,000 ml of oxygen or a resting rate of 400 ml per minute; and during a 20-minute recovery period following an exercise bout he consumed 10,000 ml of oxygen. From the recovery oxygen (10,000 ml), we subtract that amount which would have been used if the subject were resting for that particular time period; or 10,000 ml — (20 minutes × 400 ml), which equals 2,000 ml (oxygen debt).

Alactacid and Lactacid Debts. Although the oxygen debt is generally attributed to the cost of oxidation and reconversion of lactic acid (the by-product of anaerobic glycolysis), no very firm correlation of the debt volume and lactic acid content has been found. In fact, early research indicated that an oxygen debt of approximately 2.4 liters could be accumulated without significant increases in blood lactate concentration. Because these findings have been supported by other investigators working in the area, the oxygen debt has been generally accepted as having two components: *alactacid,* for which no significant lactate increment is found, and *lactacid,* which is represented by proportional increments in blood lactate (Fig. 2-6). In addition, researchers have found a tremendous difference in the repayment of these two oxygen debt components. The alactacid debt, as illustrated in Figure 2-5, accounts for the fast component of the recovery curve, and it is repaid at a rate approximately 30 times faster than the lactacid debt (the slow component of recovery).

Exercise, Energy, and Metabolism   27

The alactacid debt is generally attributed to the restoration of the ATP and CP stores in the muscles that were depleted during exercise, whereas the lactacid debt is more associated with the metabolic cost of converting lactic acid build up back to energy. More specifically, it is believed to be the direct cost of converting some of the lactic acid (approximately three-quarters) by way of the Krebs cycle and electron transport system to carbon dioxide and water with the production of ATP. Also, it is believed to be the direct cost of converting a small amount (about 10 percent) of lactic acid back to glucose in the liver and released into the blood stream as blood glucose. The remaining portion of lactic acid is unaccounted for.

As stated earlier, the lactacid oxygen debt is repaid at a rate approximately 30 times slower than the alactacid debt. This is because it takes a longer period of time to convert lactic acid back into glucose than it does to restore ATP and CP.

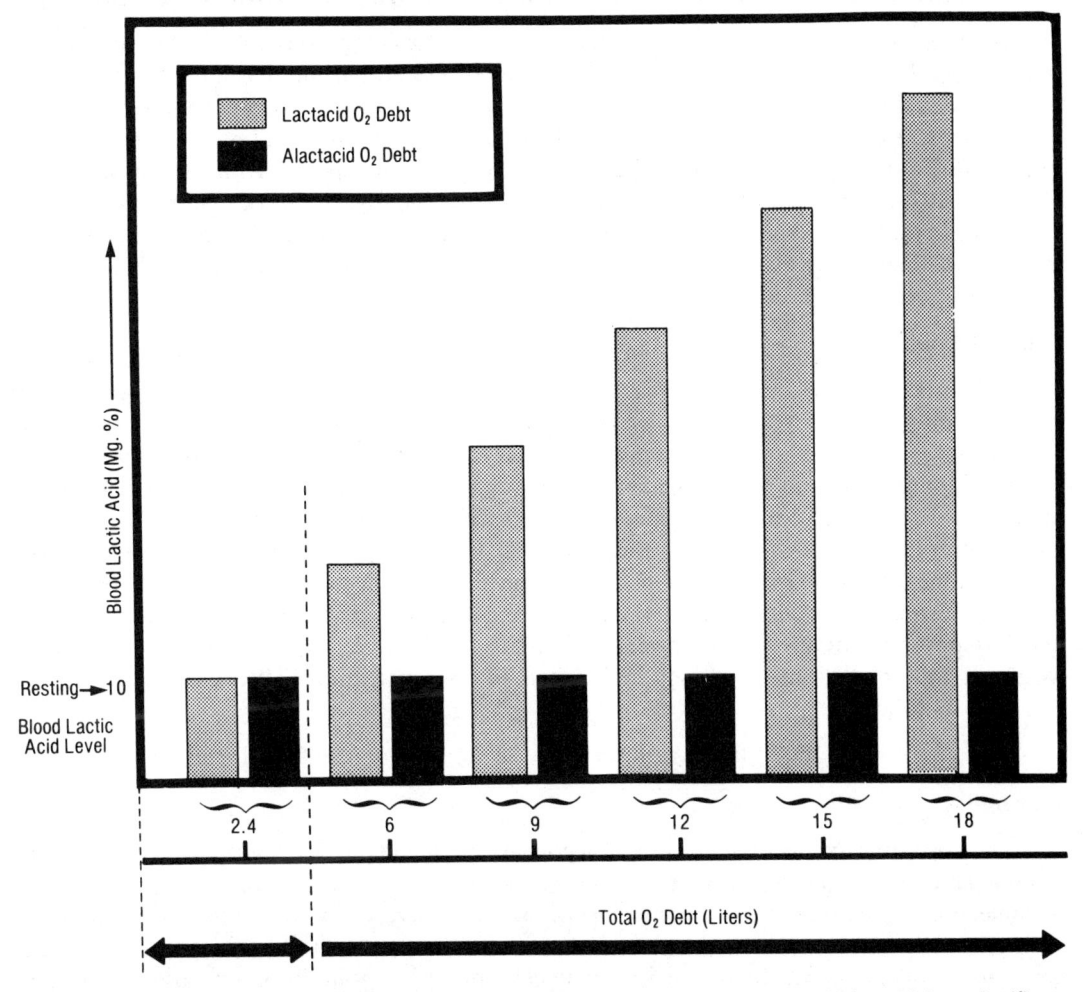

Figure 2-6 Illustration of the oxygen debt and its two components: Namely, alactacid for which no significant lactate increase is found, and lactacid which is represented by proportional increases in blood lactate.

Evidence is rather clear that lactic acid can be removed from the blood and converted into glucose and/or carbon dioxide and water at a faster rate following exercise if an individual performs light work such as walking or slow jogging or cycling rather than just sitting down and doing nothing. By keeping active during the recovery period, this not only allows for a faster conversion of lactic acid by the liver, but the heart as well as the active skeletal muscles are also using some of the lactic acid as a source of energy. Because more of the lactic acid is used as fuel under these conditions (and thus less is reconverted to glucose), the lactacid oxygen debt is reduced to about 1 to 2 liters in size. These findings support the general practice by most athletes of moving around by way of walking or jogging in between their event or matches rather than resting during recovery. This procedure obviously allows them to recover more quickly and be better prepared for their next event or match.

F. METHODS FOR ESTABLISHING A STANDARD MEASURABLE WORKLOAD

In order to collect meaningful measurements of the physiological processes during exercise, the work load must be set up in such a manner as to be measurable and repeatable, and it should demand very little skill. The majority of team sports do not lend themselves well to these requirements. For example, measuring the energy output of a basketball player would be very difficult due to the fact that his or her bursts of activity are interspersed with various periods of inactivity (free-throws, out-of-bound passes, etc.). Consequently, the work that is done changes from time to time. Listed below along with their advantages and disadvantages are three common methods that have been used in the past for establishing a standard measurable workload. They are:

Bench-Stepping

This procedure requires the subject to lift his weight a known height (height of bench) at a predetermined rate set by a metronome (Fig. 2-7). Use of this procedure requires no expensive equipment, very little skill, and is adaptable for large groups. One of the disadvantages of the bench-stepping technique is that the subject is doing both positive and negative work. Thus, negative work requires considerably less energy expenditure than positive work, and is also more difficult to measure. Another disadvantage is that once the subject becomes tired and nearly exhausted, he tends not to straighten his body at the hip and knee joint, and as a result, he has not lifted his center of gravity the full height of the bench. Work may be determined from bench-stepping by the use of the physicists' formula $W = F \times D$. Thus, a subject lifts his body weight of 140 pounds onto a 24-inch high bench 30 times per minute. Work done per minute would be as follows:

$$W = 140 \text{ lb} \times 2 \text{ ft (24-inch bench)} \times 30 \text{ steps/min} = 8,400 \text{ ft-lb/min}$$

Treadmill

The treadmill consists of a motor-driven conveyor belt and provides sufficient space for fast-running (Fig. 2-8). One end of the treadmill may be elevated so that an upgrade locomotion is possible. On some treadmills the movement of the conveyor can be reversed, making a downgrade locomotion possible. In addition, these devices are constructed so that the speed of the belt is adjustable. According to physicists, a subject running horizontally on a treadmill (0° slope) is not doing any work. He is raising and lowering his center of gravity the same distance; therefore, one destroys the other. Remember, work is moving an object through a distance, according to the physicists' formula $W = F \times D$. All energy expended by the subject when running on a treadmill at

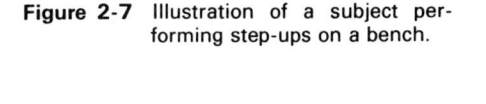

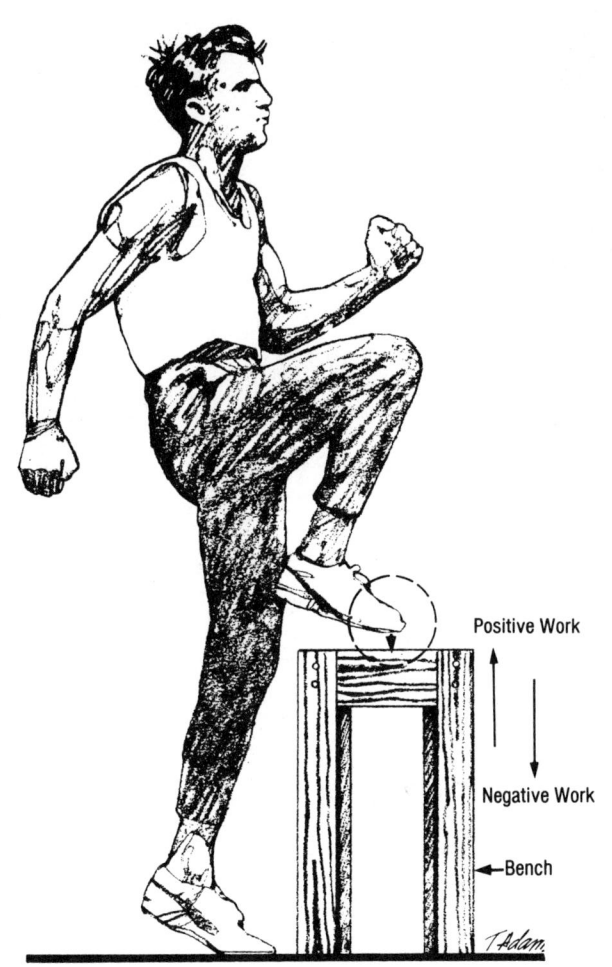

Figure 2-7 Illustration of a subject performing step-ups on a bench.

0° slope is degraded as heat without performing beneficial work. This means that in order to perform useful work on the treadmill, the slope of the treadmill must be greater than 0°. Work output is then equal to the weight of the subject times the vertical distance he would have raised himself in running up the incline of the treadmill. Mathews and Fox have recommended the following formula for computing work on the treadmill:

$$W = F \text{ (weight on subject)} \times D \text{ (vertical distance)}$$

where (1) Vertical distance = sine of angle theta (θ) times B (distance moved on the treadmill).
 (2) Sine of angle theta is measured with an inclinometer at point C in Figure 2-8. Once the degree of angle theta is found, then the next step is to find the tangent of the angle in Table 2-1. For example, assume angle θ is 1 degree, then the tangent of the angle θ is equal to 0.0175. Note that most trigonometric books will have tables similar to that of Table 2-1.

30 Essentials of Exercise Physiology

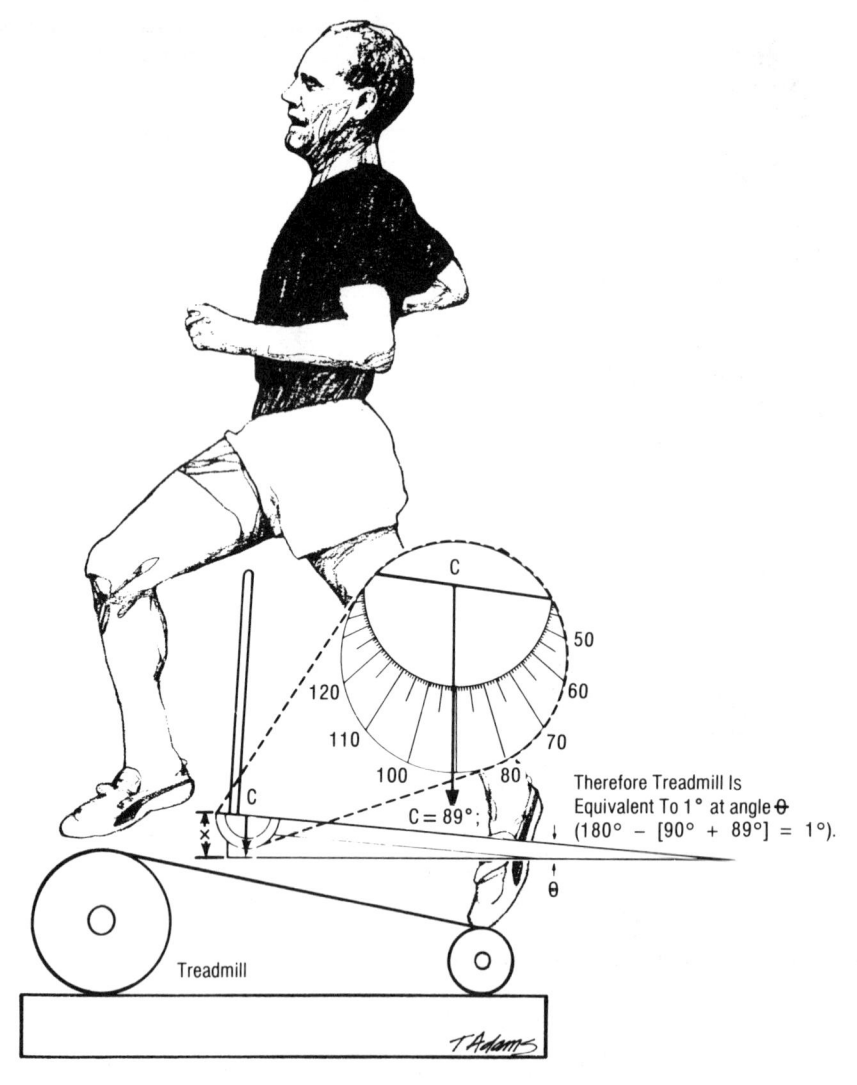

Figure 2-8 Schematic view of subject exercising by use of a treadmill.

(3) The speed of the treadmill and the time of the run are used in calculating B. An illustration of this is as follows. The speed of the treadmill is set at 4 mph. The time of the run is 15 minutes or 0.25 hours. This means that B is 1.0 mile (4 mph × 0.25 hr). Vertical distance is then calculated as 0.0175 miles (sine of angle θ = 0.0175 × 1.0 mile). Changing vertical distance in miles to feet is equal to 92.4 feet (0.0175 miles × 5,280 ft/mile). Assuming the weight of the subject is 150 pounds, then work is calculated as:

$W = F$ (150 lb) × D (92.4 ft) = 13,680 ft-lb of work accomplished during 15 minutes of running, or 924 ft-lb/min.

Table 2-1. Angles of Incline and Corresponding Per Cent Grade

θ (Degrees)	Tangent θ	Sine θ	Per Cent Grade
1	0.0175	.0175	1.75
2	0.0349	.0349	3.49
3	0.0524	.0523	5.24
4	0.0699	.0698	6.99
5	0.0875	.0872	8.75
6	0.1051	.1045	10.51
7	0.1228	.1219	12.28
8	0.1405	.1392	14.05
9	0.1584	.1564	15.84
10	0.1763	.1736	17.63

Source: Mathews, D. K., and E. L. Fox. *The Physiological Basis of Physical Education and Athletics,* 2nd edition, W. B. Saunders Co., Philadelphia, 1976, p. 64.

The treadmill is advantageous in that it allows the use of natural motions, such as walking and running, it requires no attention of the subject in keeping pace, and it brings about a greater involvement of muscle mass than either the bench-stepping or the bicycle. In fact, it is commonly believed that because larger muscle mass is involved when running on the treadmill, higher maximum oxygen consumption values are generally found when the treadmill is used than are obtained from the same subjects on the bicycle ergometer.

On the other hand, the treadmill has two major disadvantages. First, instrumentation (such as blood pressure cuffs, ECG electrodes, etc.) is difficult due to the movements of the arms and upper portion of the body. Second, it is difficult to standardize the work done, as this amount varies directly with body weight. Although it can be done, equating body weight and treadmill speed is difficult and not at all practical. Since most of the work is performed in a horizontal direction, the units of work are usually stated as running at 7 mph on a 6.6 percent slope instead of the usual standard units of foot-pounds or kilogram-meters.

Bicycle Ergometer

This ergometer is a stationary bicycle with one wheel adapted so that a belt can be passed around and attached to a spring balance (Fig. 2-9). This spring balance acts as a pendulum scale, measuring the difference in force at the two ends of the belt. The work load can be quickly and easily adjusted by changing the tension (and hence the frictional load) of the belt. Work is calculated easily from the scale, graduated in kiloponds,* which provides the frictional resistance (force), and from a counter that records the number of times the wheel has turned and thus allows calculation of distance ($D = 2\pi r \times n$). Remember that the wheel's circumference, $2\pi r$, is the distance traveled by any point on the wheel in one complete turn; n is the number of revolutions during the exercise period. Therefore, work may be written as:

$$W = F \text{ (resistance taken from scale)} \times 2\pi r \text{ (circumference of wheel)} \times n \text{ (number of wheel revolutions)}$$

*1 kilopond (kp) is the force acting on the mass of 1 kilogram(kg) at normal acceleration of gravity.

An illustrative example is as follows:
- Bicycle resistance (F) = 2 kiloponds
- Radius of wheel = .956 meters
- Pi (π) = 22/7 or 3.14
- Circumference = $2 \pi r$ or $2 \times 3.14 \times .956$ meters = 6.00 meters
- Wheel revolutions = 50

Therefore, Distance = 50 × 6.00 meters = 300 meters
Work = force × distance = 2 kiloponds × 300 meters
= 600 kilopond-meters

The advantages of the bicycle ergometer are several. First, it is an inexpensive piece of equipment—it may be built from a regular bicycle. Second, instrumentation for blood pressure, electrocardiograph, etc., is assisted since the upper portion of body is motionless during exercise. Third, the work load is expressed in standard units of work such as foot-pounds, kilopond-meters, or kilogram-meters which allows for work comparisons.

The disadvantages are that you cannot assume familiarity with this skill. Mechanical efficiency again has been shown to improve with practice; thus, you should allow at least two practice sessions before testing. In addition, as stated previously, low or maximum oxygen consumption values have been commonly found when the bicycle ergometer is used rather than the treadmill with the same subjects. Again, this may be due to the smaller muscle mass involved on the bicycle.

G. METHODS OF MEASURING THE AMOUNT OF ENERGY USED IN WORK

The sum of energy used for work can be found directly (*direct calorimetry*) by calculating the sum of heat produced, or indirectly (*indirect calorimetry*) by measuring it from the sums of oxygen absorbed and carbon dioxide eliminated. The term calorimetry is used because energy measurement (heat) is expressed in Calories (or kilocalories).

Direct Calorimetry

The direct method involves placing a subject in a specially built insulated chamber called a calorimeter with an oxygen supply (Fig. 2-10). The heat given off in response to food consumption by the subject is absorbed by water circulating around the chamber. Provided that the quantity of water and its temperature is known (upon reaching and leaving the chamber), the total sum of heat that is produced by the subject, and hence absorbed by the water, can be determined and expressed in terms of Calories or kilocalories per minute or hour.

Although this method is the basic method for research in energetics, it is very seldom used because it requires expensive equipment and is difficult to use. In addition to requiring a large staff of workers, it is also not applicable to sports activities. For these reasons, most work physiology studies with humans have been conducted by the indirect method.

Indirect Calorimetry

There are two basic subdivisions of this method: the *closed circuit* and the *open circuit*. These methods, and the subsequent determination of heat produced are based on the measurement of oxygen consumed and carbon dioxide produced. Generally, the metabolic rate is expressed in terms of either liters of oxygen per minute or Calories (or kilocalories) per minute. In order to express the quantity of oxygen absorbed in heat equivalents (i.e., Calories or kilocalories), it is

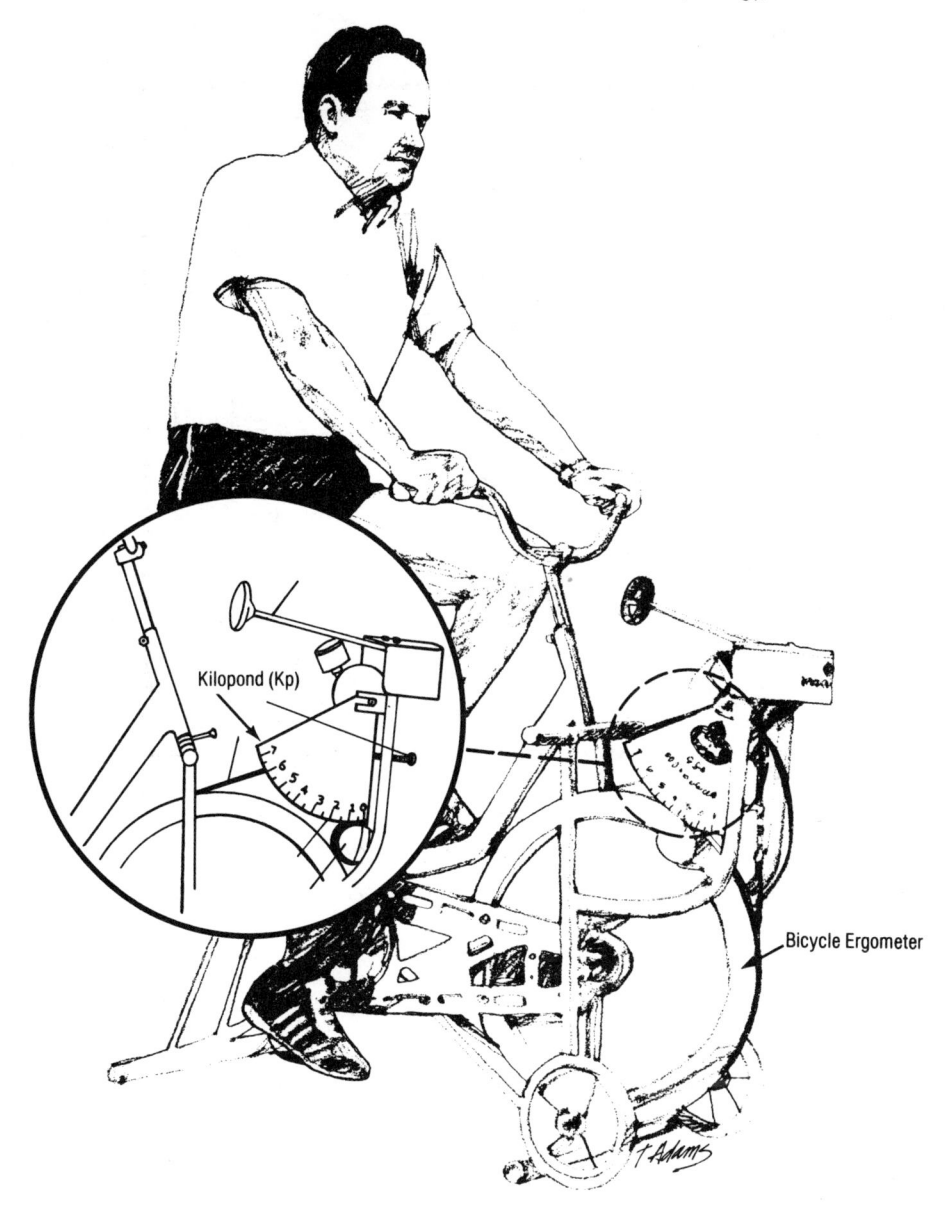

Figure 2-9 Schematic view of subject exercising by use of a bicycle ergometer.

essential that we know what type of food (carbohydrate, fat, or protein or any combination of them) is being metabolized. Note that this is made possible through the calculation of the respiratory quotient which will be discussed later in this chapter.

Closed Circuit. Figure 2-11 illustrates the closed circuit type of apparatus for measuring metabolism. The subject breathes oxygen from either a special mask or mouth piece that is connected to a special-type spirometer. The exhaled air returns to the spirometer and passes

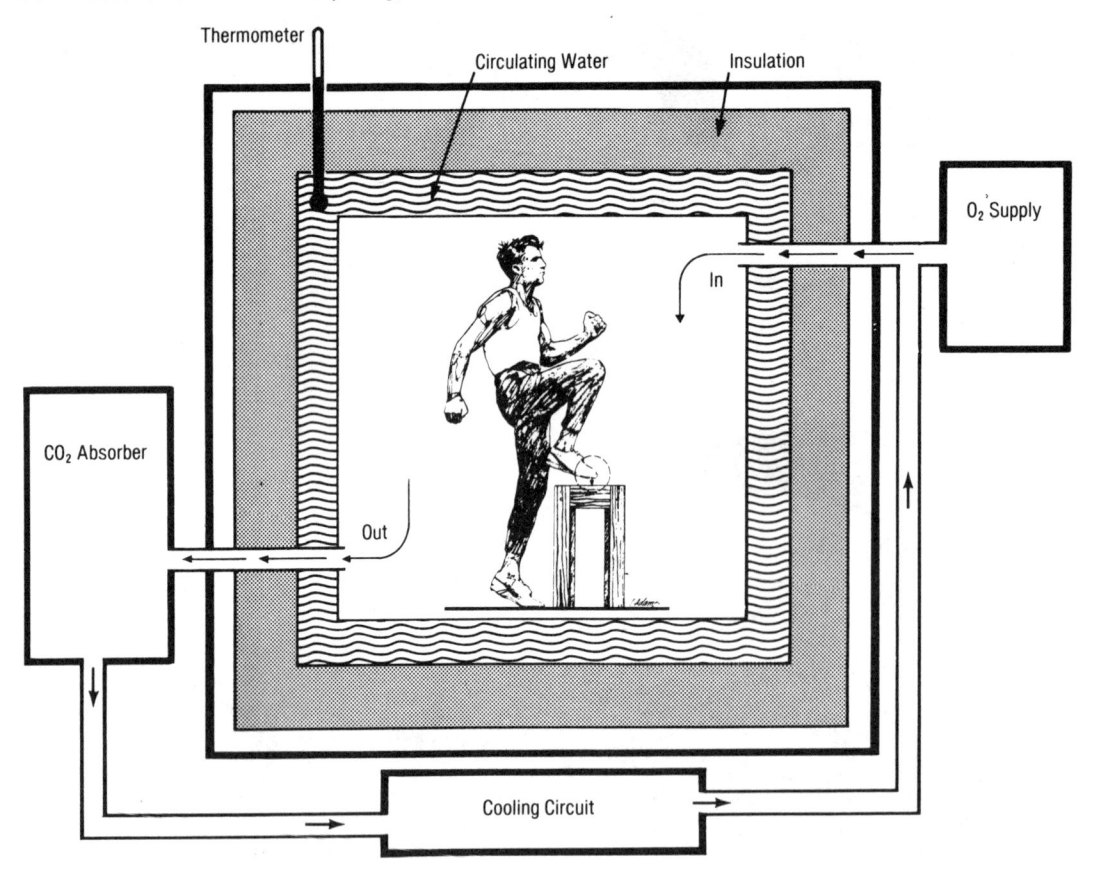

Figure 2-10 Direct calorimetry method for measuring heat energy.

through soda lime where the carbon dioxide is absorbed. As the carbon dioxide is absorbed, the changes in the volume of the oxygen that remains in the chamber are recorded from breath to breath on a revolving drum. Each peak on the kymogram, as illustrated in Figure 2-11, represents one respiration and by computing the downward slope of the lower points of the record per unit time, the amount of oxygen consumed can be determined as well as the oxygen deficit at the beginning of the exercise and the oxygen debt during recovery.

Although the closed circuit system is relatively simple to use, it has several disadvantages and they are: (1) its accuracy is only about ±10 percent of the true value; (2) the volume of the kymogram is so small until it is difficult to use during any kind of exercise; (3) the resistance is too large; and (4) since no value for the carbon dioxide produced is obtained, the respiratory quotient must be estimated.

Open Circuit. Figure 2-12 illustrates the open circuit method for determining metabolism. This is the most commonly used method in exercise physiology. In this system, the subject inhales

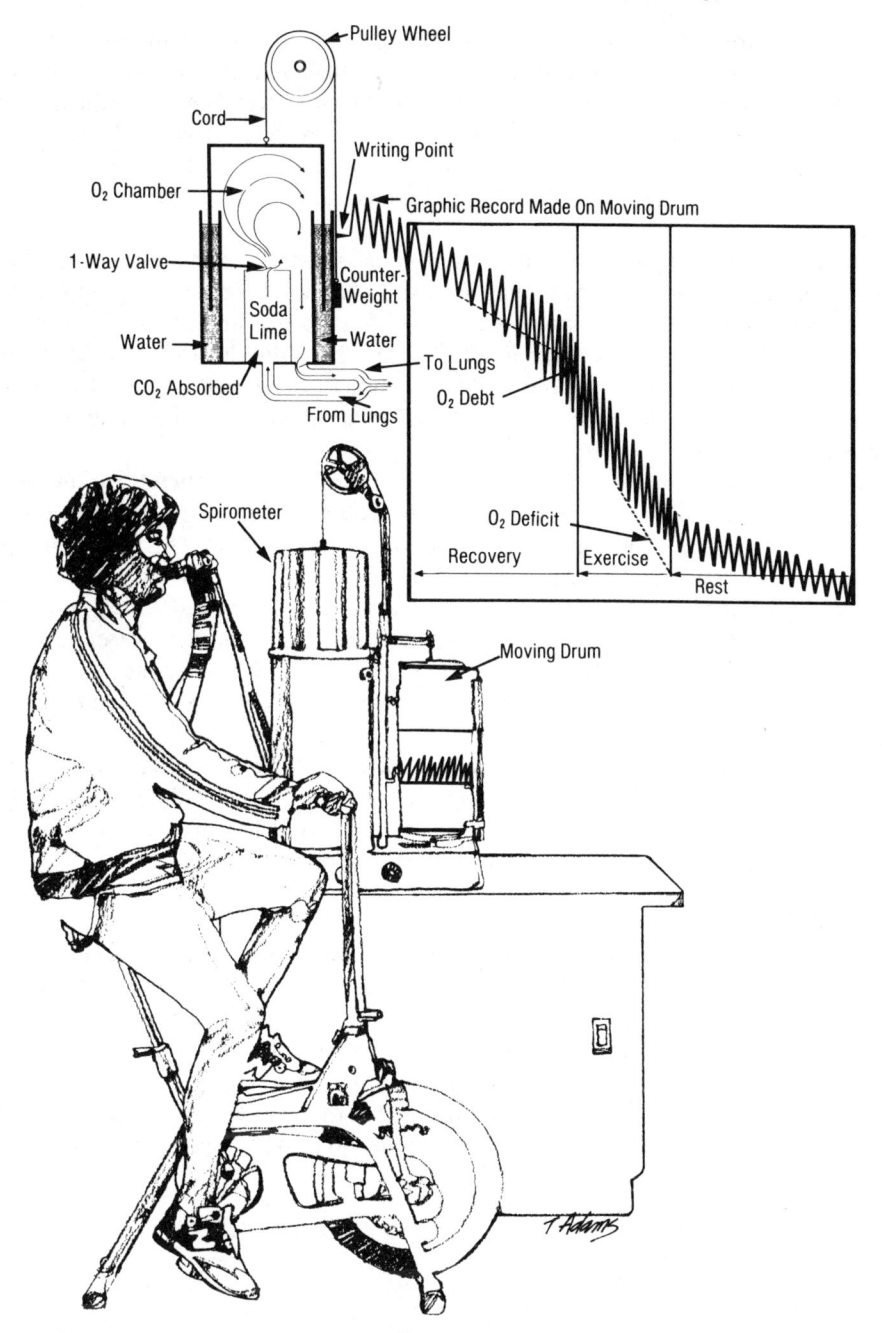

Figure 2-11 Illustration of the closed circuit (indirect calorimetry) method for measuring metabolism.

directly from the atmospheric air and exhales through a low-resistance, high-velocity type valve into some type of collecting apparatus such as a rubberized canvas bag (Douglas bag), a meteorological balloon, or a portable spirometer. Once exercise is over (during which gas collection is accurately timed), samples of the expired air are taken from the bag for oxygen and carbon dioxide analysis by either biochemical or electronic analyzers (the Haldane, the Scholander, the Beckman LB-2 and OM-11, and the Gas Chromatograph are just a few that are available).

The total volume of expired air is determined by passing it through a gas meter or by drawing it into a wet spirometer, whereas the volume of inspired air is determined from the percentage of nitrogen in the expired air (the amount remaining after oxygen and carbon dioxide have been analyzed). Since the percentage of oxygen (20.93) and carbon dioxide (0.03) in the atmosphere is always constant, the sum of oxygen consumed or carbon dioxide produced can be determined by multiplying the percentage times the volume of both inhaled and exhaled air, and thus computing the difference.

Because the amount of a gas (by weight) in a unit of volume depends on its pressure and temperature, it is generally common to reduce the volume of gases to standard conditions—temperature, 0°C; pressure, 760 mmHg; and water vapor, absent (dry). This is commonly referred to as standard temperature and pressure, dry, abbreviated STPD. In certain situations where the body temperature has to be used in the final computations, one should definitely indicate this by the abbreviation BTPD, where B stands for body. In other cases where it is essential to know the total volume of air moved, volumes are corrected to body temperature, atmospheric pressure saturated, abbreviated BTPS. Table of correction factors for both STPD and BTPS may be found in Appendix B and C, respectively.

Although the open circuit method is more involved than the closed-circuit, the accuracy is much greater. For example, the error in the open circuit system is usually less than ±1.0 percent, compared with ±10 percent for the closed circuit. Also, since the percent of carbon dioxide is calculated, it is possible to determine the respiratory quotient.

H. RESPIRATORY QUOTIENT (R.Q.)

The *respiratory quotient* (R.Q.) or *respiratory exchange ratio* (R) is equal to the volume of carbon dioxide produced to the volume of oxygen consumed. When this is calculated under resting or steady state conditions, it reflects the metabolic foodstuff being oxidized. For example, when carbohydrate (a foodstuff that in addition to carbon, consists of hydrogen and oxygen in proper proportions—two hydrogen atoms for every oxygen atom—to form water within the molecule) is oxidized, extra oxygen is required only for the oxidation of carbon. Therefore, for every molecule of oxygen consumed, a molecule of carbon dioxide is produced. This relationship can be written as:

$$C_6H_{12}O_6 + 6O_2 \text{ (sugar)} = 6CO_2 + 6H_2O$$

Thus,

$$R.Q. = \frac{6 \text{ (volumes } CO_2)}{6 \text{ (volumes } O_2)} = 1.0$$

Table 2-2 shows that for an R.Q. of 1.0, 5.047 kcal of energy per liter of oxygen will be released. On the other hand, when fat is oxidized, more oxygen is consumed than carbon dioxide is produced. This is because oxygen not only combines with carbon to form carbon dioxide, but it

Exercise, Energy, and Metabolism 37

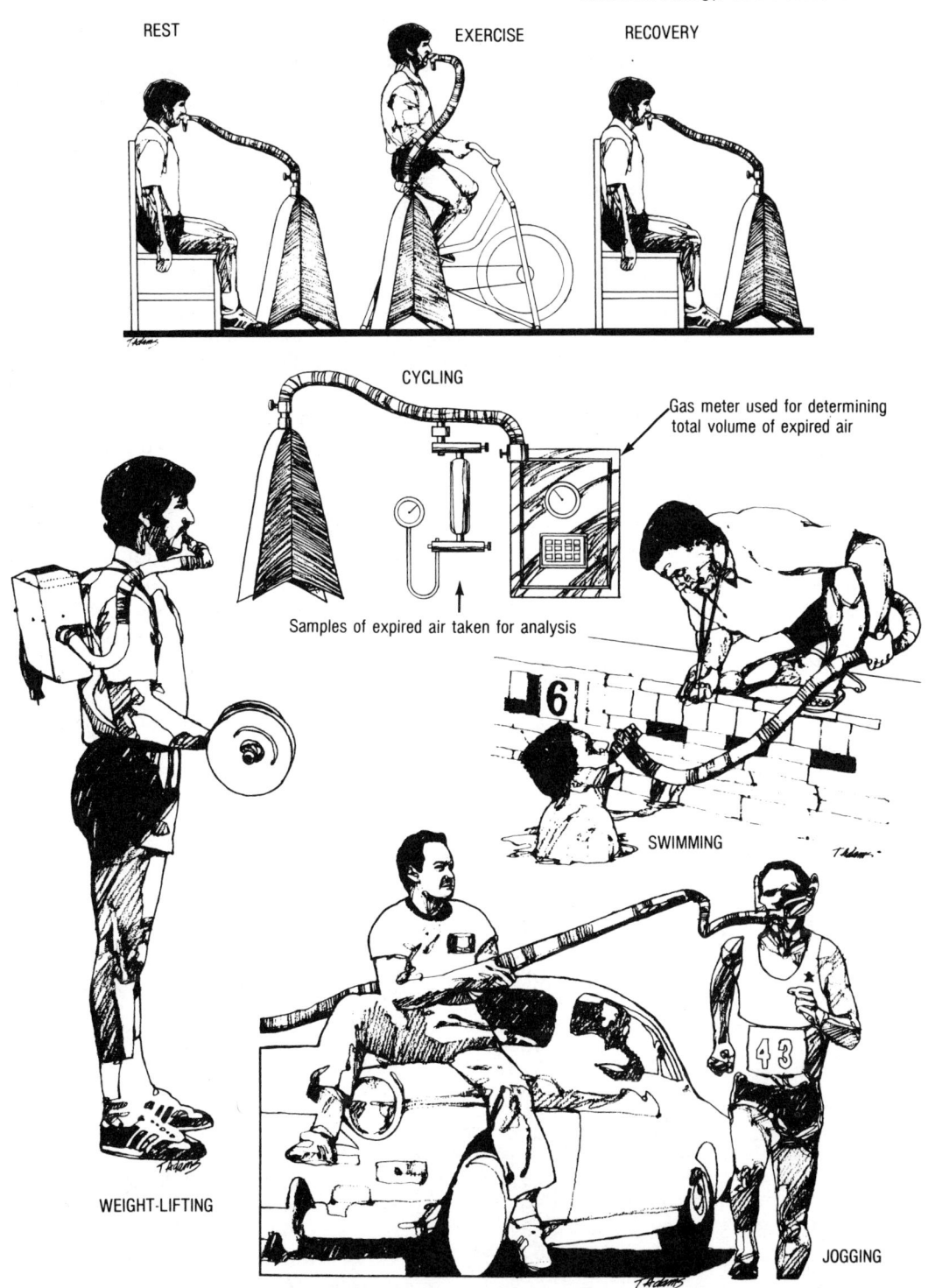

Figure 2-12 Illustration of the open circuit (indirect calorimetry) method for measuring metabolism.

also combines with hydrogen to form water. Consequently, the R.Q. will always be less than unity. Oxidiation of a typical fat molecule can be described as follows:

$$2C_{51}H_{98}O_6 + 145O_2 = 102CO_2 + 98H_2O$$

Hence,

$$R.Q. = \frac{102 \text{ (volumes } CO_2)}{145 \text{ (volumes } O_2)} = 0.70$$

Again, Table 2-2 illustrates that for an R.Q. of 0.70, 4.686 kcal of energy per liter of oxygen will be released.

Since the exact nature of the large protein molecule is not completely understood, the respiratory quotient for protein metabolism is estimated from known amino acid structures as about 0.80. However, it is generally believed that protein metabolism is not greatly increased in exercise, and is, therefore, not an important factor. Because its role can be closely determined from urine analysis (note that protein contains nitrogen in addition to carbon, hydrogen and oxygen; and when proteins are used, the body must get rid of the nitrogen and it is disposed of not as a free gas, like carbon dioxide, but instead, as urea), it is not important for the present discussion.

At this point, it should be emphasized that other factors, in addition to oxidative metabolism, can affect the R.Q. For example, just prior to exercise, some individuals show an anticipatory increase in pulmonary ventilation (hyperventilation), which results in excessive carbon dioxide loss and thus may temporarily increase R.Q. Additional increases in R.Q. may also be noticed in heavy exercise (anaerobic) as lactic acid begins to diffuse from the working cells into body fluids. The carbon dioxide is then blown off, a process that compensates for metabolic acidosis. The additional blowing off (where more carbon dioxide is being blown off than is being formed metabolically) may increase R.Q. as high as 1.6. Actually, the R.Q. may continue to increase for several minutes following exertion. The reason for this is that the amount of oxygen consumed during this period not only drops rather rapidly, but at the same time, lactic acid is still

Table 2-2. Caloric Equivalent Values Per Liter of Oxygen for Different Nonprotein Respiratory Exchange Ratios

R or RQ	kcal/liter O_2	R or RQ	kcal/liter O_2
1.00	5.047	0.84	4.850
0.99	5.035	0.83	4.838
0.98	5.022	0.82	4.825
0.97	5.010	0.81	4.813
0.96	4.998	0.80	4.801
0.95	4.985	0.79	4.788
0.94	4.973	0.78	4.776
0.93	4.961	0.77	4.764
0.92	4.948	0.76	4.751
0.91	4.936	0.75	4.739
0.90	4.924	0.74	4.727
0.89	4.911	0.73	4.714
0.88	4.899	0.72	4.702
0.87	4.887	0.71	4.690
0.86	4.875	0.70	4.686
0.85	4.862		

diffusing from the cells and thus forcing carbon dioxide formation. However, as the recovery process continues and lactic acid is eventually removed from the body fluids, these reactions are reversed. The carbon dioxide that is produced metabolically will be retained in bicarbonate to replace the lactate. Consequently, with the carbon dioxide retention, the R.Q. value may reach values as low as 0.5. Complete recovery is accepted as being a return to normal readings.

It is apparent that an R.Q. calculated under these conditions is not a reliable measure of oxidative metabolism. Thus, in some circles, it has been suggested that under these conditions, the term respiratory exchange ratio should be used instead of respiratory quotient. This has the advantage in that the ratio need not always be considered to represent a measure of oxidative metabolism, but instead, it is a ratio based simply on the rate of exchange of the respiratory gases.

I. BASIC PROCEDURES FOR INDIRECTLY DETERMINING NET AND GROSS ENERGY COST.

Computation of Energy by Way of Measuring Only the Oxygen Consumption

Suppose one is given the task of determining both the gross and net energy cost of push-ups. What basic procedures should be followed? As was pointed out by Mathews and Fox, three measurements are needed: (1) the oxygen used per minute at rest; (2) the oxygen used during the exercise under investigation; and (3) the oxygen used during the period of recovery (in other words, the oxygen debt) following exercise.

The resting oxygen consumption measurement is needed because this figure must be subtracted from the oxygen consumed during exercise and recovery in order that the *net oxygen cost of exercise* may be determined. Since the amount of oxygen taken in during exercise reflects only the energy supplied from aerobic metabolism, the recovery oxygen consumption (oxygen debt) measurement is needed because it reflects the energy supplied through anaerobic metabolism.

Prior to the exercise, the subject should be tested preferably in a basal state or, at least, two or three hours following a meal. During this time, the subject should be given a chance to get accustomed to breathing through the mask or mouthpiece. The individual should not have taken part in physical activity or smoking before the test since both may increase metabolism.

As stated earlier, some type of collection apparatus such as a rubberized canvas bag (Douglas bag) or meteorological balloon is required for collecting the exhaled gas for purposes of volume measurement and analysis. Figure 2-12 illustrates that the resting sample is obtained first, then the exercise, and finally the recovery. All three collection bags are maintained and analyzed separately. It should be pointed out that although recovery periods seldom go over 30 minutes, an exhaustive-type exercise may require a longer period of time. Thus, in some cases, more than one recovery bag may be needed. Samples of the expired air are first taken from each of the bags for oxygen and carbon dioxide analysis. The volume in each bag is then measured by either passing the gas through a gas meter or by drawing it into a wet spirometer.

Following a rest period of 10 minutes, let us assume that the subject consumed 2,500 ml of oxygen. Dividing this by 10, we obtain 250 ml, which represents the *resting oxygen consumption* per minute. During two minutes of push-ups, controlling the cadence by a metronome, the subject consumed 3,500 ml of oxygen. This represents the *exercise oxygen consumption*. Following exercise, the subject consumed 5,000 ml of oxygen for a period of 15 minutes. This represents the *recovery oxygen*. How do we determine gross and net cost of the push-ups?

Gross cost of exercise is found by adding the quantity of oxygen consumed during exercise and recovery (3,500 ml + 5,000 ml = 8,500 ml or 8.5 liters). To determine the *net cost*, it is necessary to subtract from the gross cost the quantity of oxygen which the subject would have consumed during same period if he were resting (2 min of exercise + 15 min of recovery = 17 min). For example, the net cost of the push-ups is:

$$17 \text{ min} \times 250 \text{ ml } O_2 \text{ (resting } O_2 \text{ min.)} = 4{,}250 \text{ ml}$$
$$8{,}500 - 4{,}250 \text{ ml} = 4{,}250 \text{ ml, or } 4.25 \text{ liters}$$

The net cost of the push-ups per minute would be:

$$4{,}250 \text{ ml} \div 2 \text{ min} = 2{,}125 \text{ ml/min, or } 2.125 \text{ liters/min}$$

Computation of Energy by Way of Determining the R.Q.

Although the computation of energy would be simple if the number of kilocalories produced would remain constant for each liter of oxygen consumed, however, it is well-known that the caloric equivalent of a liter of oxygen varies from 4.686 to 5.047 kilocalories, depending upon the type of food being oxidized such as carbohydrates, fats, proteins, or any combination of them (Table 2-2). Since proteins play a relatively minor role in exercise metabolism, the oxidation of them may be disregarded. Therefore, the caloric value of 1 liter of oxygen will depend on the relative amounts of carbohydrate and fat used. It is apparent that for an accurate appraisal of the amount of energy expended in doing work, it is necessary to have data on both oxygen and carbon dioxide in order that the R.Q. might be determined.

As an illustration, let us assume that 4 liters of oxygen were consumed in riding a bicycle ergometer for 5 minutes. From Table 2-2, if the individuals diet were carbohydrate (R.Q. = 1.0), the caloric value of 4 liters of oxygen would equal 20.188 kilocalories (4 × 5.047) of energy used.

In the closed circuit system, where all computations are based solely on the amount of oxygen consumed, the respiratory quotient is generally assumed to be 0.82 (1 liter of O_2 = 4.825 kcal) on a normally mixed diet.

Modified Ways of Indirectly Determining Energy Cost

At this point, it should be mentioned that during some exercises such as sprinting a 220-yd dash or swimming underwater (mainly anaerobic type work), it is nearly impossible to collect expired air during the activity without affecting the performance. For this reason, several researchers have used modified techniques for indirectly determining energy cost. For example, in determining the net cost of such exercise, the resting oxygen consumption is first determined and then, during the activity, the subject holds his breath until the exercise is completed, at which time he then directs all exhaled air into some type of collection apparatus such as a Douglas bag. In following this procedure, the net cost is based entirely on the oxygen debt. Caution should be taken when using this procedure since it has been documented that the energy expenditure of work computed primarily from the oxygen debt is generally larger than what it would be if the same work was done aerobically where a steady state could be obtained.

It should be pointed out that normally when submaximal type work is performed (aerobic work), the net cost of the work may be calculated without necessarily having to determine the recovery oxygen. This is assuming, of course, that during the submaximal exercise, a steady state is obtained. At the same time, if the work is short and exhaustive such as running a 100-yd dash, the oxygen consumption during the sprint is not really a true indicator of oxygen needs, and therefore, the oxygen debt should be determined in order to get a more accurate picture of the oxygen requirement.

Recently, the *telemetry* recording device has been incorporated in teaching and research studies for the purpose of estimating indirectly from heart rate determinations the oxygen consumption of various activities. It has been especially popular in team and individual sport activities. In order to use this method, a graph similar to that shown in Figure 2-13 should be computed for each subject separately, indicating the relationship between heart rate and oxygen consumption during submaximal-type work. For example, the subject may be asked to ride a bicycle ergometer at progressively increasing work loads; and then the oxygen consumption and heart rate is determined and recorded against each work load. The subject is then able to use this graph as his own personal instrument for estimating the energy cost of other activities. Once the graph is finished, the subject is then equipped with a small transmitter which has a set of electrodes attached to it. The transmitter is attached around the subjects waist. After the electrodes have been placed on the subject in correct positions, the small transmitter is then ready to transmit the heart rate to a recorder which may be several hundred feet away. At any time during the activity (for example, a soccer game), heart rate can be measured and oxygen consumption estimated. For example, Figure 2-13 illustrates that if heart rate were 140 beats per minute, then oxygen consumption would equal about 1.75 liters per minute at that particular time.

It should be pointed out under submaximal work loads, it is generally well known that heart rate is linearly related to the work load and the oxygen consumption values. It is because of this relationship that the telemetry system has been able to be used with fairly good success. However, it should also be mentioned that this linearity between heart rate and oxygen consumption only holds true for submaximal work. For instance, upon approaching maximum, the heart rate has a

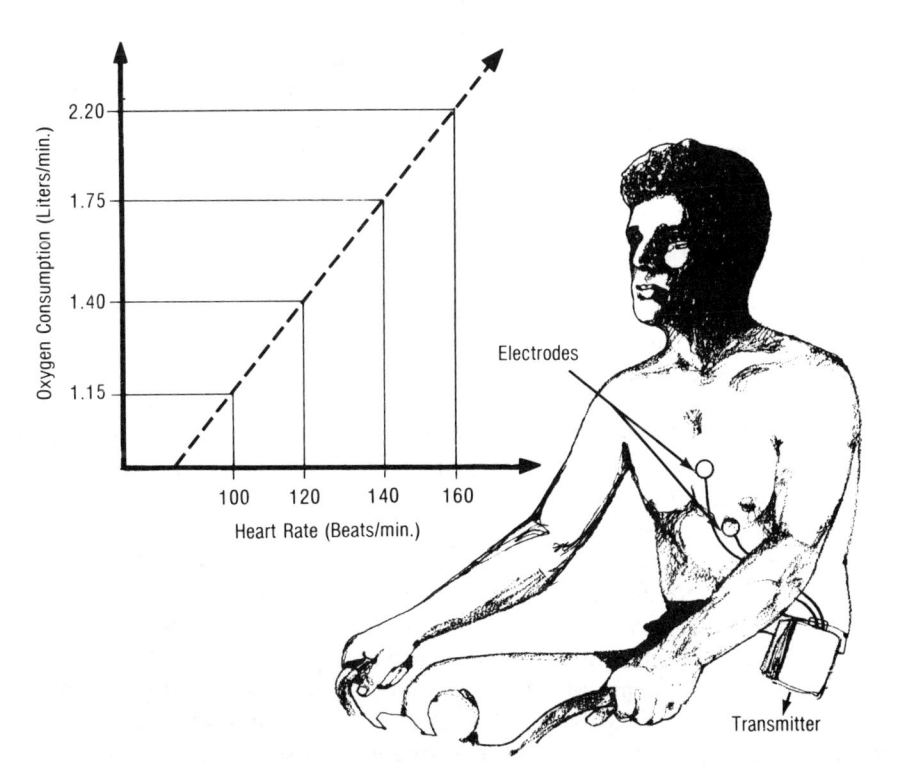

Figure 2-13 Schematic diagram illustrating the relationship between heart rate and oxygen consumption during progressively increasing submaximal-type work loads.

tendency to level off, while at the same time, the oxygen consumption may continue to climb. Consequently, if oxygen consumption is computed under these conditions on an assumption of heart rate-oxygen consumption linearity, it will generally be smaller than the true value.

It is interesting to note that telemetry equipment allows for radio transmission or telemetering of not only heart rate, but several other physiological variables including respiratory rate, blood pressure, and electromyography. The type of transmission obviously depends upon the type of transmitter and receiver that you may or may not have.

J. NEGATIVE WORK

Up to this point, the primary concern has been with positive work (concentric-type contractions in which the muscle shortens during work). However, energy is also required during *negative work* (eccentric-type contractions in which the muscle lengthens while resisting the opposing force—gravity).

In the past, it has generally been the policy to use the physicist's definition of work ($W = F \times D$) in calculating eccentric contractions and just referring to it as negative work. However, it has been demonstrated that work calculated in this manner cannot be used interchangeably with that of positive work because the amount of energy involved in performing the work is somewhat different. For example, when two bicycles were coupled together and the riders were asked to pedal against each other (one pedaled eccentrically while the other pedaled concentrically), the subject performing positive work required more than three and one-half times as much oxygen as the subject doing negative work (Fig. 2.14). Note that in this particular investigation, both riders developed the amount of force that was required to balance each other.

It is interesting to note that when both negative and positive workloads are plotted against oxygen consumption, Figure 2-15 illustrates a typical drawing showing that while both types of work are linearly related to oxygen consumption, the negative work demands less oxygen. In fact, evidence is rather clear that positive work is somewhat more costly (somewhere between 3 and 9 times) in terms of energy expenditure than negative work.

K. BASAL METABOLIC RATE (BMR)

Basal metabolic rate (BMR) is defined as the minimum amount of energy (expressed in kilocalories) required for each square meter of body surface area during a state of complete rest. The measurement is generally determined by use of the indirect calorimetry method and is usually done after a normal night's sleep and before breakfast by calculating the amount of oxygen consumed by the body for 10 to 15 minutes. It should be pointed out that there should be no voluntary muscular movement during the test and no muscular activity within half an hour to an hour prior to the test. Also, there should be no stress due to extremes of environmental temperature (note that room should be around 80° F). A cold room would have a tendency to speed up metabolism. Under these conditions, basal metabolism is the energy needed to maintain the body's internal processes such as heart beat, muscle tone, respiration, and nervous system activity.

Normally, basal metabolism is directly proportional to body surface which, in turn, is based on height and weight; thus each individual has his own basal metabolic rate. It is generally known that after the age of 5, the basal metabolic rate for females is about 5 to 10 percent lower than for males. As shown in Figure 2-16, at about the age of 20, the rate drops for both sexes and continues to decline slowly with age. Between the ages of 20 and 40, women usually average around 35 kcal/m² of body surface area per hour in caloric expenditure, which over a period of 24 hours, will result in basal rates ranging from 1,200 to 1,400 kcal. At the same time, men of comparable age

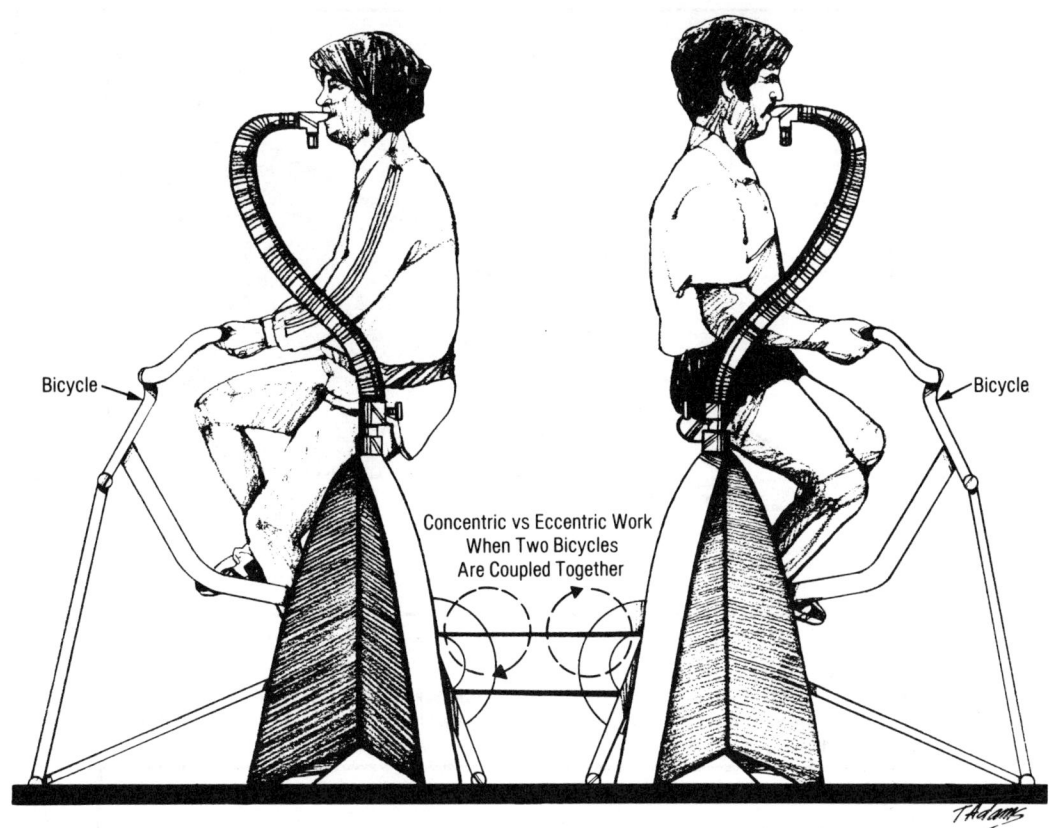

Figure 2-14 Schematic view of two subjects riding two bicycles that were coupled together. One subject is performing positive work (concentric-type work) while the other subject is performing negative work (eccentric-type work).

and body structure show values around 38 kcal/m² of body surface area and basal rates for a 24-hour period of about 1,668 kcal. A more detailed discussion of BMR between men and women can be found in Chapter 11.

A common method of reporting basal metabolic rate is in terms of the percentage deviation from the standard value. For example, if the basal metabolic rate of a female subject, age 25, is determined to be 38.2 kcal/m² per hour and compared with the standard value of 36 kcal/m² per hour:

$$\text{Percentage deviation} = \frac{38.2 - 36.0}{36.0} \times 100 = +6.1\%$$

Normally, the individual should not deviate more than ±10 percent from this standard. Any devergence beyond these limits indicates an abnormal basal metabolic rate for a subject of this age and sex.

Basal metabolic needs can be determined quickly by utilizing the body surface area calculation nomogram in Figure 2-17. For example, assuming the female subject above was 5 feet tall and weighed 110 pounds, she would have a body surface area of 1.47 square meters and

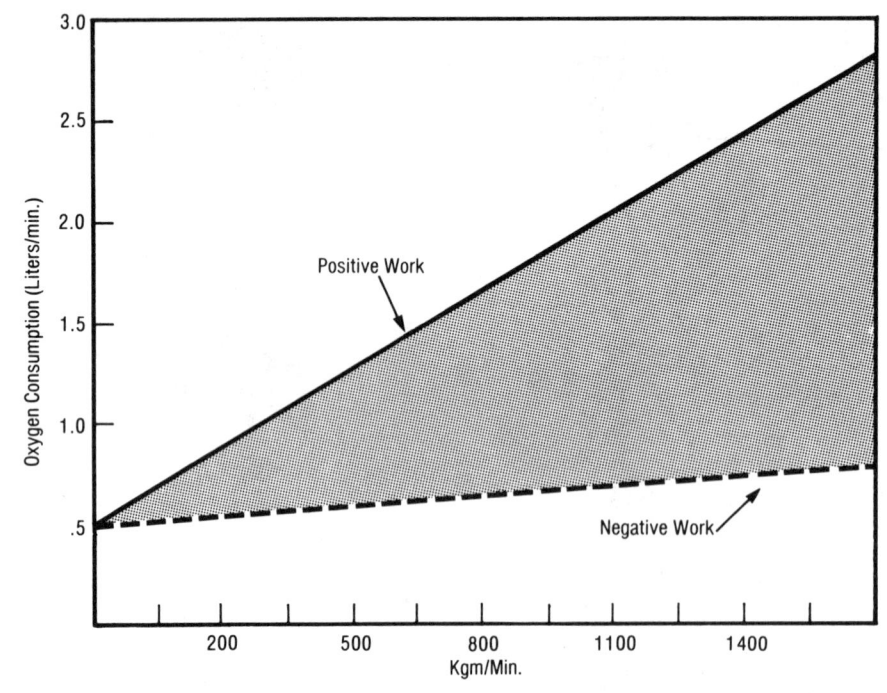

Figure 2-15 Illustration showing the relationship between positive workloads and oxygen consumption and between negative workloads and oxygen consumption.

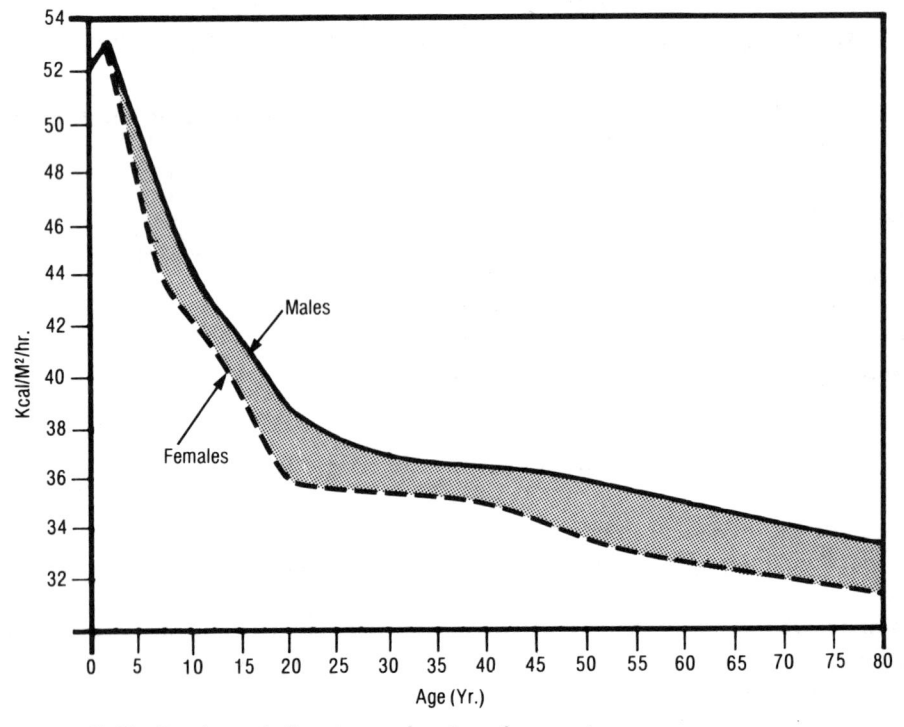

Figure 2-16 Basal metabolic rate as a function of age and sex.

corresponding basal metabolic energy need of about 56 kcal per hour (38.2 × 1.47) or 1,344 kcal for the day (24 hr × 56 kcal). It is obvious that daily caloric needs far exceed these basal requirements.

Another quick, but less reliable way of determining resting metabolism is to determine the caloric equivalent of the total amount of oxygen consumed in a 24-hr period of time. For example, recall from earlier discussion that the respiratory quotient (R.Q.) during the post-absorptive state is generally assumed to be 0.82 which results in 4.83 kcal per liter of oxygen consumed during the oxidation of a mixed diet. Therefore, basal heat production is determined on the basis of 4.83 kcal of heat for every liter of oxygen consumed. Because the average, normal resting oxygen consumption is around 0.25 liters/min (or 250 ml/min), an average resting energy cost per minute would be 1.21 kcal (4.83 kcal × 0.25 liter). When this is computed over a 24-hr period (24 hr × 60 min/hr = 1440 min), it turns out to be 1,742 kcal (1.21 kcal × 1,440 min). It should be remembered, however, that this method of computing resting metabolism does not take into account differences in an individuals overall body size such as body surface area (height and weight), and therefore, it is only a rough estimate of resting metabolism. Figure 2-18 illustrates the estimated relative energy needs (in terms of oxygen consumption) of the various organs of the body.

III. SUMMARY

(1) In order to understand and appreciate the measurements of the metabolic processes during work and recovery, the following terms are needed:

    (a) energy (in kcal): 1 kcal = 3,087 ft-lb

    (b) work: $W = F \times D$

    (c) power = $\dfrac{\text{work}}{\text{time}}$ or $\dfrac{F \times D}{t}$ or if power is defined in horsepower:
    1 hp = 33,000 ft-lb/min

    (d) gross efficiency (percent) = $\dfrac{\text{external work output}}{\text{total energy used for work}} \times 100$

    (e) net total energy used for work = $\dfrac{\text{external work output}}{\text{total energy used} - \text{basal requirements}} \times 100$

    (f) METS: 1 MET × metabolic cost during rest; 2 METS × two times the resting level; 3 METS × three times the resting level, etc.

(2) The immediate sources of energy for a muscle cell come from ATP (adenosine triphosphate) and CP (creatine phosphate). Because these sources are not dependent upon oxygen nor on a series of reactions, they are especially important for activities involving powerful quick starts of football players, high jumpers, sprinters, and basketball players as well as events taking only a few seconds to complete such as running up a flight of stairs.

(3) Anaerobic and aerobic metabolism are the two energy sources by which ATP is formed. The anaerobic pathway (also called glycolysis), while using only carbohydrates (glycogen and glucose), does not require oxygen in its production of ATP, whereas the aerobic pathway requires the presence of oxygen and may use all three foodstuffs (carbohydrates, fats, and proteins). The aerobic pathway results in a complete breakdown to CO_2 and H_2O. When compared to the aerobic pathway, the anaerobic system is very inefficient since it results in an incomplete breakdown of food to lactic acid (which causes muscular fatigue).

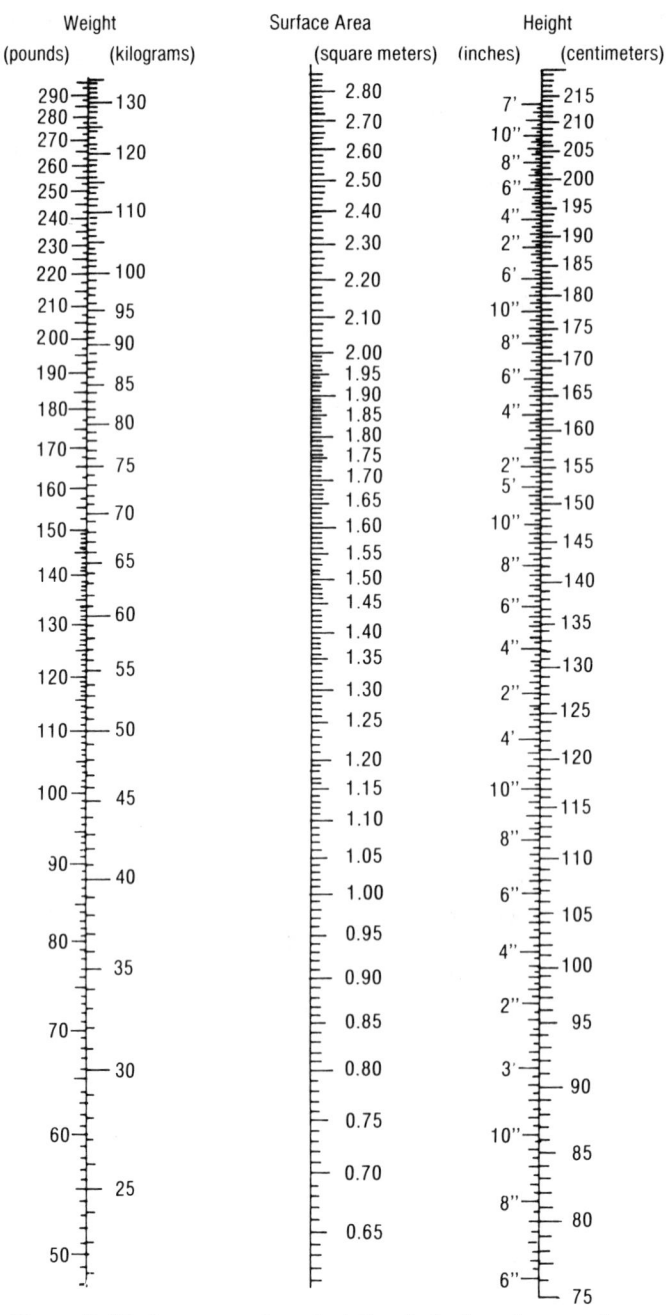

Figure 2-17 Nomogram for calculating the body surface area from height and weight.
(Adapted from the Dubois Body Surface Chart, Warren E. Collins, Inc., Braintree, Mass.)

Exercise, Energy, and Metabolism   47

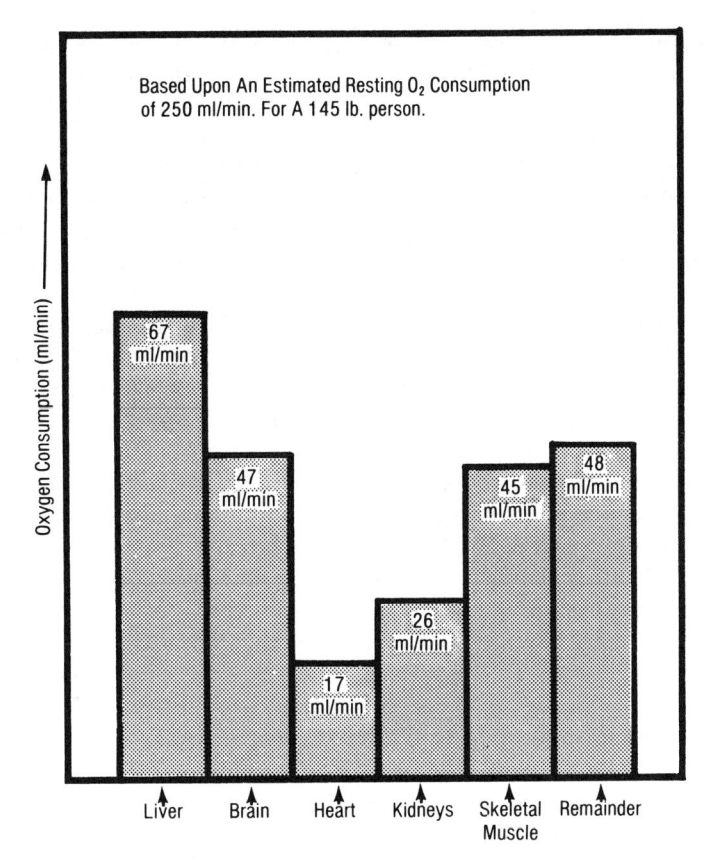

Figure 2-18 Illustration of the estimate relative energy needs in terms of oxygen consumption of the various organs of the body.

(4) During rest, aerobic metabolism supplies all the ATP needs of the body. Approximately two-thirds of the food source is contributed by fats and the remaining one-third by glucose. Protein contribution is negligible.

(5) During short-duration, high-intensity exercises (events lasting up and no more than 2 minutes), the primary food fuel is the stored ATP and glycogen. Fatty-acids may play a minor role if intervening rest periods are allowed. The predominent pathway is anaerobic with the aerobic cycle playing only a minor part.

(6) In high-intensity exercises that can last from 5 to 10 minutes, the major food fuels are stored ATP, creatine phosphate, and muscle glycogen. Oxidation of fatty-acids contribute less than 10 percent of the energy cost. Activities include middle-distance running, swimming, cycling, lacrosse, soccer, and basketball. These performances require a blend of both anaerobic and aerobic energy sources with lactic acid formation.

(7) In long duration activities of low intensity, the aerobic breakdown of fat, glycogen and glucose furnish most of the energy with very little lactic acid production. As the work is continued, and the glucose is nearly depleted, a greater contribution of the energy comes from the stored fat as well as from the fatty-acids. Activities include channel swimming, marathon running, recreational jogging, cycling, and laborers working an 8-hr day in a factory.

(8) Oxygen consumed over and above resting values following a bout of exercise is called oxygen debt. The oxygen debt has two components: (a) alactacid component which accounts for the fast component of the oxygen debt recovery curve, and (b) lactacid component which is illustrated by the slow component of the curve.

(9) Oxygen consumed during the alactacid portion of the debt is used to replenish the ATP and CP stores in the muscles, whereas the lactacid debt is attributed to (a) converting a small amount (about 10 percent) of the lactic acid produced during work back to glucose in the liver and released into the blood stream as blood glucose; (b) converting approximately three-quarters of the lactic acid by way of the Krebs cycle and electron transport system to carbon dioxide and water with the production of ATP; and (c) the remaining portion of lactic acid is unaccounted for.

(10) Three popular methods that are used for establishing a standard measurable workload are: bench-stepping, treadmill, and bicycle ergometer.

(11) Two methods are generally used in calculating the energy cost of work. They are: (a) the indirect calorimetry method whereby the sums of oxygen absorbed and carbon dioxide eliminated are measured. The indirect method utilizes either the closed-circuit or the open-circuit system.

(12) During rest or steady-state exercise conditions, the respiratory quotient (R.Q.) accurately indicates the metabolic foodstuff being oxidized. Carbohydrates yields the highest and fats the lowest.

(13) During exercise, the R.Q. may increase as high as 1.6 because of lactic acid being buffered while during recovery, the R.Q. may reach values as low as 0.5 when the lactic acid is being oxidized and bicarbonate is being reformed.

(14) When indirectly determining the energy cost of an activity, three measurements are generally required. They are: (a) the oxygen used per minute during rest; (b) the oxygen used during the activity under investigation; and (c) the oxygen used during the period of recovery following the activity. Because the caloric equivalent of a liter of oxygen varies from 4.686 to 5.047 kcal, depending upon the type of food being oxidized (carbohydrates, fats, proteins, or any combination of them), a more accurate appraisal of energy cost is possible by measuring both oxygen and carbon dioxide and determining the R.Q.

(15) Because heart rate during submaximal workloads is linearly related to workload and oxygen consumption values, a modified procedure for determining energy cost may be used during submaximal work by recording with a telemetry the heart rate and using a graph similar to that in 2-13 to predict the actual energy cost of that particular activity.

(16) Negative work is approximately 3 to 9 times more economical than positive work in terms of energy cost.

(17) Basal metabolic rate (BMR) is defined as the minimum amount of energy (expressed in kcal) required for each square meter of body surface area during a state of complete rest. It is based upon age, sex, and body surface area.

(18) Women, between the ages of 20 and 40, usually average around 35 kcal/m^2 of body surface area per hour in caloric expenditure, while men of comparable age and body structure show values around 38 kcal/m^2.

IV. REVIEW REFERENCES

(1) Edington, D. W., and V. R. Edgerton. *The Biology of Physical Activity,* Houghton Mifflin Co., Boston, 1976.
(2) Gollnick, P. D., and L. Hermansen. "Biochemical adaptations to exercise: Anaerobic metabolism," in *Exercise and Sport Sciences Reviews,* Vol 1, J. H. Wilmore, ed. Academic Press, New York, 1973.
(3) Guyton, A. C. *Textbook of Medical Physiology,* 5th ed., W. B. Saunders Co., Philadelphia, 1976.
(4) Holloszy, J. O. "Biochemical adaptations to exercise: Aerobic metabolism," In *Exercise and Sport Sciences Reviews,* Vol. 1, J. H. Wilmore, ed. Academic Press, New York, 1973.
(5) Katch, F. I., and W. D. McArdle. *Nutrition, Weight Control, and Exercise,* Houghton Mifflin Co., Boston, 1977.
(6) Knoebel, L. K. "Energy Metabolism," In *Physiology,* 4th ed., E. E. Selkurt, ed. Little, Brown, and Co., Boston, 1976.
(7) Lamb, D. R. *Physiology of Exercise: Responses and Adaptations,* Macmillan Publishing Co., Inc., New York, 1978.
(8) Mathews, D. K., and E. L. Fox. *The Physiological Basis of Physical Education and Athletics,* 2nd ed., W. B. Saunders Co., Philadelphia, 1976.

3

THE RESPIRATORY SYSTEM AND EXERCISE

KEY CONCEPTS TO BE GAINED FROM THIS CHAPTER

(1) Respiration during exercise is regulated by chemical, neural, and temperature factors as well as by the secretions of norepinephrine and epinephrine.

(2) During exercise, minute ventilation or pulmonary ventilation is regulated more to the need for carbon dioxide disposed than to oxygen consumption.

(3) Alveolar ventilation is the most important measure of the effectiveness of a person's respiration.

(4) The exchange of gases (oxygen and carbon dioxide) between the alveoli of the lungs and the blood as well as between the blood and the tissue cells is determined by pressure gradient differentials.

(5) During exercise, the diffusion surface capacity is increased at both the alveolar-capillary and the tissue-capillary membranes due to the fact that many more capillaries are now open.

(6) During exercise, the hemoglobin concentrations in the blood increases, thus resulting in an increased oxygen-carrying capacity of the blood.

(7) The oxygen dissociation curves play an extremely important part in the understanding of gas transport.

(8) The releasing of oxygen into the tissues facilitates the loading of carbon dioxide into the blood, while the releasing of carbon dioxide into the lungs facilitates the loading of oxygen into the blood.

Generally speaking, respiration refers to all of the processes that contribute to the exchange of gases between the body and the external environment. From a functional point of view, Figure 3-1 illustrates that the respiratory process can be divided into two parts: namely, the *external* and the *internal* phases. The external (or pulmonary ventilation) phase includes the following: (1) air entering the lungs, (2) oxygen leaving the lungs and entering the pulmonary blood, (3) blood

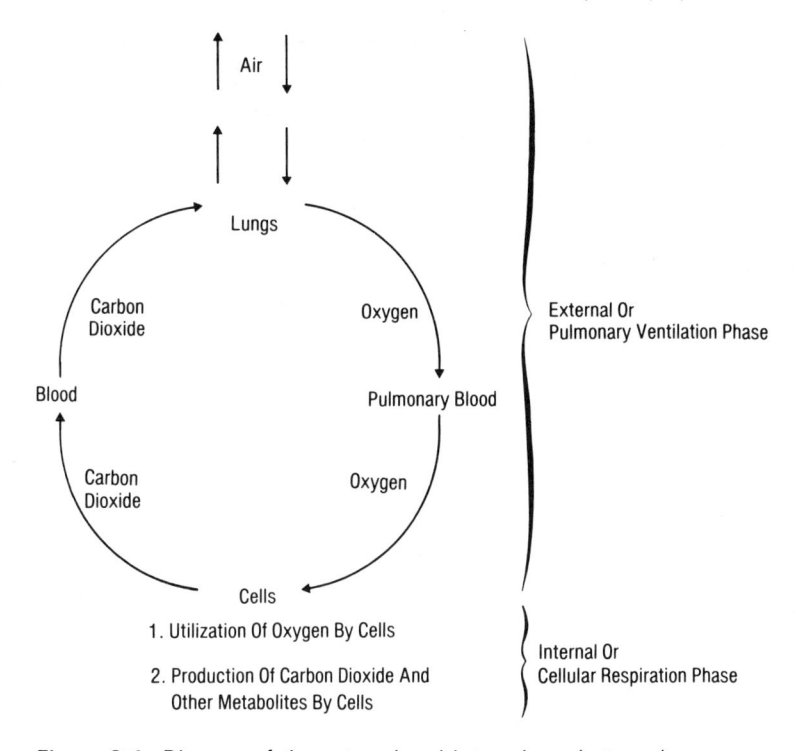

Figure 3-1 Diagram of the external and internal respiratory phases.

transporting oxygen to all the cells of the body, (4) oxygen being utilized by the cells while carbon dioxide is being produced, (5) blood transporting carbon dioxide to the lungs, (6) carbon dioxide leaving the blood and entering the lungs, and (7) carbon dioxide leaving the lungs. Internal respiration (or cellular respiration) is concerned only with the utilization of oxygen and the production of carbon dioxide and other metabolites by the cells. Thus, the purpose of this chapter is to discuss the various factors that control and regulate the respiratory process, and to present the different components of the respiratory system and their physiological responses, both at rest and during exercise.

I. STRUCTURAL PROPERTIES OF THE LUNGS

It will be recalled from basic physiology and anatomy that in order for air to enter the lungs, it must first travel through the nose and sometimes the mouth. In either case, the air ultimately flows through the *pharynx*. It should be pointed out that the nose is the preferred route, because the nasal passages are designed for this purpose. Air drawn in through the nose flows over a series of surfaces made up of the *nasal septum* and the *nasal turbinates*. These surfaces warm and moisten the inspired air. In addition, they act as baffles to its flow, causing particles of dust and other foreign bodies to settle out on the mucus films lining the nasal passages. Large parts of the surfaces are made up of *ciliated cells,* and the beating of the cilia moves the foreign products down into the throat and eventually into the stomach and destroyed. Breathing through the mouth, on the other hand, generally results in relatively cold and unfiltered air reaching the lungs.

52 Essentials of Exercise Physiology

Figure 3-2 shows that the *trachea* or wind pipe extends from the *larynx* (the voice box) and just below the base of the neck, splits into the two major *bronchi* (singular; *bronchus*); one going to each lung. Inside each lung the bronchus repeatedly branch out into smaller *bronchioles* until the *terminal bronchioles* are reached. Each terminal bronchiole subdivides into two respiratory bronchioles, which in turn, may branch again thus forming *alveolar ducts*. The alveolar ducts may or may not divide, but they eventually terminate in saclike structures called *alveoli* (singular; *alveolus*). The actual exchange of oxygen and carbon dioxide take place between the air in the alveoli and the blood which flows through very small neighboring capillaries. In addition, it is generally believed among researchers that a certain amount of gas exchange may also take place in the respiratory bronchioles. All the other structures just mentioned serve only as air passageways; no gaseous exchange takes place in them.

II. THE RESPIRATORY MUSCLES

Figure 3-3 illustrates the location of the lungs within the rib cage and the principal muscles involved in breathing. The size of the chest cavity is enlarged during inspiration as a result of the contraction of the ventilatory muscles.

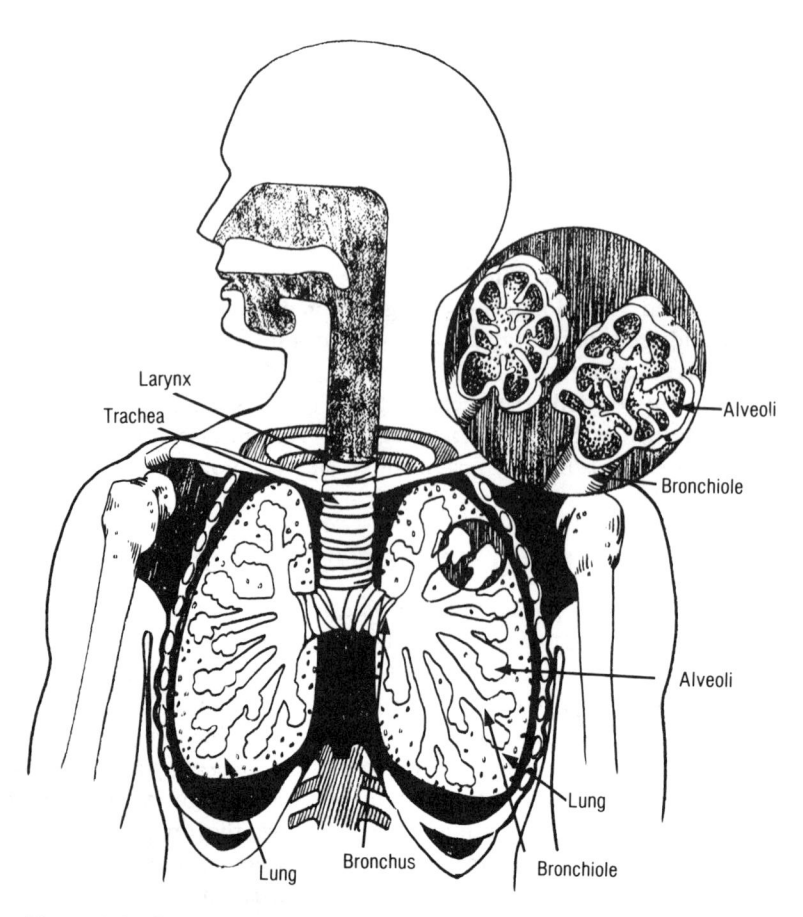

Figure 3-2 Structure of the lungs.

A. MUSCLES USED IN INSPIRATION

The *diaphragm* is believed to be the most important single muscle of inspiration. During rest conditions, it makes a dome over the liver and stomach. When it contracts, it causes the bottom of the thorax to flatten (increases the vertical dimension of the thorax). In other words, the domed area is lowered. Also, during strenuous work when heavy breathing is required, the *external intercoastal* muscles are brought into play much more extensively. They raise the ribs and sternum in order to create additional enlargement of the anteroposterior and lateral diameters of the chest cavity.

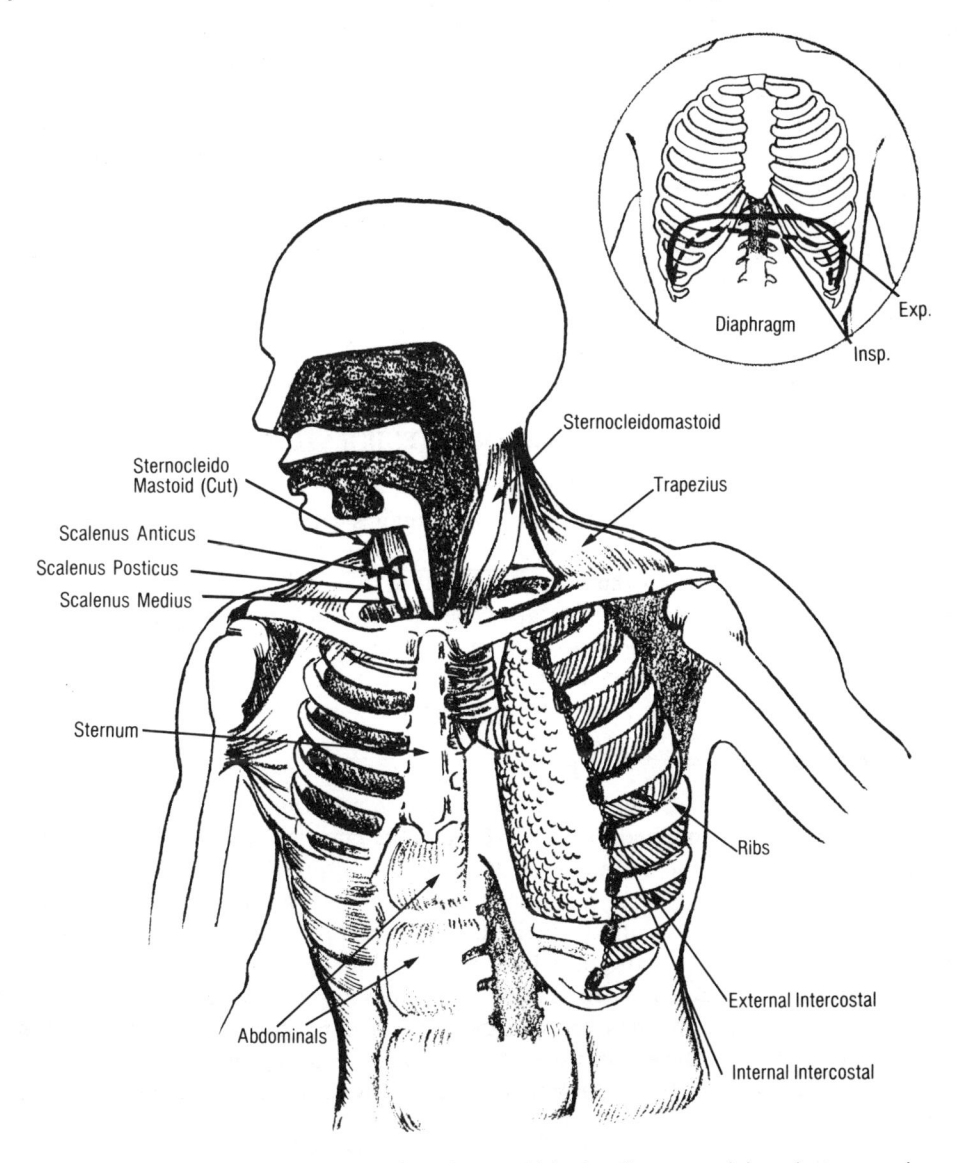

Figure 3-3 Schematic illustration of the lungs within the rib cage and the primary muscles involved in breathing.

Furthermore, during exercise, the large volume of inspired air is also aided by contraction of two other inspiratory muscles. For instance, contraction of the *scalene* and the *sternocleidomastoid* muscles helps raise the first two ribs and the sternum, respectively. It should also be pointed out that the *extensor* muscles of the back and neck, along with the large *trapezius* muscle also help facilitate inspiratory breathing during vigorous work.

B. MUSCLES USED IN EXPIRATION

During normal resting conditions, expiration is primarily due to the elastic recoil of the inspiratory muscles (diaphragm and external intercoastals) as they return to their resting positions. This means that during normal resting conditions, expiration plays a passive role while inspiration plays a more active role. However, during exercise, expiration is aided by contractions of the expiratory muscles, thus making it an active process. The *abdominals* are the most important muscles of expiration during heavy work. When these muscles contract, they not only flex the trunk, but they also press down the lower ribs. This, in turn, helps raise the pressure inside the abdomen. The diaphram is then forced upward into the thoracic region, thus reducing the overall size of the thoracic area and aiding in expiration. In addition to the abdomials, the *internal intercoastal* muscles are also brought into play during heavy breathing. Figure 3-3 shows clearly that the internal intercoastal muscle fibers are directly opposed to those of the external intercostals. This means that during their contraction, they will pull the ribs down, thus bringing them closer to each other. Hence, the combined action of the abdominals and the internal intercostal muscles aid in reducing the size of the thorax, and thus facilitate the role of expiration.

III. REGULATION OF RESPIRATION

Although the respiratory muscles play an important part in facilitating the movement of air in and out of the lungs, the ultimate control of breathing is carried out automatically (without conscious control) through rhythmical discharge of nerve impulses arising in an area of the brain called the *medulla oblongata* and the *pons*. While all of the mechanisms in respiration are not totally understood, the following factors are generally accepted. For simplicity, they will be discussed according to: (a) the reflex mechanism of respiration, and (b) the chemical, nervous, temperature, and hormone factors that control the rate and depth of respiration. It cannot be over emphasized, however, that they all function together in a "team-like" fashion.

A. THE REFLEX MECHANISM

As illustrated in Figure 3-4, there is an *inspiratory center* and an *expiratory center* located on each side of the medulla. Combined, these two centers are known as the *respiratory center*. The inspiratory center sends nerve impulses to the various respiratory muscles (primarily the intercostals and the diaphram via the intercostal and phrenic nerves, respectively), thus causing contraction or inspiration. If left to itself, the chest would remain in a state of inspiration. However, within the lung tissue themselves, are specialized nerve endings or *stretch receptors* which become stimulated when the lungs are stretched. The vagus nerve is responsible for sending the impulses from the stretch receptors to the medulla, where in turn, they bring about expiration and inhibit inspiration. When inhibited, the inspiratory center no longer sends impulses to the chest muscles; consequently, the lungs are able to empty themselves passively. After the air has been removed

The Respiratory System and Exercise   55

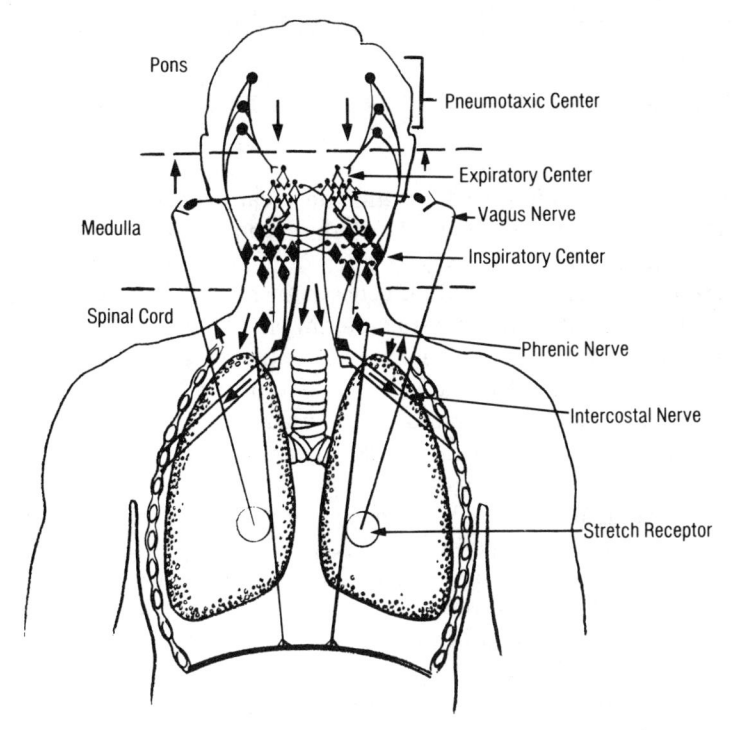

Figure 3-4 A schematic view of the nervous reflex mechanism for the control of breathing.

from the lungs, the action of the stretch receptors subsides, and thus the inhibitory effect of the expiratory center dwindles. Shortly afterwards, the impulses from the inspiratory center are renewed and the cycle starts over. This reflex action for preventing overinflation of the lungs is called the *Hering-Breuer inflation reflex*. Thus, the act of inspiration is automatically ended after it has gone so far. It should be pointed out that the Hering-Breuer reflex also works in reverse (called the *Hering-Breuer deflation reflex*) to cause inspiration when no signals are generated from the stretch receptors.

Also, there is another automatic mechanism which aids in closing off the tonic excitation of the inspiratory center. This is called the *pneumotaxic reflex*. When the inspiratory center fires vigorously, it not only transmits impulses to the appropriate muscles but also sends impulses up to the pneumotaxic center which is located in the pons, as illustrated in figure 3-4. This center, in turn, is activated and sends excitory impulses down to the expiratory center, in much the same way as do the stretch receptors in the lungs. The excited expiratory center then inhibits the inspiratory center. Following this action, the pneumotaxic center requires another series of nerve impulses from the inspiratory center in order to activate it once again.

There is some evidence to indicate that in normal, quiet breathing the pneumotaxic center does not function. Apparently, it operates only in conditions which demand maximal breathing such as an athlete running a 220-yd dash. Thus, it is generally regarded as being a second line of defense, to augment the Hering-Breuer reflex or to substitute for it if need be during strenuous work.

B. CHEMICAL, NERVOUS, TEMPERATURE, AND HORMONE FACTORS

Chemical Factors

The respiratory center is stimulated by three different chemical conditions of the blood. These are commonly referred to as the tension of the carbon dioxide, the concentration of the hydrogen ions, and the tension of the oxygen. Each of these wil be discussed separately.

Carbon Dioxide. The most powerful influence known to affect the respiratory center is a slight increase in carbon dioxide tension of the arterial blood—*hypercapnia*. When this tension begins to increase, as in exercise, the center is excited and the ventilation rate and depth is stepped up. Figure 3-5 illustrates that increased carbon dioxide in the blood can increase the rate of alveolar ventilation to as much as 10 times above normal.

According to experts working in this area, evidence shows that somewhere around 50 percent of the carbon dioxide effect on the respiratory center is the result of its direct action on the respiratory neurons. This action brings about an increased level of excitement. The remaining 50 percent is apparently the result of the hydrogen ions when they are indirectly formed by the breakdown of carbon dioxide to carbonic acid. For example, during exercise when carbon dioxide increases in the blood, a certain amount of it diffuses over into the fluid (called cerebrospinal) in which the brain is surrounded. Here, carbon dioxide combines with water to form carbonic acid (reaction is $CO_2 + H_2O \rightleftarrows H_2CO_3$). With the increased production of carbonic acid, more hydrogen ions are also formed, thus increasing its concentration in the cerebrospinal fluid. The respiratory center is specifically excited by the hydrogen ions because it is located on the anterior side of the medulla which is in immediate contact with the fluid. More will be said abut hydrogen ions in the next section as well as later in the chapter.

Hydrogen Ions. It is now generally acknowledged that the second most powerful stimulus on the respiratory center is the hydrogen ion concentration in the body fluids. For instance, when the hydrogen ion concentration becomes high as a result of a low pH (brought about by an increased carbon dioxide), the respiratory neurons are excited, and thus ventilation increases. Figure 3-5 illustrates, however, that by increasing the hydrogen ion concentration, maximum ventilation can only be increased about 5 times above normal. Thus, an increase in hydrogen ion concentration is only approximately one-half as potent (in terms of stimulating the respiratory center) as an increase in carbon dioxide concentration.

Oxygen. Surprisingly enough, the lowering of the blood-oxygen tension (*hypoxemia*) by increased consumption in work and exercise has almost no direct effect on the respiratory centers. For instance, at normal ventilatory rates the hemoglobin always becomes almost completely saturated with oxygen, and large increases or moderate decreases in ventilation make very little difference in the amount of oxygen transported away from the lungs by the hemoglobin. At the same time, however, when one goes to high altitudes where the oxygen concentration in the atmosphere is very low, then the oxygen concentration in the alveoli of the lungs may fall too low to supply sufficient amounts of oxygen to the hemoglobin molecule. This may also occur when a person contacts pneumonia or some disease. Under these conditions, there is a mechanism called the *chemoreceptor system* which invokes hyperventilation. Within the wall of the arch of the aorta and in the bifurcation of the carotid arteries of the neck, there are *chemoreceptors* (Fig. 3-6). These chemoreceptors are sensitive to the lack of oxygen in the blood, and if the arterial oxygen falls too low, they are stimulated to send impulses to the medulla, where they stimulate the respiratory

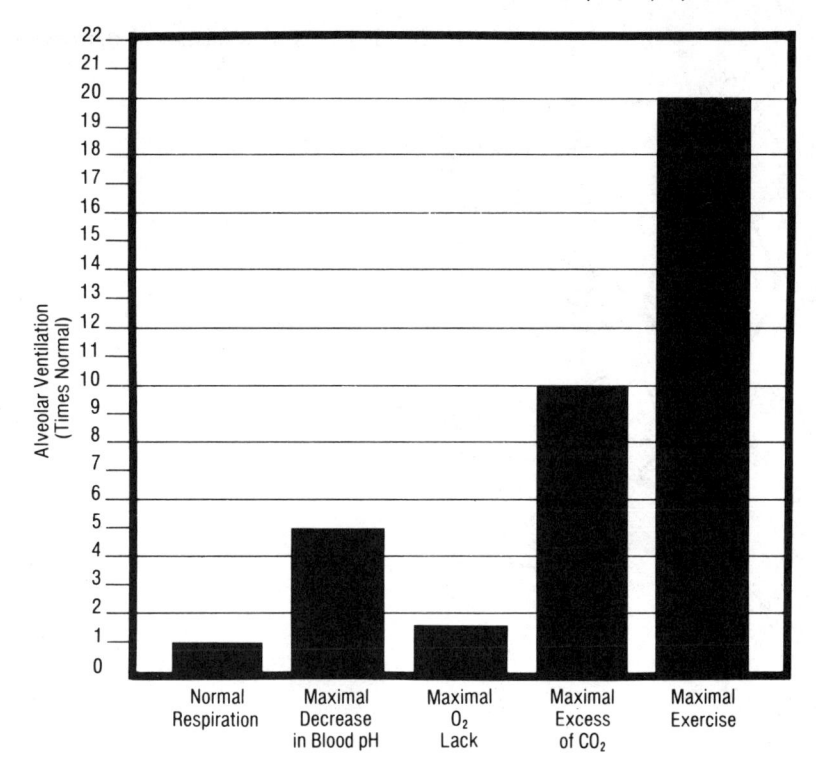

Figure 3-5 Illustration of three different chemical conditions of the blood (carbon dioxide, hydrogen ions, and oxygen) for controlling the breathing process.

center to increase the rate and depth of breathing. As illustrated in figure 3-5, the chemoreceptor system is not a powerful stimulator of respiration in comparison with the excess carbon dioxide or hydrogen ions. Figure 3-5 shows that maximum oxygen lacks can increase alveolar ventilation to about one and two-third times its normal value in comparison with an increase of 10 and 5 times caused by excess carbon dioxide and hydrogen ions, respectively.

Nervous Factors. It is interesting to note that most physiologists believe that the increase in respiration during exercise is not caused by either an increase in carbon dioxide nor to a decrease in oxygen. Instead, it is generally believed that an increased ventilation during exercise is the result of some stimulus reaching the respiratory center by way of the nervous system. For example, there is a substantial amount of evidence to indicate that during the anticipation of exercise as well as during exercise, the *cerebral cortex* transmits signals not only to the exercising muscles but also to the respiratory center to increase the rate and depth of breathing. In addition, considerable evidence exists that movement of the limbs and other parts of the body sends sensory (afferent) impulses from the *proprioceptors* up the spinal cord to excite the respiratory center. Thus, it is strongly believed that these two signals (from cerebral cortex and proprioceptors) are the primary factors that increase respiration during exercise, and that an increased carbon dioxide and hydrogen ion level along with a diminished oxygen supply are second line defenses for increase ventilation. A more detail discussion concerning the cerebral cortex and proprioceptors can be found in Chapter 6.

58 Essentials of Exercise Physiology

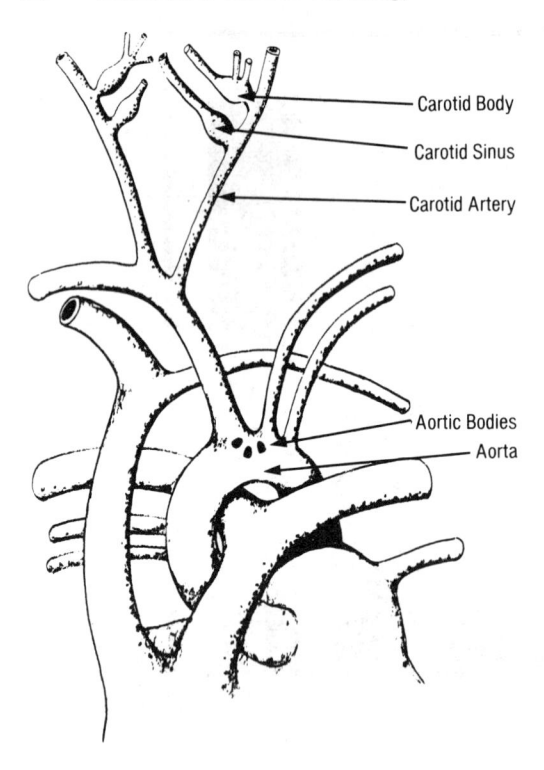

Figure 3-6 Structure of the chemoreceptor system.

Other Factors. In addition to the aforementioned factors, *temperature* increases also affect the rate and depth of respiration. As body temperature rises, the breathing rate goes up in direct proportion. At the same time, however, most authorities agree that as the body temperature drops below normal, respiration also drops in direct proportion until death eventually follows from respiratory failure. Another factor involved in controlling the rate and depth of ventilation is the secretion of the hormones *norepinephrine* and *epinephrine* from the adrenal medulla. Their action is to increase the rate and depth of breathing.

Obviously, breathing can be voluntarily controlled at least within broad ranges (for example, in speaking, coughing, straining, eating, and in holding your breath for varying periods of time). However, as stated earlier, the overall control of respiration is probably a combination of all the factors mentined above and not a result of any particular one.

IV. LUNG VENTILATION RESPONSE TO EXERCISE

A. MINUTE VENTILATION OR PULMONARY VENTILATION

Minute ventilation or pulmonary ventilation is defined as the amount of air inspired or expired per minute. At rest, this value is around 5 to 8 liters/min for the normal, healthy person. In a short period of hard work, it may exceed 130 liters/min for females and 180 liters/min for males. In well-trained athletes, it may go over 200 liters/min which is more than 30 times the resting value. Such an increase is brought about by a tremendous increase in the breathing rate (from a resting rate of 12-20 breaths/min to an exercise rate of 50-60 breaths/min) and in the tidal volume. Tidal volume is defined as the amount of air inspired or expired per breathe and it increases from a resting value of 0.5 liters to around 3 liters.

Figure 3-7 illustrates with trained and untrained subjects a typical drawing showing the relationship between minute ventilation and oxygen consumption and carbon dioxide production during exercise. It is rather clear that minute ventilation not only increases during exercise, but for the most part, there is a linear relation between this increase and the amount of oxygen absorbed, and the amount of carbon dioxide produced per minute. Figure 3-7 also indicates that minute ventilation, under maximal exercise conditions, is probably regulated more toward the removal of carbon dioxide than toward oxygen consumption. For example, in Figure 3-7 the oxygen consumption curves show that ventilation is somewhat disproportional to oxygen uptake at or near maximal values whereas the remaining two curves do not suggest this with respect to carbon dioxide production. This suggestion was made earlier by Mathews and Fox in their textbook.

When comparing the trained with the untrained in Figure 3-7, it shows that untrained subjects have lower working capacities as well as lower respiratory efficiencies. In other words, the trained subjects have a smaller V_E at a given $\dot{V}_{O_2}$ than do the untrained subjects.

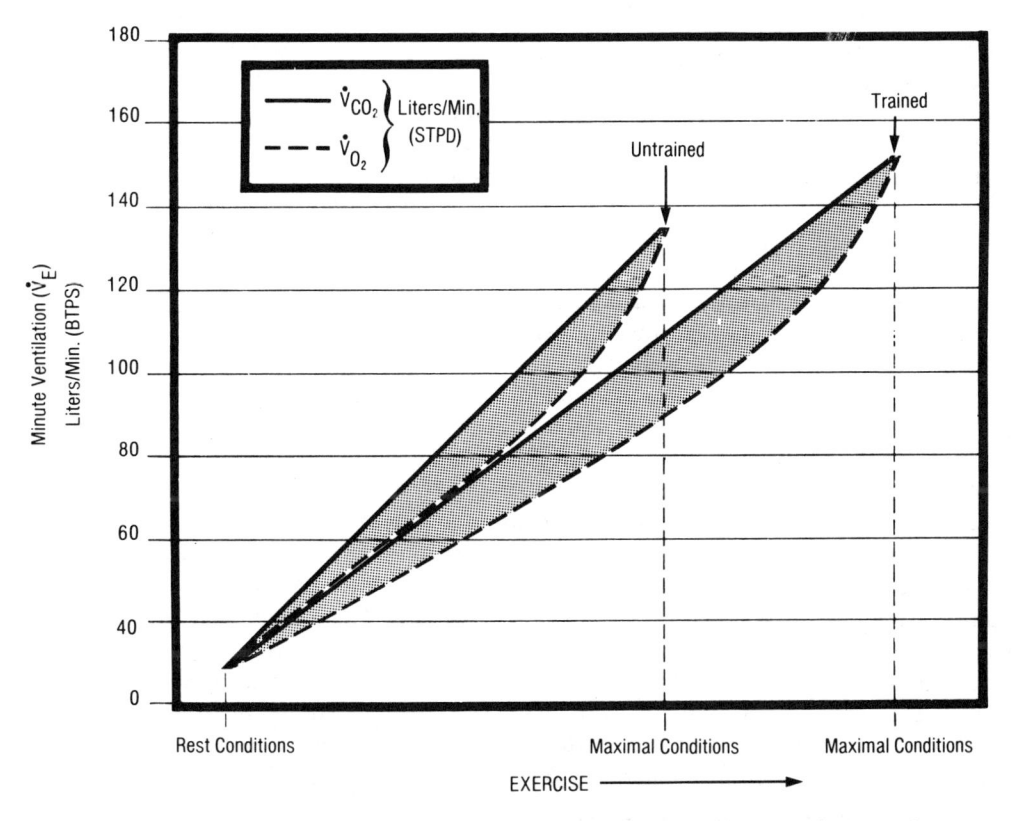

Figure 3-7 Schematic diagram illustrating the relationship between minute ventilation and oxygen consumption and carbon dioxide production during exercise for both trained and untrained subjects.

B. DEAD SPACE

At inspiration, not all of the fresh air gets down to the alveoli where the gaseous exchange can take place with the blood; some of it remains throughout areas in the respiratory passages such as the nose, mouth, pharynx, larynx, trachea, bronchi, and even the bronchioles. This air is considered to be useless from the point of view of oxygenating the blood. Thus, the air that remains in these areas is referred to as the *dead-space air*. The dead space may be calculated if the concentration of one of the respiratory gases in the expired air and alveolar air, and the volume of the expired air are known. For example, if the amount of carbon dioxide in the alveolar air is 5 percent, in the expired air 4 percent, and the volume of expired air is 800 ml, then:

$$\frac{800}{5} = \frac{x}{4} = 640 \text{ ml}$$

Thus, 640 ml represents the quantity of alveolar air in the expired air. The dead space is equal to 800 − 640, or 160 ml. It should be pointed out, however, that due to methodological difficulties, it is not easy to measure the volume of dead space, particularly during exercise. Therefore, researchers have estimated that on the average, the dead space amounts to about 150 ml for men and 100 ml for women. These figures also tend to increase slightly with age. The air that reaches the alveoli is called *alveolar ventilation*, and it is the most important measure of the effectiveness of a person's respiration.

Alveolar ventilation is equal to tidal volume times the rate of breathing minus the dead-space volume. If normal ventilation at rest is approximately 8,000 ml/min (500 ml for tidal volume × 16 breaths/min), and the dead space is 150 ml, then alveolar ventilation will be 5,600 ml/min (350 ml × 16) or 5.6 liters/min. During exercise, however, alveolar ventilation can be increased to as high as 100 liters/min, whereas at the opposite extreme, an individual can remain alive for several hours with an alveolar ventilation as low as 1200 ml/min. It should be pointed out that during exercise, even though the dead space volume may double (through dilatation), because tidal volume also increases, sufficient alveolar ventilation is generally maintained.

It is interesting to note that alveolar ventilation will be greater if the depth of breathing is increased rather than the rate. For example, if tidal volume is 500 ml, the rate of breathing is 50/min. and the dead space volume is 150 ml, then the alveolar ventilation is 500 ml − 150 ml = 50 = 17,500 ml, and the minute ventilation is 25,000 ml/min (500 ml × 50).

At the same time, if the tidal volume is increased to 1562.5 ml, the rate is 16/min, and the dead space 150 ml, the alveolar ventilation is 1562.5 ml − 150 ml × 16 = 22,600 ml, and the minute ventilation is still 25,000 ml/min (1562.5 ml × 16). The above examples indicate rather clearly that minute ventilation alone does not indicate whether or not alveolar ventilation is sufficient. In addition, the above illustrations suggest that the best means of increasing alveolar ventilation is by increasing the depth (tidal volume) rather than the rate. It is well known among the coaching circles that the trained person learns to reduce the rate of breathing while increasing the depth. At the same time, however, it should be pointed out that extremely deep breathing requires a larger energy output to overcome the elastic recoil of the lungs. Therefore, greatest efficiency is actually obtained by increasing both rate and depth.

C. LUNG VOLUMES AND CAPACITIES

Much can be learned of lung function by calculating the volume of air moved with each breath. This is generally done by using nothing more than a spirometer. Table 3-1 provides a list of

Table 3-1. Lung Volumes and Capacities and Their Definitions

Lung Volume or Capacity	Definition
Volumes	
Tidal Volume (TV)	The volume of air breathed in and out during each respiratory cycle.
Inspiratory Reserve Volume (IRV)	The maximal volume of air that can be taken in following inhalation of tidal volume.
Expiratory Reserve Volume (ERV)	The maximal volume of air that can be exhaled following the end of a normal exhalation of tidal volume.
Residual Volume (RV)	The volume of air still remaining in the lungs following a maximal exhalation.
Capacities	
Total Lung Capacity (TLC)	The volume of air contained in the lung following a maximal inspiration.
Vital Capacity (VC)	The maximal volume of air that can be forcefully exhaled from the lungs following a maximal inspiration.
Inspiratory Capacity (IC)	The maximal amount of air that can be taken in following a normal exhalation of tidal volume.
Functional Residual Capacity (FRC)	The amount of air remaining in the lungs at the resting expiratory level.

8 lung volumes or capacities along with a statement explaining each term. Furthermore, Figure 3-8 provides illustrations of these volumes and capacities at rest for both men and women. It should be mentioned that residual volume cannot be measured directly with a spirometer. Instead, the subject breathes for approximately 6 minutes from a tank of pure oxygen, and the expired air is collected. Once the lungs have been "washed out," the percentage of nitrogen is then calculated from the expired air. By determining the percentage of nitrogen in the expired air, the total air in the lungs (including residual volume) can be easily calculated since nitrogen is always 79.03 percent of the air we take in. Final lung volumes and capacities are generally corrected to body temperature and pressure, saturated with water vapor, abbreviated BTPS.

It is generally well known that during strenuous exercise, tidal volume may be increased several times over its resting value. This change in tidal volume is brought about primarily from a decrease in the inspiratory reserve volume, although the expiratory reserve volume is also lowered somewhat. Also, as Mathews and Fox has pointed out, since blood flow increases in the capillaries of the lungs during exercise, the available gas volume space is reduced, and as a result, there is generally a slight decrease in vital capacity as well as in total lung capacity. As a result, this obviously means that during exercise, residual volume and functional residual capacity will both be slightly increased over their resting values. Although it has been demonstrated that body size is proportional to vital capacity and total lung capacity, with the exception of tidal volume, men and women in training tend to have larger resting lung volumes than those individuals who are not in training.

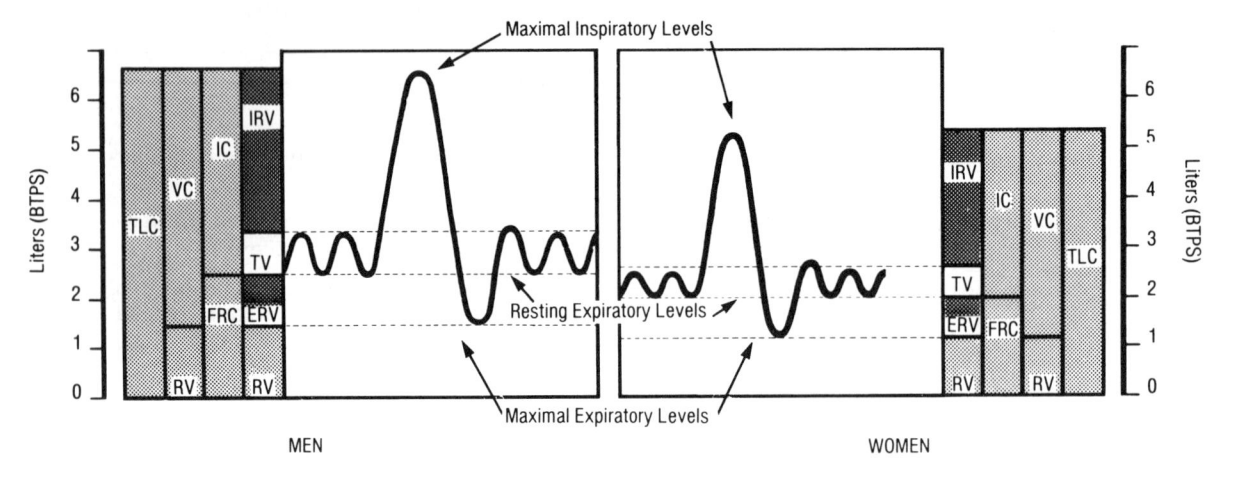

Figure 3-8 Schematic illustration of lung volumes and capacities for both men and women during rest conditions.

V. GASEOUS EXCHANGE

The exchange of gases (oxygen and carbon dioxide) between the alveoli of the lungs and the blood as well as between the blood and the tissue cells is due entirely to the physical force of *diffusion*. Gases move from one point to another only because of differences in pressure, called pressure gradients. This means that gases move from a point of high pressure to one of low pressure. Thus, oxygen moves from the alveoli of the lungs into the blood if the oxygen pressure is smaller in the blood than it is in the alveoli. In addition, carbon dioxide moves from the blood into the alveoli if the carbon dioxide pressure in the alveoli is smaller than that in the blood. Similar processes take place between the blood and the tissue capillaries. For example, because of the metabolism of the tissue cells, oxygen is used (thus lowering the oxygen pressure) and carbon dioxide is produced (thus increasing the carbon dioxide pressure). Consequently, as the blood moves past the tissue cells, oxygen moves from the blood into the cells, and carbon dioxide moves from the cells into the blood. Figure 3-9 illustrates the flow of oxygen and carbon dioxide throughout the various parts of the body as previously described.

It is well known that a gas molecule has no particular shape or volume, and that it conforms to the shape and volume of its holder. Gas molecules are constantly in a state of motion at high velocities. It is also known that a gas molecule exerts a pressure depending upon the activity and number of molecules in its volume. Thus, pressure of a gas can be increased by confining it in a smaller volume, or by increasing the activity of each molecule. In addition, if gas is heated, the velocity of the molecules increases, and increased pressure results. Unlike gases, liquids are made up of molecules that are very close together which results in their having a definite, independent volume, which fluctuates very little with temperature or with the size and shape of the holder.

A. LAWS GOVERNING THE BEHAVIOR OF GASES

To understand the taking up and setting free of oxygen and carbon dioxide by the blood, it is necessary to discuss briefly the laws governing the behavior of gases. They are: (1) Boyle's law, (2) Charles' law, (3) Henry's law, and (4) Dalton's law of partial pressure.

Boyle's Law

This law states that the pressure of a gas is inversely proportional to its volume so long as the temperature is kept constant.

Charles' Law

This law states that the pressure of any gas is directly proportional to its absolute temperature so long as the volume remains constant. Boyle's law and Charles' law may be combined to describe the relationship between pressure, temperature, and volume as follows:

$$\text{Pressure} = \frac{\text{temperature}}{\text{volume}}$$

Henry's Law

This law states that with a constant temperature, the amount of a gas that will dissolve in a liquid is directly proportional to its partial pressure.

Dalton's Law of Partial Pressure

This law states that in a mixture of gases, each gas exerts a pressure proportional to its percentage in the total mixture. The partial pressure (P), or tension of the gas is expressed quantitatively in mmHg. For example, if the total atmospheric (or barometric) pressure was 760 mmHg, the partial pressure of the gases that primarily make up the atmospheric air (oxygen, carbon dioxide, and nitrogen) would be as follows:

(1) Oxygen concentration = 20.93%
    $P_{O_2} = 20.93/100 \times 760 = 159.1$ mmHg
(2) Carbon dioxide concentration = 0.04%
    $P_{CO_2} = 0.04/100 \times 760 = 0.3$ mmHg
(3) Nitrogen concentration = 79.03%
    $P_{N_2} = 79.03/100 \times 760 = 600.6$ mmHg

The partial pressure of a gas is dependent on the total atmospheric pressure, and the fractional concentration of that gas. In addition, if a gas mixture is moist, the water vapor also exerts a pressure proportional to its concentration as well as to the temperature of the gas. For example, the alveolar air in the lungs is normally completely saturatd with water vapor (approximately 6.2%) at body temperature (37°C), which contributes a partial pressure of 47 mmHg ($P_{H_2O} = 6.2/100 \times 760 = 47$ mmHg). Theoretically therefore, the partial pressure of oxygen in the lungs at a barometric pressure of 760 mmHg should be $20.93/100 \times (760 - 47)$ or about 149 mmHg if it was possible to completely exchange the air in the lungs. Obviously, this is not possible since alveolar air in the lungs is a mixture of atmospheric air and old air (air already taken part in the respiratory exchange). Instead, the partial pressure of alveolar oxygen as well as carbon dioxide and nitrogen are as follows:

(1) Oxygen concentration = 13.6%
    $P_{CO_2} = 5.3/100 \times (760 - 47) = 40.0$ mmHg
(2) Carbon dioxide concentration = 5.3%
    $P_{CO_2} = 74.90/100 \times (760 - 47) = 569.0$ mmHg

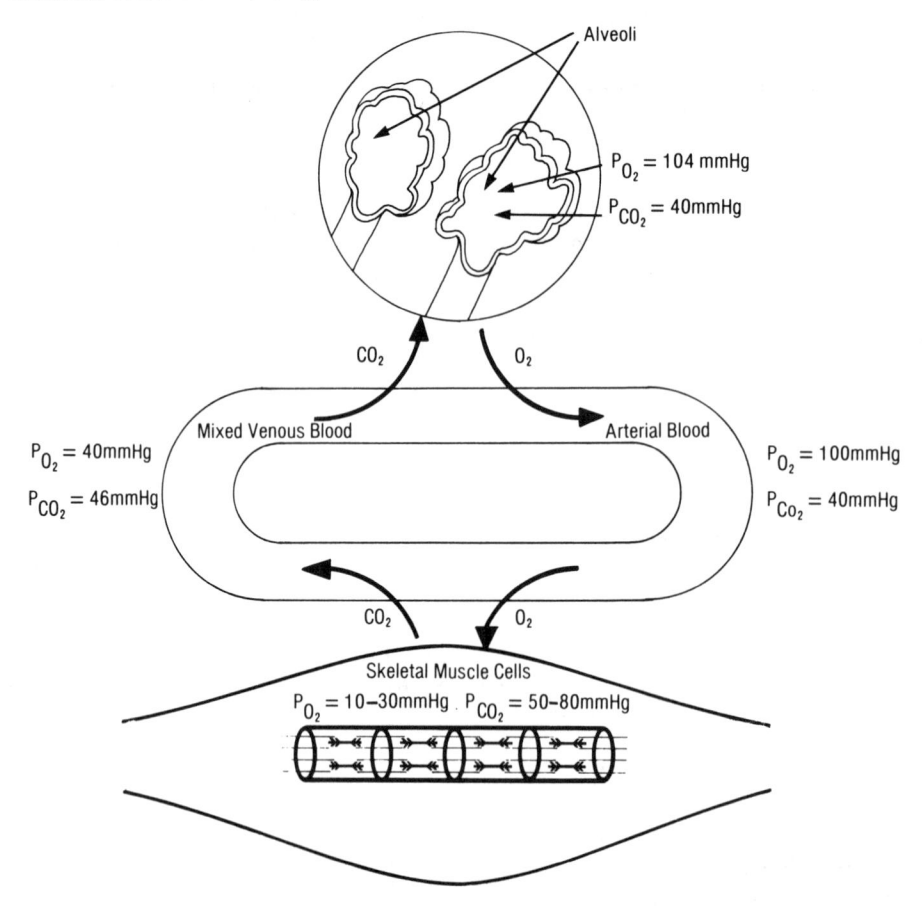

Figure 3-9 Schematic view of the flow of oxygen and carbon dioxide throughout the various parts of the body.

(3) Nitrogen concentration = 74.90%
P_{N_2} = 74.90/100 × (760 − 47) = 569.0 mmHg

It should be mentioned that the above partial pressures are generally constant during rest, however, these values change greatly during work depending on the rate and depth of alveolar ventilation as well as the rate of oxygen and carbon dioxide transfer into and out of the blood. For example, a high alveolar ventilation furnishes large amounts of oxygen to the alveoli, thereby increasing the alveolar oxygen pressure. At the same time, high alveolar ventilation takes away carbon dioxide from the alveoli more rapidly than usual, thus decreasing the carbon dioxide pressure.

As stated earlier, the exchange of gases between the alveoli and the blood as well as between the blood and the tissue cells is due entirely by diffusion. The data in Figure 3-9 explains why this is true. The oxygen partial pressure (P_{O_2}) of venous blood entering the lungs is only 40 mmHg in comparison with the alveolar air of P_{O_2} of 104 mmHg, which causes extremely rapid diffusion of oxygen into the blood. In addition, the P_{O_2} of arterial blood flowing from the lungs to the tissue cells is 100 mmHg in comparison with the cell P_{O_2} of only between 10-30 mmHg. The concentration of oxygen in the cell rarely rises above 30 mmHg because when oxygen enters a cell it reacts very readily with sugar, fat, and protein to form carbon dioxide and water. Thus, the oxygen diffusion gradient of approximately 70 mmHg causes it to diffuse rapidly into the tissue cells.

Although the diffusion gradient for CO_2 *is only about 5 to 6 mmHg, it is sufficient to maintain the necessary homeostatic relation for CO_2 levels.* This can be explained by the fact that diffusion of gases across a membrane depends not only upon the pressure gradient but also upon the ease with which the membrane can be penetrated by the gases. Since this, in turn, depends upon the solubility of the gas in the membrane (primarily water), and since carbon dioxide in water is approximately 20 or more times soluble than that of oxygen, this obviously explains the need for a greater diffusion gradient for oxygen.

It should also be pointed out that because red blood cells transport both oxygen and carbon dioxide, any alteration in their number will obviously affect gas exchange. In other words, a greater amount of red blood cells will increase gas exchange while a decrease in red blood cells will lower the gas exchange. An increase in the number of red blood cells is one of the more important physiological changes that occur from cardiorespiratory endurance training.

And finally, one other important factor that affects gas exchange is the amount of area available at both the lung and muscle site for diffusion. The number of capillaries functioning at both sites play an extremely important part in determining the surface area available for diffusion. Because exercise increases the number of active capillaries at each site, it should be easy to understand that the diffusion surface capacity for oxygen and carbon dioxide exchange is increased at both tissue sites during exercise as compared to rest conditions. For the person who is performing exhaustive-type work and needs high levels of oxygen, while at the same time, avoiding high levels of carbon dioxide build-up, this mechanism, along with the others previously mentioned, play an extremely important part (especially during exercise and physical labor).

VI. GASEOUS TRANSPORT

A. TRANSPORT OF OXYGEN

Oxygen is transported not only by the iron-protein molecule called *hemoglobin* which is found in the red blood cells, but a small amount is also carried by the liquid portion of the blood called *plasma*. Because the plasma-carried oxygen does not take part in any chemical changes, it is dissolved and carried in a physical solution. Only about 3 percent is transported in this manner. The remaining 97 percent diffuses into the red blood cells and combines chemically and reversibly with the iron portion *heme* of hemoglobin (Hb) to form what is called *oxyhemoglobin* (HbO_2). The reaction is as follows:

$$\text{Hemoglobin (Hb)} + \text{oxygen (O}_2) \rightleftarrows \text{oxyhemoglobin (HbO}_2)$$

The maximum amount of oxygen (oxygen capacity) which the blood can carry is determined by the amount of hemoglobin present. One gram of hemoglobin can combine with 1.34 ml of oxygen. The blood of the average person at rest and at sea level contains approximately 15 grams of hemoglobin per 100 ml of blood (16 grams per 100 ml for males and 15 grams per 100 ml for females). Therefore, under these conditions, the average person carries about 20 ml of oxygen per 100 ml of blood (15 × 1.34) or 20 volumes percent of oxygen. Note that volumes percent refers to milliliters of oxygen per 100 ml of blood.

It is interesting to note that during exercise, as a partial result of fluid shifting from the blood into the active muscle cells, the hemoglobin content may increase as much as 10 percent which is a definite advantage for people performing work (especially aerobic-type work). For example, a 10 percent increase would mean that there will be approximately 16.5 grams of hemoglobin per 100 ml of blood or 22.1 volumes percent of oxygen instead of the normal 15 grams or 20.1 volumes percent.

B. OXYGEN DISSOCIATION CURVES OF HEMOGLOBIN

As stated earlier, oxygen unites with hemoglobin in a chemical and reversible manner. The amount of oxygen which combines this way is determined primarily by the partial pressure of oxygen. For example, if the pressure is increased, more oxygen and hemoglobin combine; when the partial pressure of oxygen falls, the hemoglobin molecule gives up a portion of the oxygen. At the same time, there are other important factors that affect the saturation of hemoglobin with oxygen besides the partial pressure. For example, the temperature and pH (acidity) of the blood as well as the level of carbon dioxide in the blood all play important roles in determining the amount of saturation of hemoglobin with oxygen.

Oxygen dissociation curves in Figure 3-10 illustrates the typical relationships of these factors to percent saturation of hemoglobin with oxygen. The dissociation curves in Figure 3-10 are extremely important in the understanding of gas transport. Figure 3-10A represents normal resting conditions. That is, the arterial blood partial pressure of oxygen (P_{O_2}) is 100 mmHg; mixed venous blood P_{O_2} is 40 mmHg; blood pH is 7.4; and body temperature is 37°C. In Figure 3-10A the values on the right ordinate represent the amount of oxygen combined with hemoglobin at the various percent saturations, and these values are based on an hemoglobin concentration of 15 grams per 100 ml of blood.

The curve in Figure 3-10A shows that the higher the P_{O_2}, the greater is the association of oxygen with hemoglobin, whereas the lower the P_{O_2}, the greater is the dissociation of oxygen from hemoglobin. For instance, at a P_{O_2} of 100 mmHg, the hemoglobin in arterial blood is saturated about 97.5 percent with oxygen. At this point, as Mathews and Fox stated in their text, the arterial blood contains about 19.5 volumes percent of oxygen (20 × 0.975). This indicates that for each 100 ml of arterial blood, 19.5 volumes percent of oxygen is taken (via hemoglobin) to the muscular tissues. In addition, at a P_{O_2} of 40 mmHg, the hemoglobin in the mixed venous blood returning from the various tissues is only saturated about 75 percent. At this point, the venous blood contains somewhere around 15 ml per 100 ml of blood or 15 volumes percent of oxygen (20 × 0.75). the term *arteriovenous oxygen difference* (a-$\bar{v}_{O_2}$ diff) is used to describe the difference between the two. The a-$\bar{v}_{O_2}$ diff tells us how much oxygen is actually taken on by the tissues from each 100 ml of blood flowing to them. Figure 3-10A shows that the resting a-$\bar{v}_{O_2}$ diff is 4.5 ml of oxygen. This means that the remaining 15 ml of the original 19.5 ml of oxygen can be used in an emergency situation at a later time when needed (such as in exhaustive exercise).

The curve in Figure 3-10A also illustrates that increasing the oxygen partial pressure in the arterial blood beyond 100 mmHg such as breathing 100 percent pure oxygen at sea level conditions is of no particular advantage, contrary to popular opinion. The blood-oxygen saturation may be pushed to 100 percent, but since it is generally already 97 percent saturated, the gain is of no significance. This means, of course, that the use of pure oxygen at sea level during exercise will not increase oxygen delivery. Conversely, however, as authorities have found, the partial pressure of

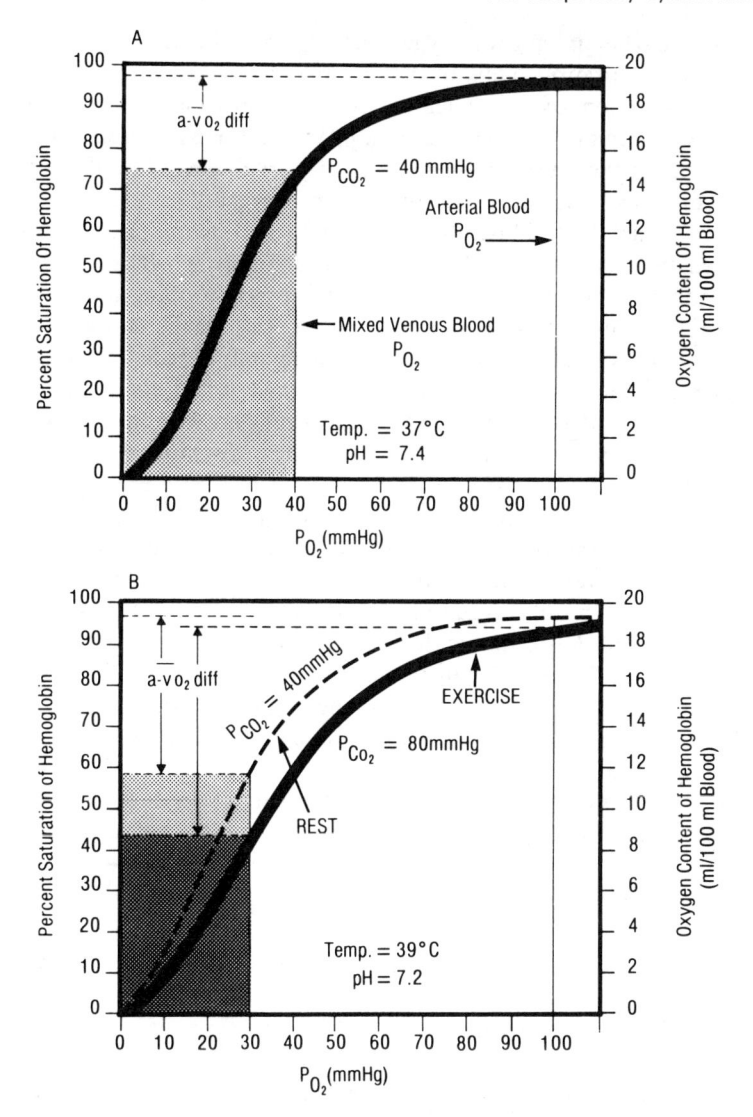

Figure 3-10 Diagram of the oxygen dissociation curves. The curve in illustration *A* represents normal resting conditions, while the curve in illustration *B* represents the effects of exercise, pH, temperature, and carbon dioxide on oxygen-hemoglobin dissociation.

oxygen can be reduced considerably below normal without depriving the blood of much of its oxygen load. For example, even when the partial pressure is cut in half, or reduced to 50 mmHg (such as going to high altitude), the oxygen saturation of the blood is still over 80 percent, a saturation which certainly serves most functions. In other words, the oxygen partial pressure in the lungs can vary over a somewhat wide range and still the blood will be adequately saturated.

Another interesting feature of the curve is that it is very steep (nearly vertical) when the partial pressures of oxygen are in the normal range of 40 mmHg or lower. This means that even the slightest change in partial pressure of oxygen on this part of the curve is associated with a large decrease in hemoglobin saturation. Thus, a small drop in tissue P_{O_2} apparently allows the tissues to take on a sufficient supply of oxygen when the need is greatest (such as during exercise). It has been suggested that this area of the curve (from the 40 to 50 mmHg P_{O_2} range on down) serves as a protective mechanism for the muscle tissues since it favors dissociation of oxygen from hemoglobin in spite of small decreases in partial pressure of oxygen.

The solid line in Figure 3-10B illustrates how exercise, pH, temperature, and carbon dioxide influence the oxygen dissociation curve. It is quite clear in Figure 3-10B that during exercise when body temperature and lactic acid levels are increasing (with pH dropping and P_{CO_2} increasing), the oxygen dissociation curve moves to the right. In essence, this means that when the blood shifts toward acidity, the affinity of hemoglobin for oxygen is actually reduced. This is referred to as the *Bohr effect*. The greatest amount of movement takes place in the middle and lower portions, whereas very little is seen at the upper end. These shifts are extremely important as other investigators have already pointed out (particularly during heavy work), since it means that more oxygen is unloaded to the working tissues at a given tissue P_{O_2}. At the same time, the loading of blood with oxygen is not generally affected in any great amount. For instance, if one examines Figure 3-10 closely at the 100 mmHg arterial blood P_{O_2} line and the 30 mmHg mixed venous blood P_{O_2} line, and if there were no change in the oxygen dissociation curve during exercise, the a-$\bar{v}_{O_2}$ diff would only be 7.9 ml of oxygen per 100 ml of blood flow (19.5 − 11.6). On the other hand, it can be seen in Figure 3-10B that with the curve moving to the right as a result of exercise, the a-$\bar{v}_{O_2}$ diff increases to 10.7 ml of oxygen per 100 ml of blood (19.5 − 8.8). It is well known that during extremely heavy exercise, the a-$\bar{v}_{O_2}$ diff can increase to as much as about 15 ml of oxygen per 100 ml of blood. In fact, following severe exercise, blood returning from the muscles may be almost completely depleted of oxygen.

The term *coefficient of oxygen utilization* is used quite often in describing the fraction of hemoglobin that gives up oxygen and it is written as:

$$\text{Coefficient of oxygen utilization} = \frac{\text{a-}\bar{v}_{O_2} \text{ diff (vol. \%)}}{\text{arterial O}_2 \text{ (vol. \%)}}$$

An illustrative example of the coefficient of oxygen utlization is as follows:

$$\text{Coefficient of oxygen utilization} = \frac{95\% - 70\%}{95\%} = 26\%$$

Normally, during rest this coefficient is around 26 percent. However, during severe exercise, it can rise to over 77 percent.

C. TRANSPORT OF CARBON DIOXIDE

The majority of carbon dioxide is carried in chemical combination (68% as *bicarbonate ions*—HCO_3 and 25% as *carbaminohemoglobin*—HbNHCOOH). The remaining 7 percent is carried in physical solution and is relatively unimportant as far as being a transporting mechanism.

Bicarbonate Ions

Once carbon dioxide diffuses into the tissue-capillary blood, it combines with blood water and the erythrocytes (red blood cells) to form carbonic acid (H_2CO_3). The formation of carbonic acid is accelerated tremendously by the action of an enzyme called carbonic anhydrase (found in red blood cells). Thus, the formation of carbonic acid occurs primarily within the red blood cells. At the same time, however, as quickly as carbonic acid is formed, it dissociates into a *hydrogen ion* (H+) and a bicarbonate ion (HCO_3). This dissociation is so thorough that very little carbonic acid remains. The complete reversible reaction is written as:

$$\text{Carbonic anhydrase enzyme}$$
$$CO_2 + H_2O \leftrightarrows H_2CO_3 \leftrightarrows H_+ + HCO_3$$

Thus, carbon dioxide, as indicated by this reaction is transported in the blood in the form of bicarbonate ions. The reaction, as indicated by the arrows, moves to the right as carbon dioxide diffuses into the tissue-capillary blood, and it reverses and moves to the left when carbon dioxide leaves the blood and enters the alveoli of the lungs.

It is rather interesting to note that even though bicarbonate ions are formed mainly in the red blood cells, they are transported principally by plasma because as the amount of bicarbonate ions increase in the red blood cell, the excess tends to diffuse out into the plasma. Note that this is only possible if the same amount of chloride ions (Cl-) diffuse over into the red blood cells from the plasma. This move of chloride ions is known as the "chloride shift" and its function is to preserve the ionic equilibrium between the plasma and the red blood cells.

At the same time, the few hydrogen ions that are formed in plasma are buffered by the plasma protein, whereas inside the red cell where the majority of the hydrogen ions are formed, hemoglobin serves as the acid buffer. It should be pointed out that if the hydrogen ions were not buffered, they would tend to raise the acidity level of the blood. An important point concerning the buffers should be emphasized at this time, and that is, that it is a well-known fact that the hemoglobin molecule is a much better buffer than the oxyhemoglobin (HbO_2) molecule. The importance of this is that as oxygen separates from the oxyhemoglobin molecule and diffuses over into the tissues, the buffering of hydrogen ions by the hemoglobin molecule is actually aided. This means that more bicarbonate ions can be created for transport of carbon dioxide without necessarily raising the acidity level of the blood. Another important point in carbon dioxide transport deals with the oxygen dissociation curve in Figure 3-10. Notice in Figure 3-10 that an increase in carbon dioxide (with a drop in pH) which is associated with an increase in acidity actually favors the removal of oxygen from the hemoglobin molecule for tissue utilization. It also means that greater amounts of hemoglobin will be available for buffering of hydrogen ions. More will be said about buffers in the next section.

Carbaminohemoglobin

As stated earlier, about 25 percent of carbon dioxide entering the blood is carried in a loose, reversible chemical combination with hemoglobin called *carbaminohemoglobin*. The reaction is:

$$HbNH_2 \leftrightarrows HbNHCOOH$$

It should be mentioned that this reaction does not occur at the same point on the hemoglobin molecule as the reaction between oxygen and hemoglobin. Instead of reacting with the heme component of hemoglobin, it reacts primarily with the *globin* protein component. While both oxygen and carbon dioxide can be transported by hemoglobin during the same period of time, reduced hemoglobin is capable of combining with carbon dioxide and forming carbaminohemoglobin much more readily than oxyhemoglobin (HBO_2) can. This explains why the entry of oxygen into the tissues helps with the loading of carbon dioxide into the blood for transport to the lungs where it is voided to the atmosphere. The reverse is also true in the lungs: the entry of carbon dioxide into the lungs helps with the loading of oxygen into the blood for transport to the tissues.

VII. ACIDS AND BASES AND THEIR REGULATION

Acids and *bases* are generally defined as chemical compounds that produce positively charged hydrogen ions (H^+) and negatively charged hydroxyl ions (OH^-) in various solutions. Thus, when one speaks of *acid-base balance,* they actually mean the constancy of hydrogen ion concentration in the body fluids. The normal hydrogen ion concentration is generally kept at an exact value of around 4×10^{-8} Eq/liter. This figure can fluctuate from a low of 1.6×10^{-8} to as much as 1.2×10^{-7}. For the sake of simplicity, the hydrogen ion concentration is normally expressed in terms of the pH by the following formula (when the hydrogen ion concentration is expressed in equivalents per liter):

$$pH = \log \frac{1}{H^+ \text{ conc.}} = -\log H^+ \text{ conc.}$$

It can be seen from this formula that a high pH results from a low hydrogen ion concentration (called *alkalosis*), whereas a low pH results from a high hydrogen ion concentration (called *acidosis*). The pH values may vary from 0 to 14.0. The normal pH of blood is between 7.3 to 7.5. During exercise, when the by-products of cellular activity (such as carbon dioxide, lactic acid, phosphoric acid, etc.) are being produced, the pH becomes more acid, around 7.05. It is interesting to note that some olympic athletes have been known to tolerate pH's as low as 6.8. Generally, a healthy untrained person cannot tolerate pH values below 7.0 and above 7.8 longer than a few minutes.

It should be pointed out that while exercise and work may bring about a decrease in pH values, it is also possible to raise the pH values. For example, during recovery following an exhaustive-type exercise, it is possible to "blow off" by breathing deep and fast some of the carbon dioxide from the blood and thus bring about a temporary alkalinity condition. The pH has been shown to increase to values as high as 7.85. However, these are exceptions and not the generally rule. At the same time, certain illnesses and diseases may also affect the pH by either lowering it to extremes of 6.0 or by raising it to as much as 7.8.

It is well known that one of the most important functions of the human body is the control and regulation of acid-base balance (pH) in the body fluids. Since slight pH changes beyond the range of 7.30 to 7.50 are inconsistent with good health, it is quite clear that the human body must be able to regulate the hydrogen ion concentration. Several systems are involved in this. They are: (1) the blood buffer systems, (2) the respiratory system, and (3) the kidneys. The *buffer system* of the blood acts as the first line of defense against pH changes. They are partically ionized formed by the combination of a strong acid and a weak base, or vice versa. One of the buffer systems in the blood is the bicarbonate buffer. A typical bicarbonate buffer system consists of a mixture of carbonic acid (H_2CO_3) and bicarbonate ion (HCO_3), as illustration in the following reaction:

$$HL + NaHCO_3 \rightarrow NaL + H_2CO_3$$

In this illustration, lactic acid (HL) which is a relatively strong acid reacts with sodium bicarbonate ($NaHCO_3$) which is a relatively weak acid to form sodium lactate (NaL) and a very weak carbonic acid (H_2CO_3). Thus, the net result is that a strong acid has been replaced for a relatively weak acid. Therefore, in this situation, lactic acid lowers the pH of the blood only slightly instead of what could have been a significant drop. It should be pointed out that in the blood there are several other bicarbonate salts such as potassium bicarbonate, calcium bicarbonate, and magnesium bicarbonate which fulfill the same basic function as sodium bicarbonate.

It has been known for a long time that *proteins* can act as both acid and alkaline buffers. They are extremely important for maintaining normal hydrogen ion concentrations in the intracellular fluids (whereas the bicarbonate buffer is more important in body fluids) because their concentration in the cells are several times as great as the concentration of the bicarbonate buffer. The major acid to be buffered is the carbonic acid that results from the respiratory exchange. The buffer systems primarily responsible for this are hemoglobin and oxyhemoglobin, each of which can perform as a weak acid or as a potassium salt.

The *respiratory center* in the medulla plays an important role in regulating the acid-base balance by it being able to automatically adjust to certain hydrogen ion situations by either increasing or decreasing the rate and depth of breathing (thus either reducing or increasing the hydrogen ion concentration back to normal).

The third and last line of defense for regulating the hydrogen ion concentration is the excretion of urine through the *kidneys*. The kidneys can remove either an acidic or alkaline urine to help readjust the proper acid-salt ratio to normal hydrogen ion concentrations.

VIII. SUMMARY

(1) The respiratory process is made up of two phases: external (or pulmonary ventilation) and internal (or cellular respiration).

(2) While the diaphragm is the principal muscle of inspiration during rest, the following muscles are especially important during exercise: the external intercoastals, the scalene and the sternocleidomastoids, the traqezius and extensors of the back and neck may also facilitate inspiratory movements during heavy work.

(3) Although expiration plays a passive role during resting conditions, it is quite active during exercise. Important muscles during this period are the abdominals and the internal intercostals.

(4) Respiration is regulated by a combination of several factors interacting upon the respiratory center in the medulla:
    (a) carbon dioxide increase,
    (b) hydrogen ion increase (resulting from a low pH),
    (c) a considerable decrease in oxygen tension,
    (d) cerebral factors,
    (e) proprioceptors,
    (f) the Hering-Breuer and pneumotaxic reflexes
    (g) body temperature increase, and
    (h) secretion of norepinephrine and epinephrine.

(5) Minute ventilation or pulmonary ventilation is the amount of air inspired or expired per minute which is at rest 5-8 liters/min, and may exceed in a short period of exercise 180 liters/min. In athletes during exhaustive work, it may exceed 200 liters/min.

(6) Alveolar ventilation (air that reaches the alveoli) is the most important measure of the effectiveness of a person's respiration. It is dependent upon three factors: (a) depth of breathing; (b) frequency of breathing; and (c) size of the dead space (dead space air is air that does not reach the alveoli, but instead, remains in the respiratory passages such as the nose, mouth, pharynx, larynx, trachea, bronchi, etc.

(7) Training improves pulmonary function as illustrated by larger resting and exercising lung volumes and capacities of athletes than of nonathletes.

(8) The exchange of oxygen and carbon dioxide between the alveoli of the lungs and the blood as well as between the blood and the tissue cells is determined by pressure gradient differences.

(9) At sea level with a barometric pressure of 760 mmHg, the partial pressure of alveolar oxygen is approximately 104 mmHg, while the venous oxygen pressure is around 40 mmHg, thus resulting in a diffusion gradient of 64 mmHg. For CO_2, the alveolar and venous figures are around 40 and 45 mmHg, respectively, with a diffusion gradient of 5 mmHg. Because CO_2 in water is about 20 times more soluble than that of O_2, it requires a lesser diffusion gradient.

(10) Several other factors besides partial pressure gradients can affect gas exchange including the number of red blood cells and the amount of tissue surface area in the lungs and muscles available for diffusion to take place.

(11) About 97 percent of oxygen is transported in the blood in combination with hemoglobin, while about 3 percent is carried in physical solution.

(12) Carbon dioxide is transported primarily within the erythrocytes in the form of bicarbonate ions (about 68 percent) and carbaminohemoglobin (about 25 percent). The remaining 7 percent is carried in physical solution.

(13) During rest, the hemoglobin in arterial blood is saturated about 95 to 97 percent with oxygen, while the venous blood returning from the tissues is only about 70 to 75 percent saturated. The term coefficient of oxygen utilization is used to describe this difference. These figures may be 97 percent and near zero percent, respectively, during exercise, thus yielding a tremendous increase in oxygen utilization.

(14) In addition to partial pressure, other factors that affect saturation of hemoglobin with oxygen are: (a) the temperature of the blood; (b) the pH of the blood; and (c) the amount of carbon dioxide in the blood. During work, fluctuations in these factors may aid in the release of oxygen to the active muscles. The oxygen dissociation curve illustrates the relationship among these factors.

(15) Regulation of the acid-base balance (pH) in the body involves the blood buffer system, the respiratory system, and the kidneys. The blood buffer system acts as the first line of defense against pH changes and it includes a weak acid and a salt of the acid. It operates by changing strong acids to relatively weak acids and neutral salts. Secondary line of defense against an abnormal pH concentration is the excretion of acids and bases by the lungs and kidneys.

IX. REVIEW REFERENCES

(1) Clarke, D. H. *Exercise Physiology,* Prentice-Hall, Inc., Englewood Cliffs, New Jersey, 1975.
(2) Comroe, J. H. *Physiology of Respiration: An Introductory Text,* 2nd edition, Year Book Medical Publishers, Chicago, 1974.
(3) Dempsey, J. A., D. A. Pelligrino, D. Aggarwal, and E. B. Olson, Jr. "The Brain's Role in Exercise Hyperpnea," *Medicine and Science in Sports,* 11:213-20, 1979.

(4) deVries, H. A. *Physiology of Exercise for Physical Education and Athletics,* 2nd edition, Wm. C. Brown Company, Dubuque, Iowa, 1974.
(5) Guyton, A. C. *Textbook of Medical Physiology,* 5th edition, W. B. Saunders Co., Philadelphia, 1976.
(6) Langley, L. L. *Physiology of Man,* 4th edition, Van Nostrand Reinhold Co., New York, 1971.
(7) Mahler, M. "Neural and Humoral Signals for Pulmonary Ventilation Arising in Exercising Muscle," *Medicine and Science in Sports,* 11:191-97, 1979.
(8) Mathews, D. K., and E. L. Fox. *The Physiological Basis of Physical Education and Athletics,* 2nd edition, W. B. Saunders Co., Philadelphia, 1976.
(9) Sutton, J. R., and N. L. Jones. "Control of Pulmonary Ventilation During Exercise and Mediators in the Blood; CO^2 and Hydrogen Ion," *Medicine and Science in Sports,* 11:198-203, 1979.
(10) Whipp, B. J., and J. A. Davis. "Peripheral Chemoreceptors and Exercise Hyperpnea," *Medicine and Sports,* 11:204-12, 1979.

4

THE HEART AND EXERCISE

KEY CONCEPTS TO BE GAINED FROM THIS CHAPTER

(1) The cardiac cycle includes three phases:
  (a) *diastasis* which represents the period that the entire heart is completely relaxed,
  (b) *systole* which represents the contraction of the atrial and ventricle, and
  (c) *diastole* which represents the relaxation of the atrial and ventricle.
(2) Functionally, cardiac output is the most important aspect of heart function, and it is determined by the product of heart rate times stroke volume.
(3) In addition to exercise, there are several other factors that affect heart rate including posture, sex, age, emotion, and environmental factors.
(4) The heart enlarges (hypertrophies) as a result of long-term endurance training.
(5) The electrical excitation characteristics of the heart muscle is represented by the electrocardiogram (ECG) which may, in turn, reveal information such as heart rhythm, size of the hearts chambers, and cardiac muscle damage.
(6) Neural and chemical factors regulate heart rate during work.

The total work an individual can accomplish is restricted largely by the heart, for this organ pumps blood, which in turn, carries oxygen and nutrients to the cells of the body and transports away the waste products such as carbon dioxide, lactic acid, etc. In this chapter, the various components of the heart and its functions as well as its physiological responses, both at rest and during exercise conditions are examined. In addition, the different means by which these responses are brought about and regulated are also discussed.

I. STRUCTURAL PROPERTIES OF THE HEART

Under the microscope, the cells of cardiac muscle are striated and the arrangement of actin and myosin protein filaments is assumed to be similar to that in skeletal muscle (Fig. 4-1). The

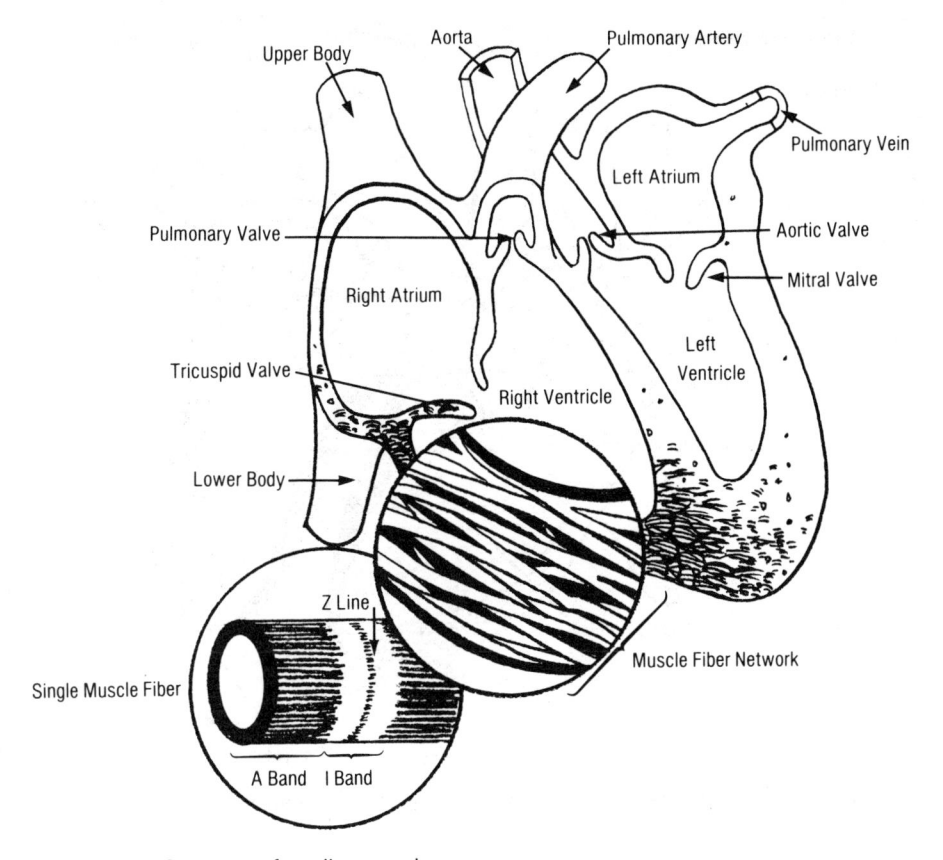

Figure 4-1 Structure of cardiac muscle.

cardiac or *myocardium* muscle is composed of three separte muscle fibers: the *atrial* and *ventricular* muscles; and the *specialized excitatory* and *conductive* structures. These fibers are joined by surface connections called *intercalated discs* which run transversely across the fibers. Because of this *syncitial* arrangement (where the fibers interweave and are connected together) as shown in Figure 4-1, an impulse originating at one point in the heart spreads throughout the muscle mass and the entire heart contracts with every beat, whereas in skeletal muscle each fiber is a separate entity, and can contract individually.

Unlike the skeletal muscle, the cardiac muscle is not normally considered to be under voluntary control. The muscle tissue of the heart possesses *authorhythmicity* which means that it does not need nervous impulses to start each contraction. The contraction of the heart is due to a wave of depolarization originating from a small area of specialized tissue in the right atrium known as the *sino-atrial* (S-A) *node,* or the *pacemaker* (Fig. 4-2). The S-A node depolarizes spontaneously at regular intervals.

The wave of excitation is transmitted from the S-A node by way of the syncytium of muscle fibers in the auricle to all areas of the heart muscle by a specialized conducting system called the *atrioventricular* (A-V) *node* or the secondary pacemaker and the *Purkinje system* (Fig. 4-2). When the wave of excitation reaches the A-V node, there is a slight pause, then the A-V node fires

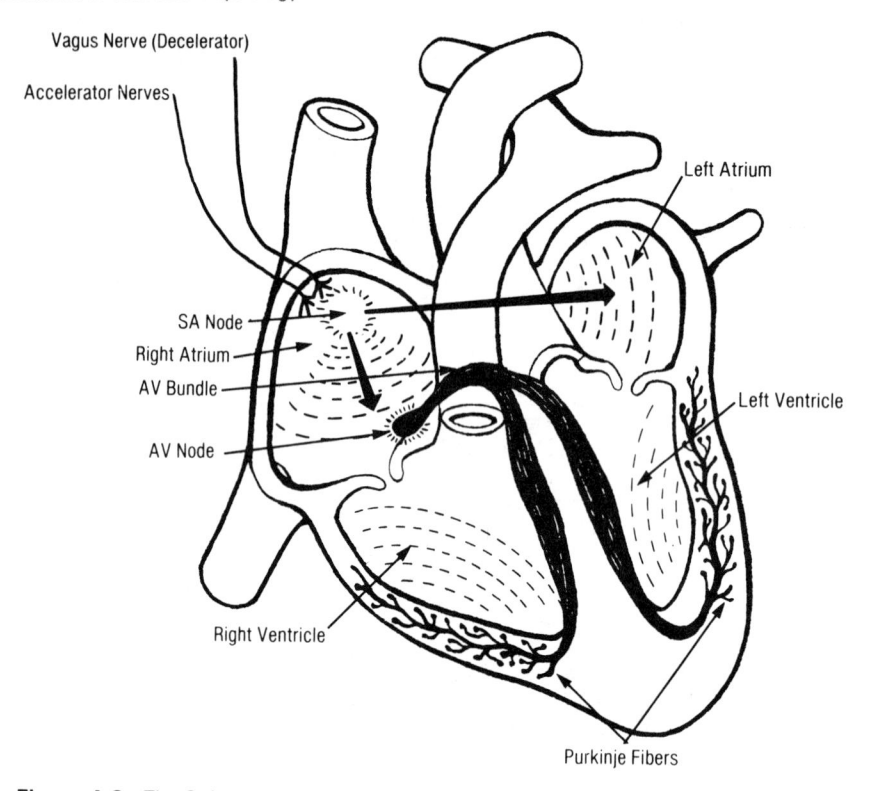

Figure 4-2 The S-A node, the A-V node and the purkinje system of the heart.

sending the wave of excitation (or impulse) into the A-V bundle. At this point, the A-V bundle conducts the impulse down the left and right bundle branches of Purkinje fibers, which eventually transmits the impulse to all parts of the ventricles. The pause at the A-V junction is valuable in that it allows time for the blood to flow from the atria into the ventricles before the ventricles contract.

It should be mentioned that if the S-A node's rate of impulse should be slowed down by an abnormal condition, then any area of the heart that has a faster inherent rate may take over the role of pacemaker. This is possible since all cardiac tissue has the property of authorhythmicity. Generally, this is what happens in abnormal heart rhythms.

Figure 4-3 illustrates an overall scheme of the heart and circulation. It shows rather clearly that the heart contains 4 chambers, the right and left *auricles* or *atria* (singular, *atrium*) and the right and left *ventricles,* all weighing less than a pound. The right atrium receives blood from the *superior* and *inferior vena cava veins* and pumps it via the *pulmonary arteries* to the lungs. Here it flows through *capillaries* where oxygen is absorbed and carbon dioxide removed. The oxygenated blood enters the left atrium of the heart from the lungs via the *pulmonary veins.* It then flows into the left ventricle which pumps it out through the *aorta,* and through the *systemic arterial system* to the capillary beds of the various tissues. After passage through the capillaries, the blood flow is returned through veins of increasing size and eventually reaches the right atrium again via the two great veins: one from the *anterior* or *upper regions* (the superior vena cava), and the other from *posterior* or *lower regions* (the inferior vena cava). Note briefly that a vessel carrying blood from

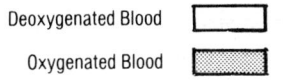

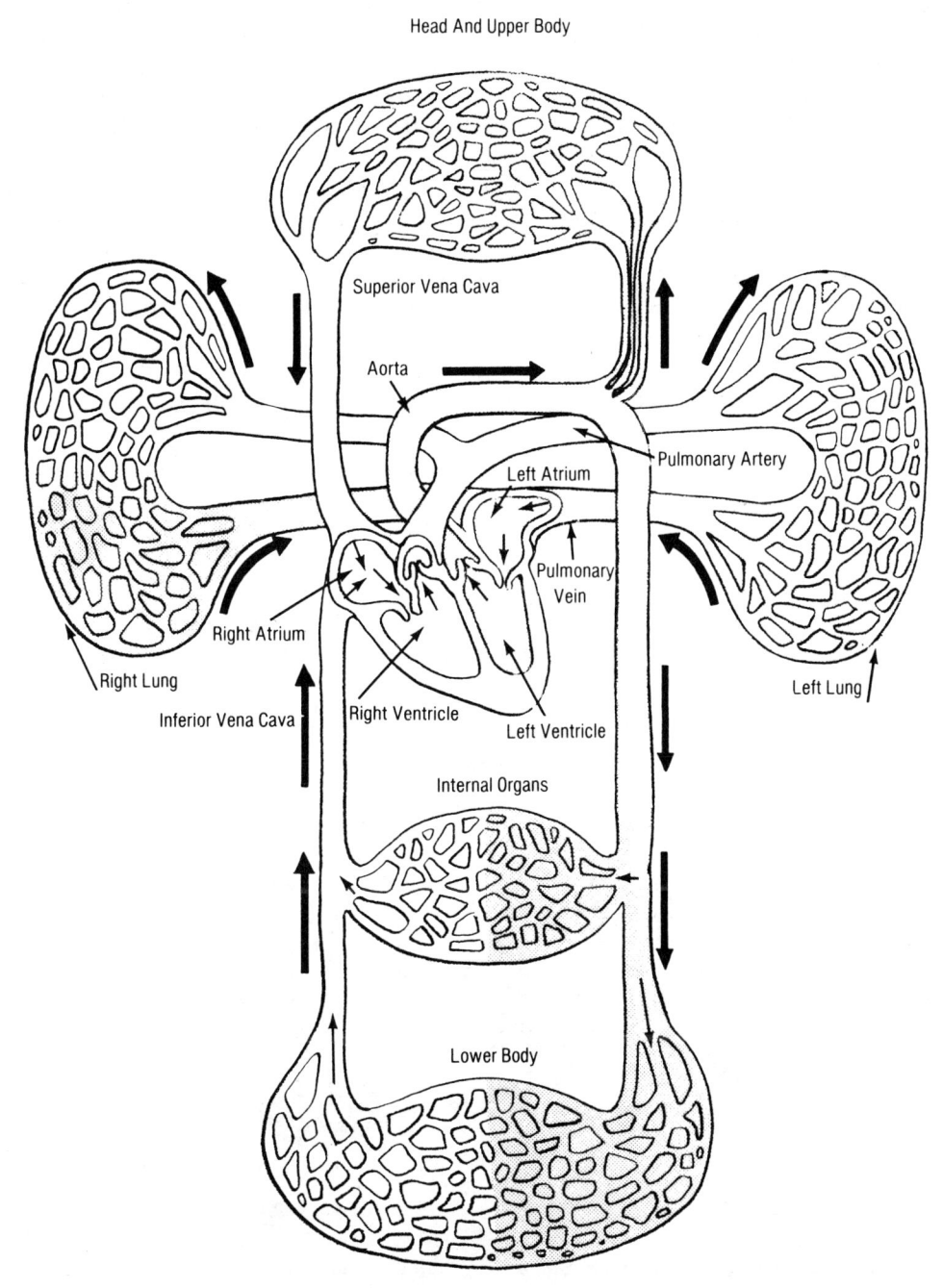

Figure 4-3 Schematic view of the heart, the pulmonary circulation, and the systemic circulation.

the heart is referred to as an artery and one carrying blood to the heart is known as a vein. More will be said about these vessels and the vascular system in the next chapter.

The systemic arteries contain *oxygenated* blood which is bright red in color and often referred to as *arterial* blood, whereas *venous* blood is much darker in color and it contains *deoxygenated* blood. Thus, we see that there are two parallel circulations, each with its own pump. The *pulmonary circulation* for allowing gas exchange in the lungs, and the *systemic circulation* for maintaining a relatively constant internal environment for the cells in the other tissues. The right heart is the pump for the pulmonary circulation and the left heart for the systemic circulation. Note, however, that all the blood passes through both systems.

It should be pointed out that the heart muscle itself is not nourished by the blood contained within its cavities, but instead, is supplied by its own *coronary circulatory system.* Figure 4-4 illustrates that the heart muscle has two small *coronary arteries* that branch out from the aorta immediately above the heart. The left vessel supplies the left atrium and ventricle, whereas the right supplies the right atrium and ventricle. A portion of the oxygenated blood that leaves the left ventricle by way of the *coronary sinus* with each heart beat passes through the two coronary arteries and is then distributed throughout the entire area of the heart. The blood returns to the right atrium by way of the *coronary veins.* Sufficient blood and oxygen supply to the heart muscle

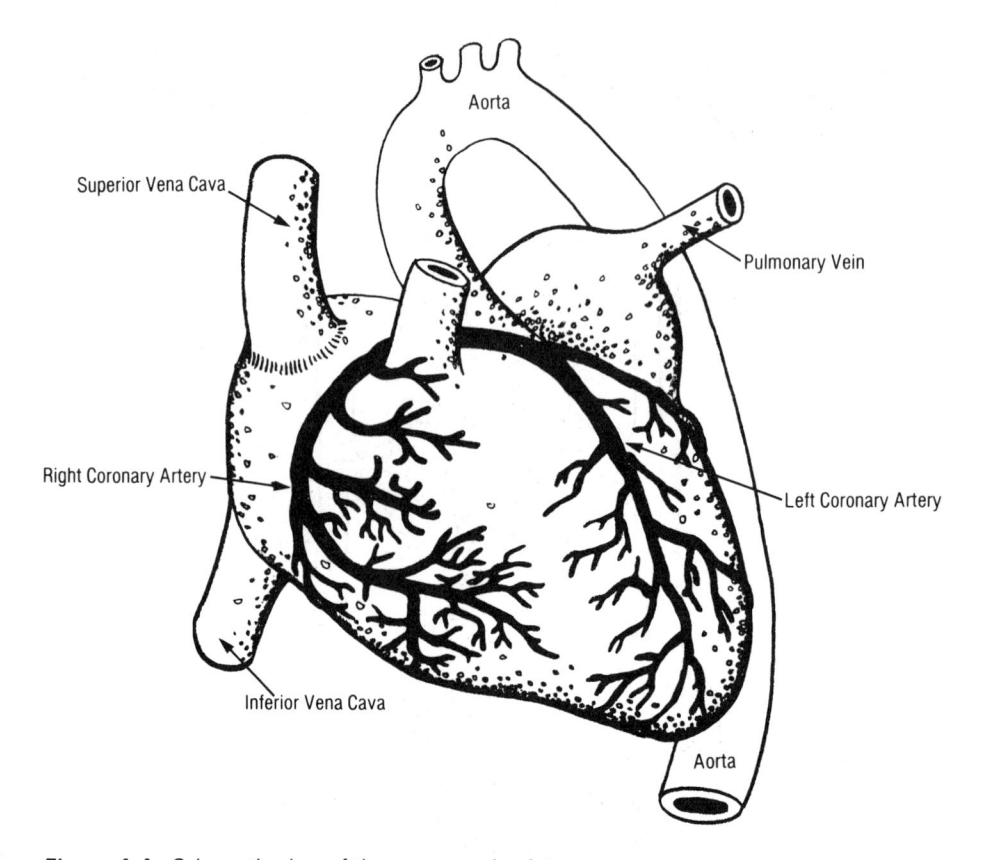

Figure 4-4 Schematic view of the coronary circulatory system.

is so critical that even the slightest reduction (as a result of perhaps a tiny clot or a progressive build-up of fatty substances) will bring about chest pains or *angina pectoris*. If the reduction is severe enough and the normal heart function is interrupted, death could result. The various cardiac abnormalities will be covered later in this chapter.

Because of this need for nutrients, the heart muscle receives a much greater supply of blood than does the remaining body parts. Recall from the previous chapter that the coefficient of oxygen utilization is somewhere around 26 percent for the whole body. For the heart, this figure is around 75 percent which means that the extraction of oxygen for the coronary circulation is around three times greater than that for the systemic circulation. Exercise produces an even greater flow of oxygenated blood into the coronary circulation.

II. THE CARDIAC CYCLE

The *cardiac cycle* involves all the pressure changes, volume changes, and valve actions that take place during one complete phase of contraction and relaxation of the heart (Fig. 4-5).

The contraction of the atrial and ventricle is known as *systole* and the relaxation as *diastole*. The period during which the entire heart is completely relaxed is termed *diastasis*. Therefore, a typical cardiac cycle includes three phases: (1) diastasis (resting period), (2) systole (contraction period), and (3) diastole (relaxation period).

A discussion of the cardiac cycle may begin at any one of the three phases. For convenience the present discussion will start with the period in which the whole heart is completely relaxed (the diastasis period). Venous blood from the superior and inferior venae cavae flows into the right atrium, and at the same time, oxygenated blood from the pulmonary veins flows into the left atrium. The valves between the atrium and the ventricle (atrioventricular—A-V) on each side are open so that the blood that enters the atria is able to flow freely through the relaxed ventricles. Meanwhile, the valves between the right ventricle and the pulmonary artery and the left ventricle and the aorta are closed so that none of the blood entering the ventricles is able to escape. Then, atria systole (contraction) occurs thus filling the ventricles more completely than they would be by passive inflow of blood. Very shortly after atria systole is completed, ventricle systole begins. The rising blood pressure in the ventricle exceeds the atria pressure and thus causes a sudden closure of the A-V valves through which the last blood has just been pumped by atrial contraction.

Note that the vibrations set up in the heart and vessels by the closure of these valves result in the *first heart sound*. Since all the valves of the heart are closed and no blood is being pumped out during this period, the ventricles are in a state of *isometric contraction*. That is, the heart muscle cannot shorten during this phase. However, as the ventricular pressure continues to rise above the pressure in the pulmonary artery and the aorta, the valves at the entries of these vessels open and blood is immediately pumped out into the circulation. Since the heart (ventricular chamber) muscle is able to shorten during the ejection period, this represents an *isotonic type contraction*. When ventricle systole is completed, this marks the beginning of ventricle diastole (relaxation). During this period of relaxation, intraventricular pressure falls markedly. In fact, when it drops below the pressure in the pulmonary artery and the aorta, the valves guarding these vessels close, thus allowing the *second heart sound* to be heard. When the ventricles are completely relaxed and the intraventricular pressure continues to fall and thus drops below the intra-atrial pressure, the A-V valves open again. Blood then begins to flow through to refill the ventricles and the period of diastasis is reached once again. The *third heart sound* recorded by the phonocardiogram in Figure 4-5 is the vibrations of the chamber walls caused by movement of blood into the relaxed ventricles.

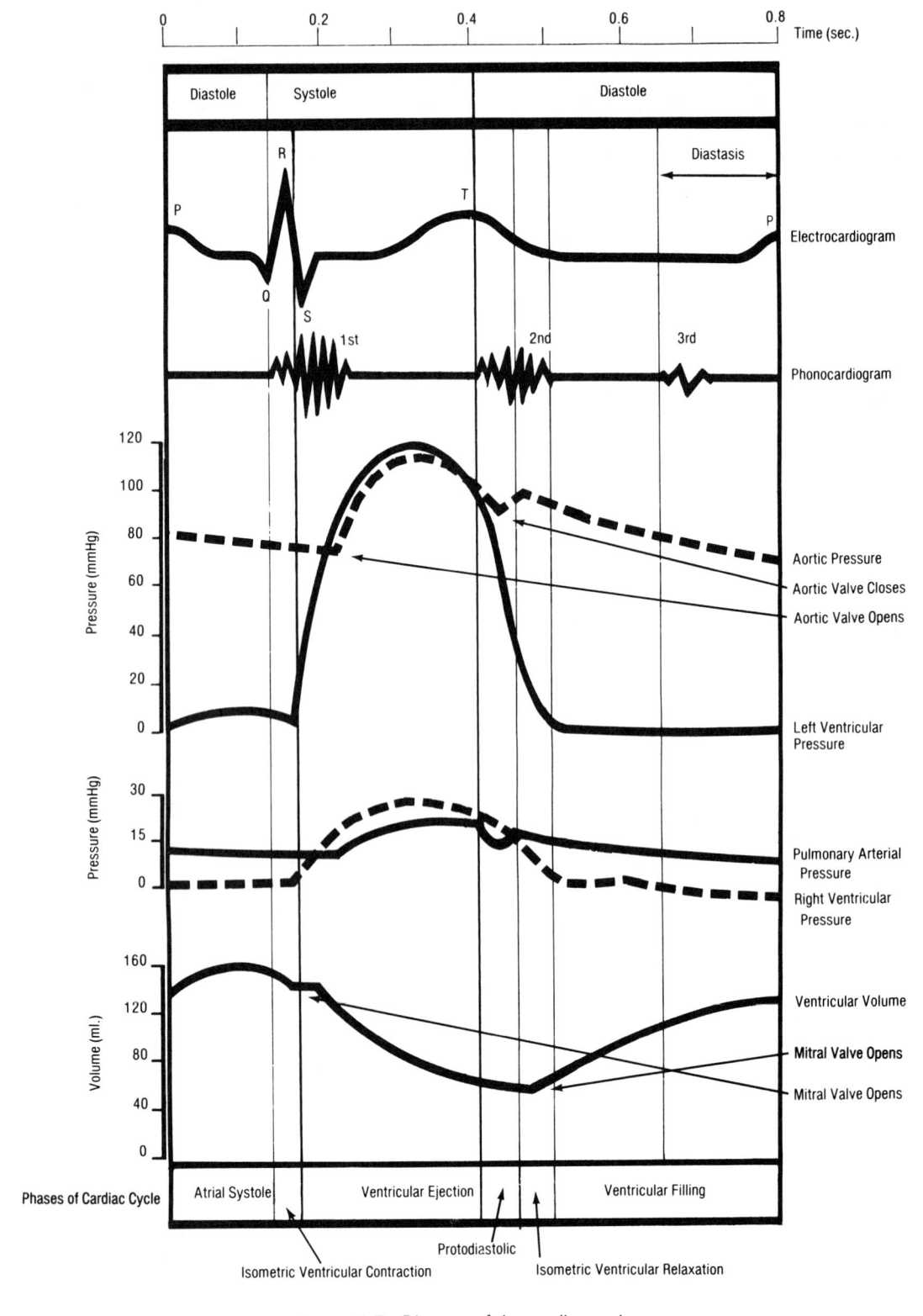

Figure 4-5 Diagram of the cardiac cycle.

The electrocardiogram (ECG), as illustrated in Figure 4-5, is a recording of the electrical impulses of the heart muscle. The ECG and its significance will be discussed in a separate section later in this chapter.

III. CARDIAC OUTPUT

From a functional viewpoint, *cardiac output* is generally considered by most exercise physiologists as the most important aspect of heart function. Cardiac output is defined as the volume of blood pumped by the heart in one minute, and is generally expressed in liters per minute or milliliters per minute. Cardiac output is the product of heart rate times stroke volume (the amount of blood pumped with each beat of the heart). For example, if heart rate equals 72 beats per minute and stroke volume equals 70 ml of blood, then cardiac output is equal to 5,040 ml/min, or 5.04 liters/min (72 × 70). Cardiac output can also be calculated from the amount of oxygen consumed per minute and the amount of oxygen taken up by the blood as it flows through the lungs. These relationships are expressed by the *Fick* principle as follows:

$$\text{Cardiac ouput} = \frac{\text{oxygen consumed per minute by the body (ml/min)}}{\text{arterial } O_2 \text{ content} - \text{venous } O_2 \text{ content (ml } O_2 \text{ 100 ml blood)}} \times 100$$

For example, if the oxygen content of the venous blood entering the lungs is 16 volumes percent (16 ml of O_2/100 ml of blood), that of the arterial blood leaving the lungs is 20 volumes percent (20 ml of O_2/100 ml of blood), and the oxygen consumption of the body 200 ml per minute, the amount of oxygen used per minute equals the amount of oxygen taken up by the lungs per minute. From the above data we can see that each 100 ml of blood flowing through the lungs picks up 4 ml of oxygen. And, since the total amount of oxygen absorbed into the blood from the lungs each minute is 200 ml, a total of fifty 100-ml portions of blood must flow through the lungs each minute to absorb this amount of oxygen. Thus the cardiac output is:

$$200/20 - 16 \times 100 = 5{,}000 \text{ ml}$$

In applying the Fick procedure, a sample of arterial blood (for the determination of arterial content) is drawn from any artery in the body since all arterial blood is thoroughly mixed before it leaves the heart and thus has the same oxygen concentration. On the other hand, because the oxygen content is not the same in the blood of all the veins, the so-called *mixed venous blood* must be used. To obtain an accurate determination of venous oxygen it is highly recommended that the blood sample be taken from the right ventricle or the pulmonary artery. Such a sample is obtained by *cardiac catheterization*. A catheter is introduced into the brachial vein of the forearm, through the subclavian vein, down to the right atrium, and finally into the right ventricle or pulmonary artery. It should be mentioned that this procedure is generally performed only under medical supervision.

The rate of oxygen consumption by the body is usually measured by a respirometer apparatus where the subject breathes from a known volume of oxygen for a period of about 6 to 10 minutes. Then by ascertaining the oxygen remaining, the amount consumed can be determined.

Since cardiac catheterization introduces some difficulties and objection, the *dye dilution method* is now widely used instead of the Fick principle. In this method, a known amount of dye is injected into an arm vein and its concentration is then obtained in serial samples of arterial blood. Once the concentration of dye is determined from the arterial blood samples, it is plotted on a graph against time to form a time-concentration curve. Cardiac output is then obtained from this curve and calculated from a formula since the area under the curve is inversely related to the cardiac output. Other methods including the carbon dioxide rebreathing test and the radioisotope test have been used over the years to determine cardiac output. While it is beyond the scope of this text to cover all the methods, the interested reader may consult almost any general physiology textbook for more information.

It should be pointed out that the Fick technique is considered to be the most accurate of all the methods in determining cardiac output only in the resting state or when steady state conditions are being used in exercise. Otherwise, when the cardiac output is changing rather rapidly, then the dye dilution technique is more accurate.

A. CARDIAC OUTPUT DURING REST

At rest in the supine position, the normal cardiac output in adults is approximately 5 liters per minute. This is generally achieved with a heart rate of 70 beats per minute for the untrained person and 45 beats per minute for enduranced trained person. Since the trained person's cardiac output at rest is also about 5 liters, then the decrease in heart rate must be offset by an increase in stroke volume if the cardiac output is to remain normal. Substituting the heart rate values in the cardiac output formula, the calculated stroke volume for the untrained person would be around 71.4 milliliters of blood per beat, whereas the stroke volume for the trained person would be about 111.1 milliliters per beat.

$$
\begin{aligned}
\text{Rest cardiac output} &= \text{heart rate} \times \text{stroke volume} \\
\text{Untrained } 5{,}000 \text{ ml} &= 70 \text{ beats/min} \times 71.4 \text{ ml} \\
\text{Trained } 5{,}000 \text{ ml} &= 45 \text{ beats/min} \times 111.1 \text{ ml}
\end{aligned}
$$

At this point, it should be mentioned that since blood generally pools in the lower portions of the body under the influence of gravity when assuming a sitting or standing position, this results in a drop in venous return to the heart and thus a 1 to 2 liters per minute reduction in cardiac output. Since the heart rate is usually increased, it is generally believed that this reduction is due entirely to a decrease in stroke volume. In recent years, much of the controversy concerning stroke volume changes in exercise and work has been the neglect of researchers to take into account the postural changes in stroke volume. Therefore, it is highly recommended that resting stroke volume be determined with the subject in the same position as that assumed during exercise.

B. CARDIAC OUTPUT DURING EXERCISE

During exercise up to 40 to 60 percent of maximal capacity, cardiac output in trained athletes may be increased to 40 liters per minute, whereas untrained subjects may attain outputs of about 20 liters per minute (Fig. 4-6). At this level of work, it is known that this 5 to 7-fold increase in cardiac output is due to increases in both heart rate and stroke volume. At levels beyond 40 to 60 percent of maximum, increases in cardiac output are mainly a function of heart rate increases. At the same time, it should be emphasized that since heart rate in strenuous exercise increases approximately the same in both athletics and non-athletics, the greater changes in cardiac output attained by the trained athletes is due to their greater ability for increasing the stroke volume of the heart. In fact, highly trained cross-country skiers have reported to have stroke volume values as high as 210 milliliters per beat. This is more than double the size of the stroke volume for untrained subjects. Again, substituting the heart rate values in the cardiac output formula, the calculated stroke values for the untrained person would be around 100 milliliters of blood per beat, whereas the stroke volume for the trained person would be approximately 200 milliliters per beat.

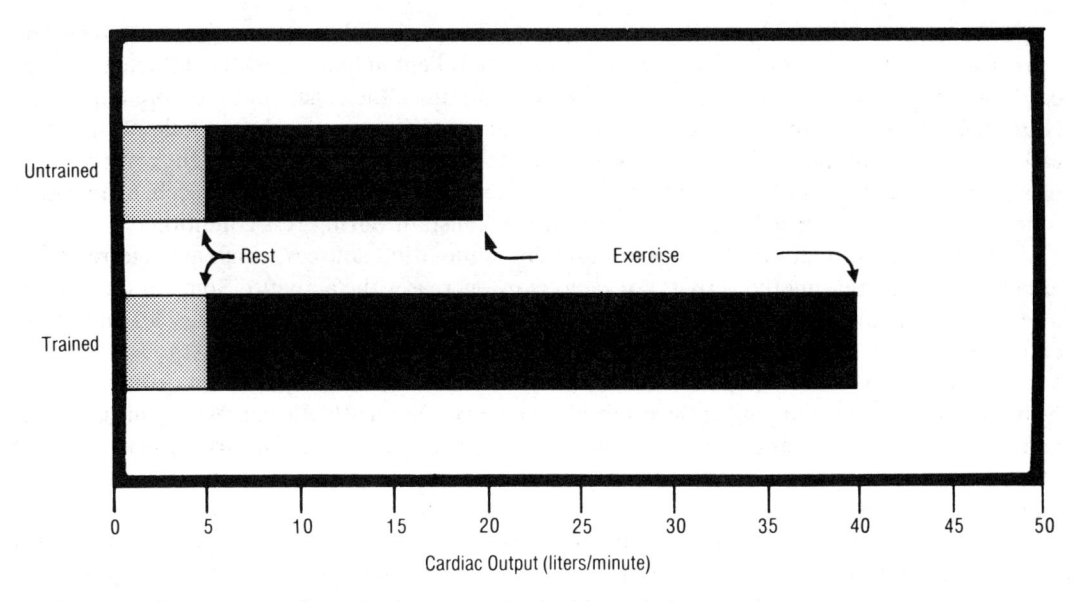

Figure 4-6 Cardiac output for trained and untrained subjects during exercise.

$$\text{Exercise cardiac output} = \text{heart rate} \times \text{stroke volume}$$
$$\text{Untrained } 20{,}000 \text{ ml} = 200 \text{ beats/min} \times 100 \text{ ml}$$
$$\text{Trained } 40{,}000 \text{ ml} = 200 \text{ beats/min} \times 200 \text{ ml}$$

The regulation of cardiac output involves the regulation of both heart rate and stroke volume. Because of their importance to exercise and performance, they will be examined separately.

IV. HEART RATE

A. CONTROL OF HEART RATE

As was stated earlier, the impulse that causes the heart to contract rhythmicly originates within the heart muscle itself, in the right atrium known as the pacemaker or S-A node. Also, as was mentioned earlier, the heart muscle, unlike the skeletal muscle, possesses authorhythmicity: that is, it does not need nervous impulses to start each contraction. However, the nerve supply to the heart does play an important role in modifying its activity. In fact, both *nervous* and *chemical* factors are involved in the regulation of heart rate during rest and exercise.

The *autonomic nervous system* which supplies the *parasympathetic* or *vagus nerves* and the *sympathetic* or *accelerator nerves* to the S-A node play a prime role in regulating the heart rate. Stimulation of the parasympathetic fibers cause the release of *acetylcholine* (Ach) from their ends. The acetylcholine slows the rate of impulse formation in the S-A node and also slows the rate of conduction through the A-V bundle which slows the impulse into the ventricles. Such impulses are called *cardio-inhibitory,* and the final result is a slower heart rate.

Stimulation of the sympathetic fibers cause the release of *norepinephrine* from their ends. The norepinephrine speeds up both the S-A node rates and the conduction rates. Such impulses are called *cardio-acceleratory* which results in a faster and more stronger heart rate.

Because of the different effects of the two nerves, we speak of the *reciprocal innervation* of the heart muscle. Although the normal, resting heart rate is kept in balance by the influence of both cardio-inhibitory impulses and cardio-acceleratory impulses, the vagal inhibition predominates. Note that the nerves controlling the heart arise from specific areas in the medulla of the brain called the cardio-inhibitory and the cardio-acceleratory centers. In other words, the control of the heart rate is predominantly through reflexes. The centers control a feedback mechanism which functions to keep the mean arterial blood pressure constant during rest conditions.

These centers are affected by several afferent stimulation sources which are referred to as either *pressor* (increasing the activity) or *depressor* (decreases the activity). Some of the pressor afferent sources are: (1) proprioceptive reflexes originating in the working muscles and joints contribute to increases in heart rate, (2) impulses arising in the chemoreceptors of the carotid body and the aortic body as a result of decreased pH or increased carbon dioxide results in an increased heart rate, (3) impulses arising in the cerebral cortex prior to an athletic contest or during frightening situations cause an anticipatory increase in heart rate, and (4) impulses arising in the adrenal medulla causes a discharge of norepinephrine and epinephrine hormones into the blood stream and an increase in heart rate.

The primary sources of depressor afferent activity are from the stretch receptors in the carotid sinus and the aortic arch. The activity from these receptors tend to slow heart rate down.

In addition to the nervous and hormonal sources that control heart rate, at least two other factors are of considerable importance. An increase in body temperature and a fall in the blood oxygen content also play a large role in the increased heart rate. However, the extent to which these changes contribute to the heart rate increase in exercise is not clear.

B. HEART RATE RESPONSE TO EXERCISE

The relationship of heart rate to exercise oxygen consumption per minute (V_{O_2}) is shown in Figure 4-7. Heart rate increases linearly with increasing oxygen consumption in both trained and untrained individuals. Figure 4-7 shows that during exercise, the heart rate of a well-trained person is consistently lower at any given workload or V_{O_2} than that of the untrained person.

In addition, it can be seen in Figure 4-7 that endurance training also tends to lower maximal heart rate from about 200 to somewhere around 185 to 190 beats per minute. That this rate becomes lower with training does not necessarily imply a reduction of the heart's capability to increase its rate of contraction. Instead, it merely means that since training also increases work capacity (and max. $\dot{V}_{O_2}$), maximal heart rates in trained individuals are obtained at relatively higher workloads and $\dot{V}_{O_2}$ levels than in untrained subjects.

Endurance training also tends to lower the resting heart rate (bradycardia). For instance, resting heart rates in highly trained athletes may be as low or lower than 40 to 45 beats per minute. On the other hand, in healthy but untrained subjects, resting heart rates may be as high as 90 to 100 beats per minute. Thus, the trained subject is generally characterized as having a low resting heart rate and the untrained as a high resting heart rate.

The highest attainable heart rate during performance of strenuous work not only depends upon the state of conditioning, but also upon age. For instance, Figure 4-8 illustrates clearly that at the age of 20 the maximal heart rate is about 200 which is reduced to approximately 155 at the age of 70. The exact mechanism involved in this age reduced maximal heart rate is not fully understood. Apparently, it is just one of the biological changes in the human body that comes with old age.

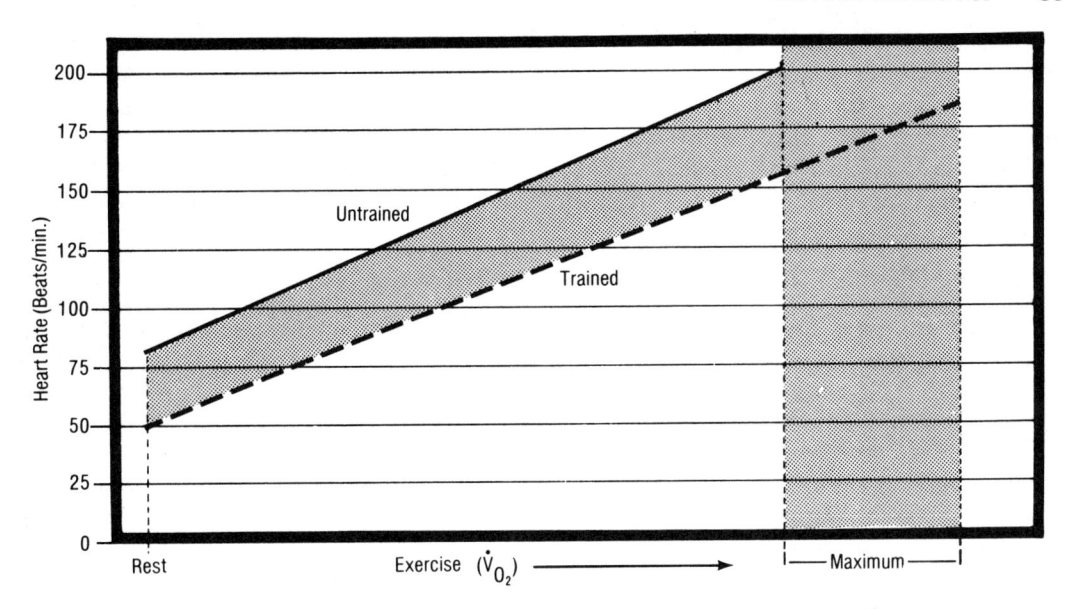

Figure 4-7 The relationship between heart rate and oxygen consumption per minute ($\dot{V}_{O_2}$) for trained and untrained subjects during exercise.

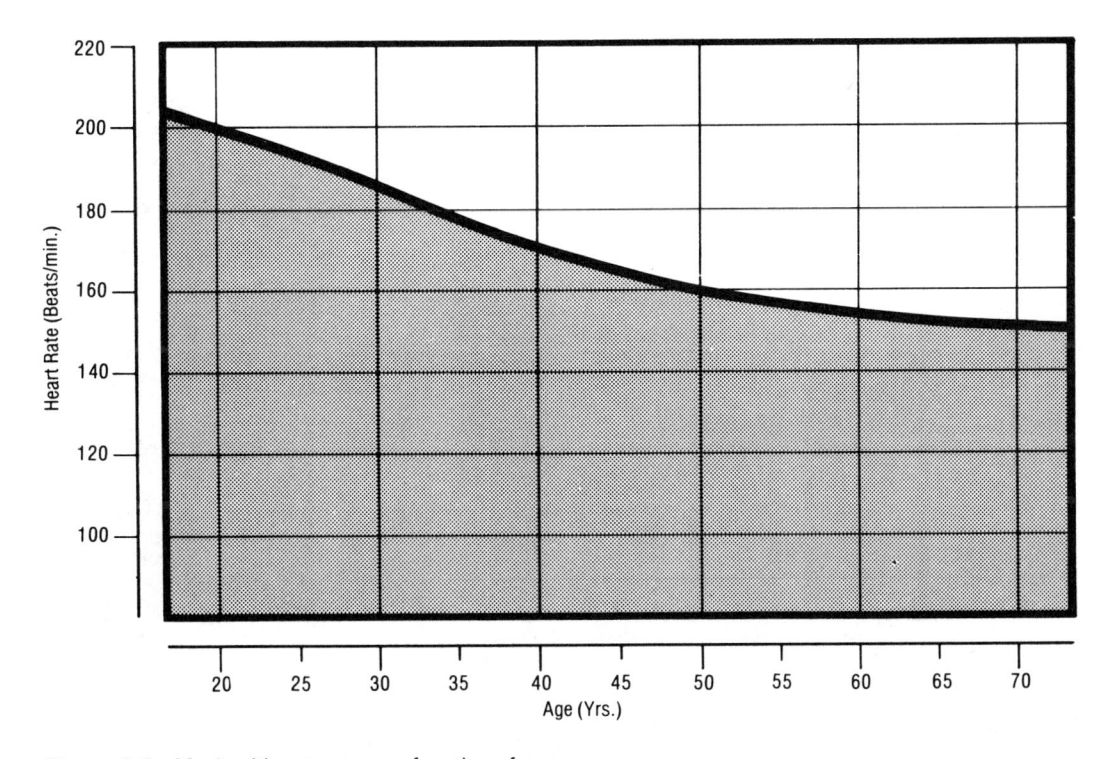

Figure 4-8 Maximal heart rate as a function of age.

86 Essentials of Exercise Physiology

It should be pointed out that the type of exercise also definitely influences the increase in heart rate. For example, the greatest acceleration of the heart occurs in exercises of speed such as sprint running, wheres the smallest increase takes place in exercises of strength such as weight lifting and throwing. This is illustrated in Figure 5-8 in Chapter 5. Also, in exercises that are classified as endurance such as distance running, the heart rate increase is somewhere between those of speed and strength exercises. At the same time, however, heart rate recovery takes longer following cessation of the endurance exercise.

C. SELECTED FACTORS AFFECTING HEART RATE

There are several factors, as illustrated in Figure 4-9, that affect the resting heart rate besides exercise and training. Briefly, these include posture, sex, age, emotion, and environmental factors.

Posture

Although the extent of variation differs with each individual, body position has a definite effect upon the heart rate. Generally, the rate is lowest in the recumbent followed by the sitting and standing. It appears that the typical response from the recumbent to the standing position is an increase of around 10 to 12 beats per minute. This is due to the influence of gravity which lowers the volume of blood returning to the heart (and thus stroke volume) when one goes from a

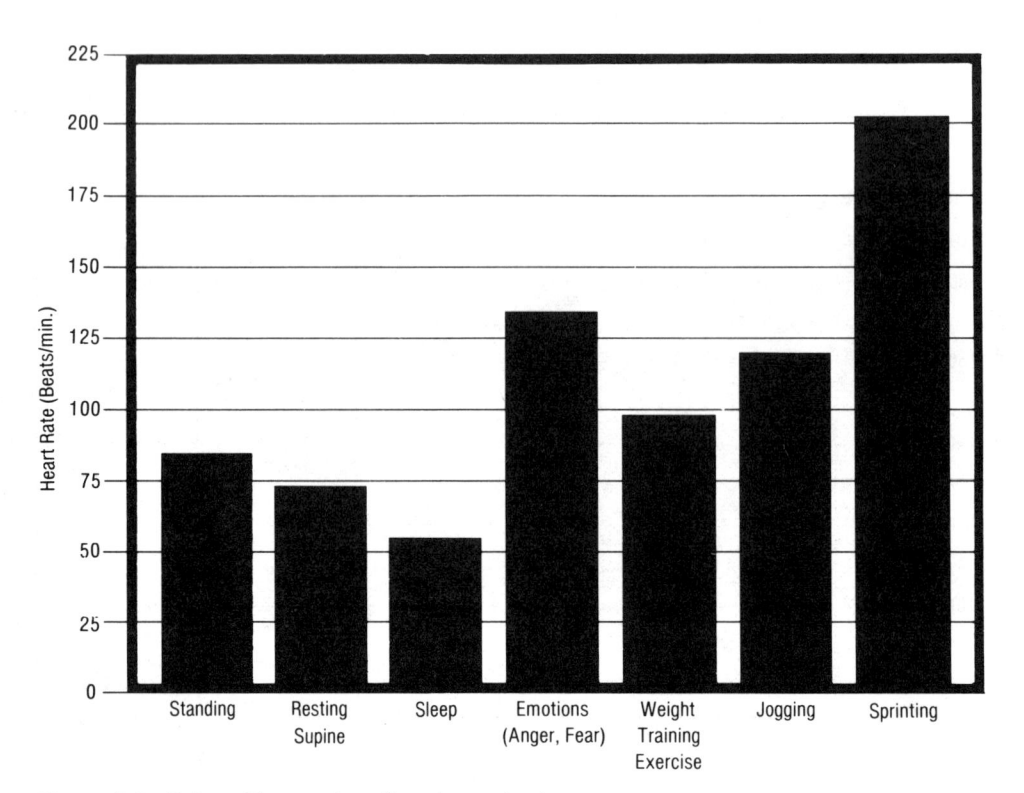

Figure 4-9 Selected factors that affect the resting heart rate.

reclining position to a sitting or standing position. Individuals who are physically fit show a smaller increase between lying and standing than do sedentary individuals.

Sex

The adult female's resting heart rate is some 5 to 10 beats per minute faster than that of the adult male under any given situation. The average resting heart rate is approximately 78 beats per minute for adult men and 84 beats per minute for adult females. A more complete comparison between men and women can be found in Chapter 11.

Age

The resting heart rate drops progressively from birth (when it is approximately 130 beats per minute) to adolescense but in old age it again increases slightly. Also, maximum heart rate decreases at a rate of not quite one beat per year. Chapter 13 has a thorough discussion on how age affects various physiological measurements.

Emotion

Emotional stress accelerates the resting as well as the exercise heart rate. Although an increased heart rate is most easily observed during rest in people as an anticipatory reaction, emotions may also result in an excessive cardiorespiratory adjustment during light exercise. For instance, under these conditions the response of the heart rate to a given work load (light) may be somewhat greater because of the combined efforts of both exercise and emotional stress (the anticipation of the event). On the other hand, emotion probably has little effect on the maximal heart rate. This anticipatory response is believed to be due to a stimulation of the cardio-acceleratory nerve centers in the medulla of the brain and also to an increased amount of norepinephrine and epinephrine hormones released from the adrenal medulla into the blood stream.

Environmental Factors

The influence of environmental factors on heart functions is considered in greater detail in Chapters 7 and 8. It is sufficient to point out here that a high temperature and altitude may greatly increase the heart rate. In addition, for any standard temperature and workload, the increase in heart rate will be significantly greater if the air is still and the humidity is high.

V. STROKE VOLUME

A. CONTROL OF STROKE VOLUME

For several years, it was generally believed that stroke volume was a direct function of the end diastolic volume of the ventricle. This was based on the well-known principle known as *Starling's law of the heart*. This law states that the greater the initial length of the cardiac muscle fiber, the stronger the myocadium contraction. It also states that the initial length of the cardiac muscle fiber is actually determined by the amount of blood which passes into the ventricle during diastole. This means that the force of the contraction determines the amount of blood pumped by the ventricles during systole. This implies, therefore, that stroke volume is directly related to the diastolic volume up to a critical point.

Recently, however, X-ray pictures and X-ray kymograms of the heart taken during rest and under exercise conditions indicate quite clearly that the size of the heart recorded at the end of diastolic does not increase during exercise over that which occurs during rest. In addition, the systolic size is also reduced somewhat below that recorded at rest. As a result of these findings, the significance of Starling's law of the heart with respect to controlling the stroke volume is now open to question and does not appear to be nearly as important as was once believed. The X-ray pictures and kymograms evidence cited above simply means that the ventricles apparently do not empty entirely during rest, and that the degree of emptying is perhaps increased during exercise. Thus, the increased stroke volume is due to a greater emptying of the heart with each beat and not to a greater diastolic filling as was once believed. This increased stroke volume implies a greater force of ventricular contraction during exercise. It is believed that the greater force of contraction is caused in part by an increased stimulation of the heart muscle from the sympathetic nervous system and by an increased amount of norepinephrine and epinephrine hormones released from the adrenal glands.

It should be pointed out that although Starling's law of the heart is not considered nearly as important in the control of stroke volume as was once believed, it still apparently plays an important role in controlling stroke volume when nervous activity to the heart is impeded.

B. STROKE VOLUME RESPONSE TO EXERCISE

Figure 4-10 shows the relationship of stroke volume to exercise in both trained and untrained subjects. This graph indicates clearly that stroke volume increases progressively from rest to moderate work and then it levels off at about 30 to 40 percent of the maximum aerobic power. Here it is interesting to note that the dynamics of adjustment are very similar in the trained and untrained subject. At the same time, however, the trained person operates at a higher level. Figure 4-11 shows similar findings for the arteriovenous oxygen difference (a-$\bar{v}_{O_2}$ diff), which represents

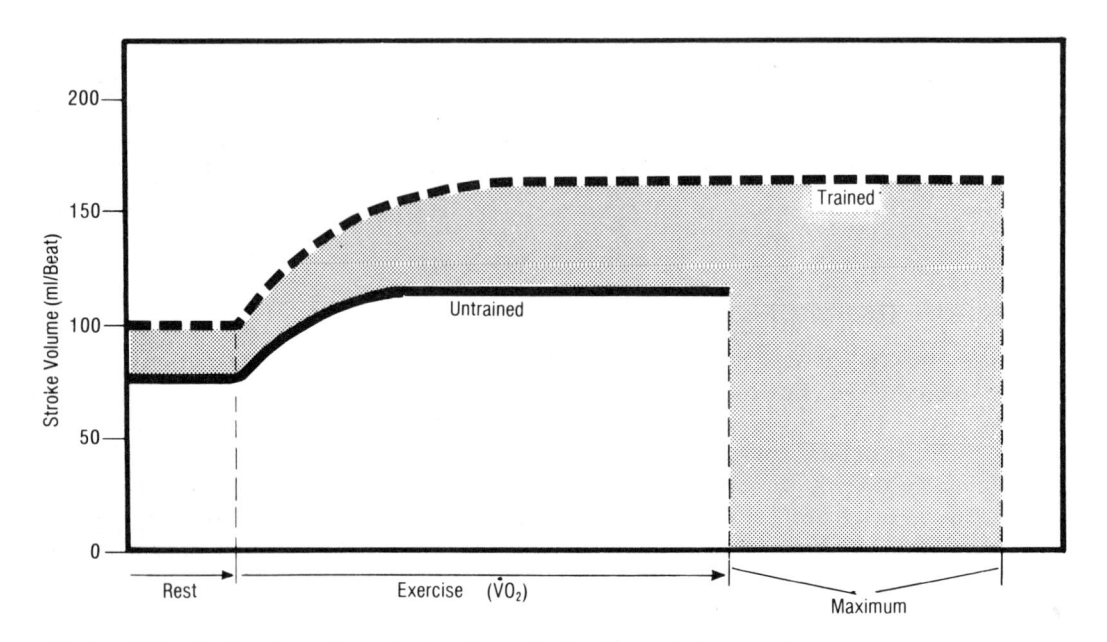

Figure 4-10 Stroke volume for trained and untrained subjects during exercise.

The Heart and Exercise   89

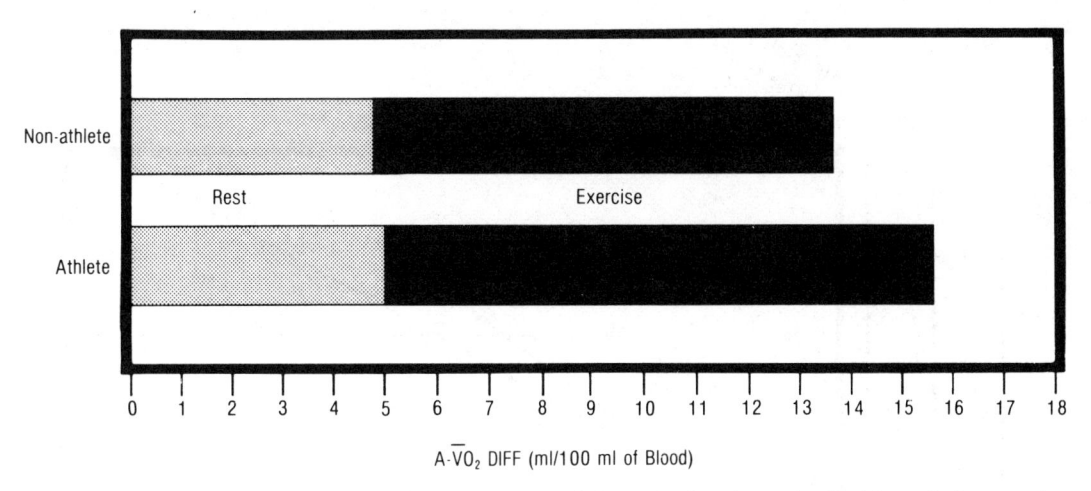

Figure 4-11 Arteriovenous oxygen difference (a-$\bar{v}_{O_2}$ diff) for trained and untrained subjects during exercise.

how much oxygen is extracted or consumed by the tissues from each 100 ml of blood perfusing them. It is rather obvious that trained athletes have a greater capacity for not only pumping more blood by the heart per beat, but they also have a greater capacity for extracting more oxygen from the blood into the muscle tissues than sedentary subjects.

Figure 4-12 illustrates the relationship between cardiac output, stroke volume, and heart rate as a function of oxygen uptake. It shows that once stroke volume reaches its maximum level (which is usually at a workload requring 30 to 40 percent of maximum aerobic power, or at a heart rate of about 110 to 120 beats per minute), any additional increases in cardiac output are obtained only through increases in heart rate. It should be noted that during maximum work when the heart rate may reach values as high as 200 beats per minute, the stroke volume is generally maintained at its maximum level. This means that the time available for the filling of the ventricles at heart rates up to 200 is sufficient to allow maximal stroke volumes.

At rest and in the supine position the stroke volume of an adult untrained man is around 70 to 100 ml per beat depending upon the body size. Maximal values range between 100 and 120 ml per beat. For trained adult men, resting values are around 100 to 120 ml, whereas maximal values fall somewhere between 150 to 200 ml per beat. In some cases, the highly trained endurance athlete may even exceed maximum values of 200 ml per beat. Hence, a relatively slow resting heart rate, coupled with a relatively large stroke volume, is characteristic of the trained person and thus indicates an efficient circulatory system. Because of the smaller size of the heart in women, their stroke volume is usually 25 percent lower. As stated earlier, since blood normally pools in the lower portions of the body under the influence of gravity when assuming a sitting or standing position, this results in a drop in venous return to the heart and thus about a 30 percent reduction in stroke volume.

It is interesting to note that there is a definite relationship between maximum aerobic work and cardiac output, and that stroke volume, to a large degree, determines the limits of cardiac output. As was pointed out earlier, this statement is true since nearly everyone has about the same maximal heart rate levels. Thus, the importance of stroke volume in long endurance type activities cannot be overemphasized. In fact, it is generally agreed among exercise physiologists that stroke volume is the difference between an individual with a large cardiac output and one with only a normal output.

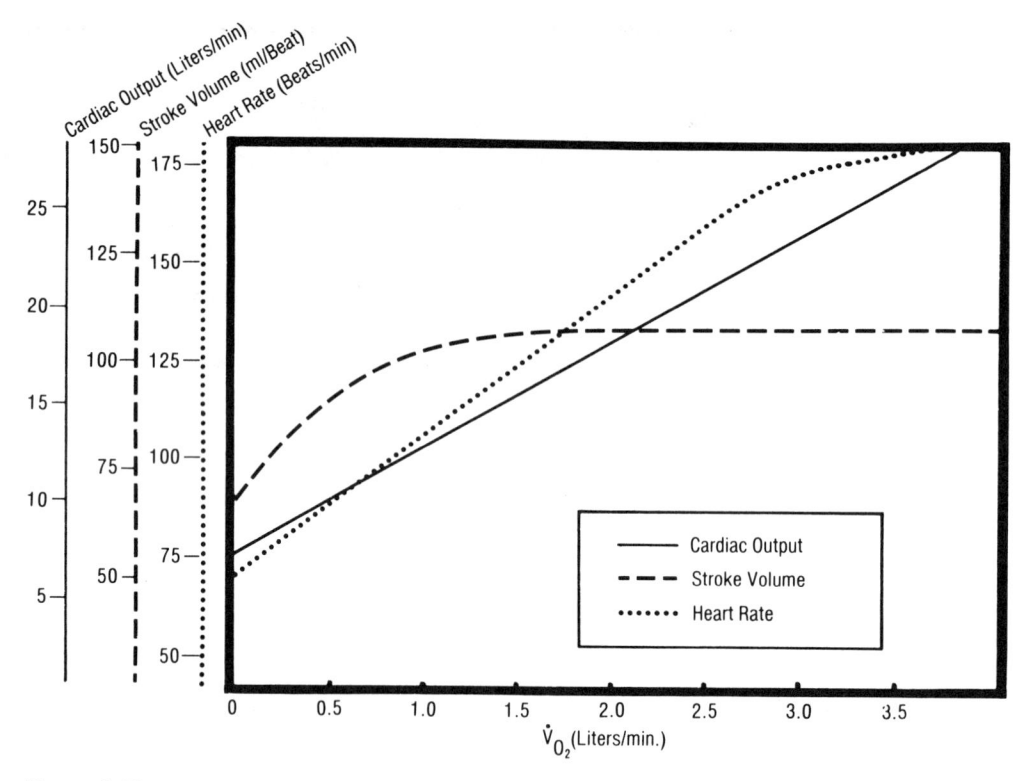

Figure 4-12 Schematic diagram illustrating the relationship between heart rate, cardiac output, and stroke volume as a function of oxygen consumption.

VI. CARDIAC HYPERTROPHY

It is well known that a period of endurance exercise training results in cardiac hypertrophy. That is, the heart itself enlarges. In the past, this change in heart size along with the slow resting heart that is normally observed in the trained athlete led some observers to believe that strenuous exercise was deleterious to the healthy heart. In fact, some felt that it brought about heart enlargement similar to that normally seen in cardiac disease.

Long-term clinical and physiological studies of endurance athletes (cyclists, cross-country skiers, and marathon runners), however, have shown no detrimental effects on the heart as a result of endurance work. In fact, all available evidence suggests that the normal heart of the trained endurance person has a greater pumping capacity and is able to provide more oxygen to the body tissues at strenuous work loads than the normal untrained heart. Recall from earlier discussion that cardiac output for the trained person may be increased from 5 liters per minute at rest to 40 liters per minute during maximum exercise. This compares to a maximum of 20 liters per minute for the untrained person. The increased capacity of the trained heart to supply blood and oxygen to the working muscles is apparently due to not only an increase in the number of capillaries and in the amount of blood flow, but also to an increase in the mitochondrial size, their content, and their related enzymes.

VII. THE ELECTROCARDIOGRAM (ECG)

The electrocardiogram (ECG), as illustrated in Figures 4-5 and 4-13, is a recording of the electrical impulses of the heart muscle. This recording represents the actual electrical sum of all the cardiac muscle fibers in the spread of depolarization and repolarization. The P wave is brought about by the spread of depolarization through the atrium (state of depolarization lasts for about 0.18 or 0.2 sec.), which causes an increase in atrium pressure as the atrium contracts. Following the P wave, the QRS complex shows up on the recording and it reflects depolarization of the ventricles (thus causing the ventricular pressure to rise) as well as repolarization of the atrium. The ST segment and the T wave represents the repolarization of the ventricles, at which time their muscle fibers begin to relax.

The ECG is not only an excellent tool for determining the beating rate of the atria and the ventricles, but it is also excellent for determining whether or not the various heart chambers are enlarged. This is possible by determining the amount of voltage generated (or the height) of the P and QRS waves. By using certain electrodes and by placing them in specific positions, it can be determined which chamber is enlarged. For instance, specific electrodes placed in front of the chest near the heart will ascertain if the left ventricle is enlarged. If the left ventricle is enlarged, the QRS waves recorded near this chamber will record a signal that may be double the normal height of the QRS wave for that particular location.

In addition, the ECG may be used for detecting people with possible cardiac damage. For instance, it is well known that Myocardial Ischemia or a reduced blood supply to the heart (which may suggest a narrowing of the coronary blood vessels) brings about changes in the rate and size of depolarization and repolarization of the heart. This occurrence generally changes the characteristics of the normal ECG, as illustrated in Figure 4-13B. The QRS wave indicates evidence of damage to the muscular wall of the chambers by the presence of a Q wave. Also, cardiac damage is indicated by an elevated ST segment and an inverted T wave. Once a heart attack has occurred, if an electrode is placed on the chest near the damaged area of the heart, the ECG may record a large downward deflection, as illustrated in Figure 4-13B, instead of the normal upright QRS wave. This recording occurs because the damaged or "dead" muscle tissue has lost all of its voltage; therefore, it leaves an electrical area from which the normal voltage is not generated.

Figure 4-13C illustrates a typical transcient change in the ECG called angina pectoris (chest pain). This type of condition is generally developed from physical or emotional factors. As can be seen in Figure 4-13C, this temporary change is an abnormality in the repolarization of the heart muscle. It involves a lowering of the ST segment and indicates a temporary reduced blood supply to the cardiac muscle.

It should be pointed out that cardiac abnormalities are more likely to be noticed if the heart is under physiological stress such as running on a treadmill or riding a bicycle. For example, it has been pointed out that approximately one-half the changes noticed during an exhaustive-type exercise will go unnoticed if the work does not exceed about 85 percent of the maximal heart rate.

VIII. SUMMARY

(1) The cardiac cycle involves all the pressure changes, volume changes, and valve actions that take place during one complete phase of contraction (or period of emptying called systole) and relaxation (or period of filling called diastole) of the heart.

(2) From a functional viewpoint, cardiac output (ml/min) is the most important aspect of

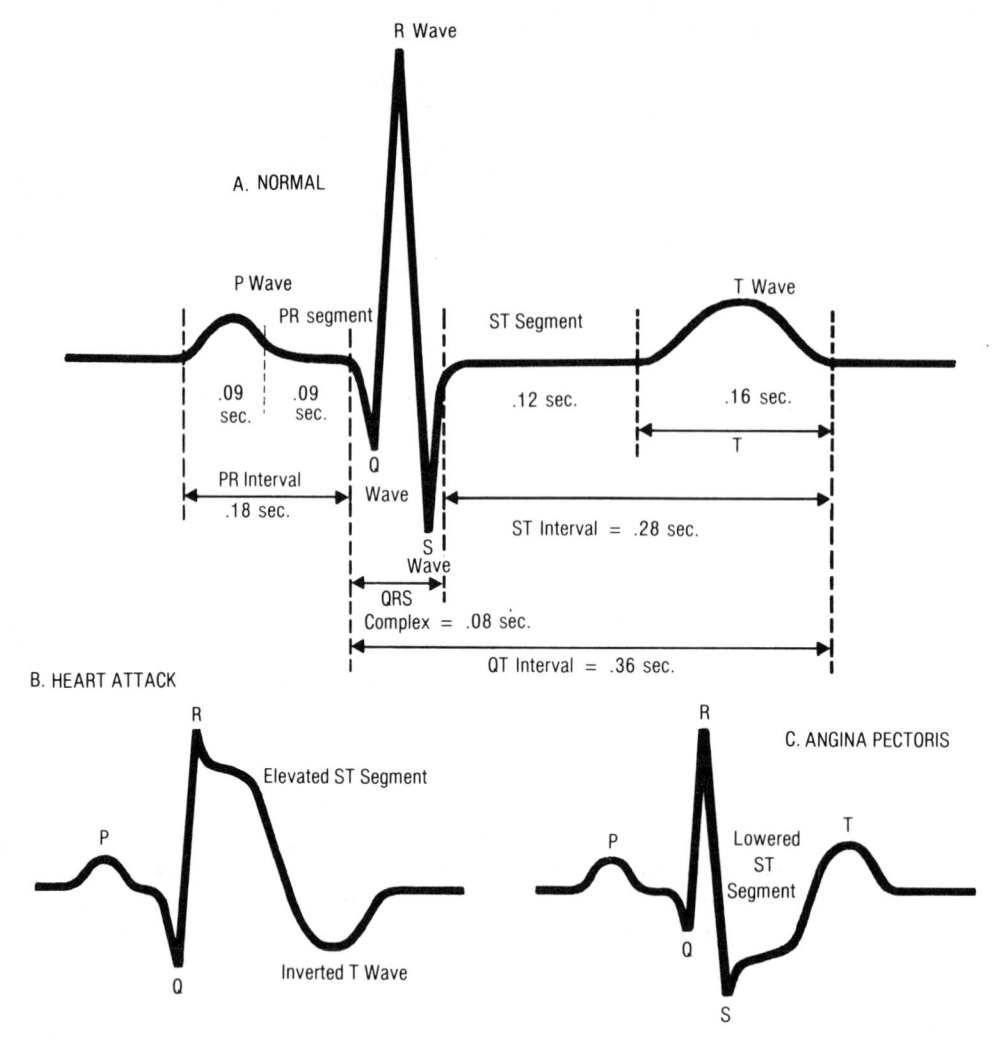

Figure 4-13 The electrocardiogram (ECG). *A*, A normal ECG. *B*, An ECG indicating a heart attack. *C*, An ECG indicating angina pectoris (chest pain).

heart function. It is determined by the product of heart rate (beats/min) times stroke volume (ml/beat). Endurance training brings about a greater working cardiac output and stroke volume.

(3) While the nerve impulse that causes the heart to contract rhythmicly originates within the S-A node of the right atrium, the rate is controlled by a balance effect of the parasympathetic (vagus) and sympathetic (accelerator) nerves of the autonomic nervous system.

(4) In both trained and untrained individuals, heart rate increases linearly as work load and oxygen consumption per minute (V_{O_2}) increases.

(5) The heart rate reacts differently to certain kinds of exercise. For example, the greatest acceleration of the heart occurs in exercise of speed such as sprint running, whereas the smallest

increase takes place in exercise of strength such as weight lifting. Endurance exercises such as distance running increases the heart rate somewhere between those of speed and strength exercises. Heart rate recovery, however, takes longer following endurance exercises.

(6) In addition to specific types of exercise and training, several other factors must also be taken into consideration when studying the effects of exercise upon heart rate. They are: age, sex, posture, emotions, and environmental factors.

(7) In the control of stroke volume, Starling's law of the heart is the principal determinant only when the venous return is altered due to postural and other gravitational changes. During exercise, however, the increase in stroke volume is due to a greater emptying of the left ventricle.

(8) A slow heart rate combined with a large stroke volume is characteristic of the trained subject and thus indicates an efficient circulatory system.

(9) While endurance exercise training may result in an enlarged heart, there is no evidence that exercise is detrimental to the healthy heart.

(10) Evidence suggests that the normal heart of the trained endurance person has a greater pumping capacity and is able to provide more oxygen to the working muscles than the untrained heart. This increased capacity of the trained heart is due to: (a) an increase in the amount of blood flow; (b) an increase in number of capillaries; and (c) an increase in the mitochondrial size and their content, and in their related enzymes.

(11) The electrical excitation characteristics of the heart is represented by the electrocardiogram (ECG), and it may detect the size of the chambers as well as muscle damage.

IX. REVIEW REFERENCES

(1) Astrand, I. "ST Depression, Heart Rate, and Blood Pressure During Arm and Leg Work," *Scandinavian Journal of Clinical Laboratory Investigation,* 30:411-14, 1972.
(2) Edington, D. W., and V. R. Edgerton. *The Biology of Physical Activity,* Houghton Mifflin Co., Boston, 1976.
(3) Guyton, A. C. *Textbook of Medical Physiology,* 5th edition, W. B. Saunders Co., Philadelphia, 1976.
(4) Katch, F. I., and W. D. McArdle. *Nutrition, Weight Control, and Exercise,* Houghton Mifflin Co., Boston, 1977.
(5) Katz. A. M. *Physiology of the Heart,* Raven Press, New York, 1977.
(6) Mathews, D. K., and E. L. Fox. *The Physiological Basis of Physical Education and Athletics,* 2nd edition, W. B. Saunders Co., Philadelphia, 1976.
(7) Roskamm, H. "Myocardial Contractility During Exercise," In J. Keul (Ed.), *Limiting Factors of Physical Performance,* Georg Thieme, Publishers, Stuttgart, 1973.
(8) Ross, J., Jr., and R. A. O'Rourke. *Understanding the Heart and its Diseases,* McGraw-Hill Book Co., New York, 1976.

5

THE SYSTEMIC CIRCULATION AND EXERCISE

KEY CONCEPTS TO BE GAINED FROM THIS CHAPTER

(1) Systemic blood flow is regulated by chemical and neural mechanisms during exercise.

(2) Potassium and low oxygen tensions are considered to be the most important local vasodilator agents in active muscle.

(3) The type of exercise performed plays an important role in influencing the increase in blood pressure. For example, isometric-type work generally causes a greater increase in blood pressure than isotonic exercises.

(4) Prolonged physical work in the untrained subject leads to a much quicker fall in systolic blood pressure (which indicates nearing fatigue) than for the trained person. Endurance training also improves the blood pressure recovery process after exercise. In other words, the blood pressure for the trained person returns to the pre-exercise level sooner than it does for the untrained person.

(5) Several other factors affect blood pressure besides exercise and training. They are: age, sex, posture, and emotion.

Recall from the previous chapter that the blood is pumped from the heart to all parts of the body. As the blood leaves the left ventricle of the heart, it flows through various peripheral blood vessels and eventually back into the right atrium of the heart. Upon returning to the right atrium, this completes a full circuit of the blood. This circuit is called the *systemic* or *peripheral circulatory system*. Thus, the purpose of this chapter is to discuss the flow of blood as it passes through this system.

I. STRUCTURAL PROPERTIES OF THE SYSTEMIC CIRCULATORY SYSTEM

A. ARTERIES AND ARTERIOLES

The *arteries* are the larger vessels which carry the blood away from the heart. They have low resistance and large diameters. The arteries have more elastic tissue and more smooth muscle as well as thicker walls than the other vessels. This difference is due to the higher pressure of blood in the arteries. Also, this elasticity is of vital importance in maintaining a steadier flow of blood than the pumping action of the heart could accomplish alone. For instance, as the blood is forced into the aorta during systole, the tremendous pressure stretches the arteries which temporarily absorbs some of the pumping energy. Afterwards, when the pressure drops during diastole (time the heart is relaxed), the elastic rebound of the arterial walls compresses the blood and continues to force it into the tissues. Thus, the elastic tissue in the arterial walls tends to more or less "smooth out" the fluctuations of blood flow through the cardiac cycle. The expansion of the arterial wall during the systolic ejection period extends all the way out to the periphery and can be detected as a pulse in several arteries (radial artery in the wrist, the femoral artery in the leg, and the carotid artery in the neck) near the surface. Figure 5-1 illustrates the differences in the cross-section appearance of the various vessels.

The *arterioles* (small arteries) are found between the arteries and the capillaries. In arterioles the resistance to blood flow is quite high, thus resulting in a marked pressure drop. Figure 5-2 shows how the arterioles are arranged in a series of parallel channels joining the capillary bed (and veins) with the arterial side. Since it is well known among exercise physiologists that arterioles can change the total resistance against the blood flow from the arteries and thereby the arterial blood pressure and work of the heart, they definitely have a significant influence on the distribution and regulation of the blood flow to the various organs. Much of this control is brought about by vasoconstriction and vasodilatation adjustments (via the sympathetic nervous systems control over the smooth muscles of the arteriolar walls) in the diameters of the arterioles. Note that vasoconstriction is when the diameters of the blood vessels gets smaller, whereas vasodilatation is when the diameters get larger.

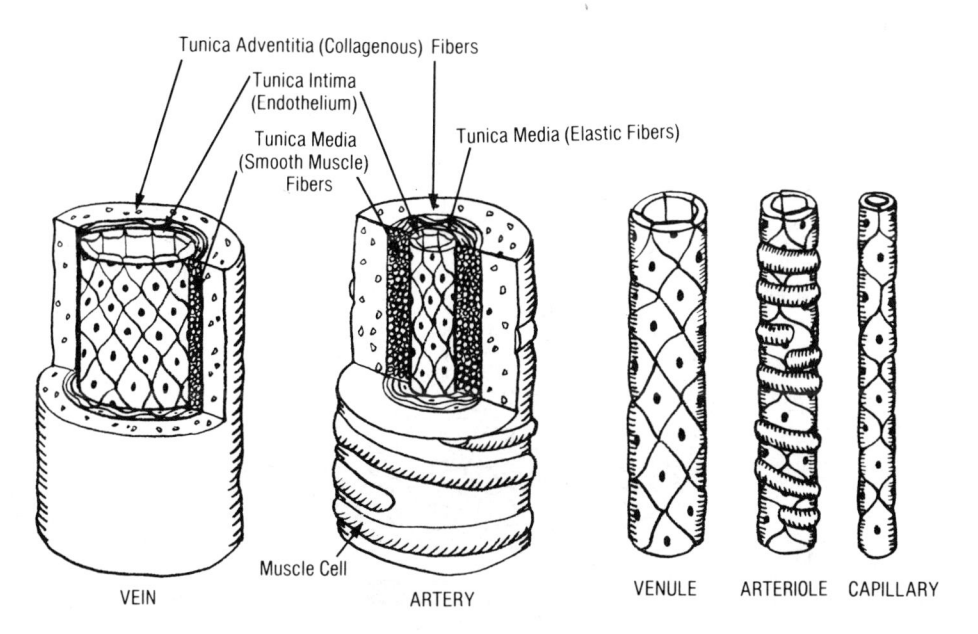

Figure 5-1 Structures of the various blood vessels.

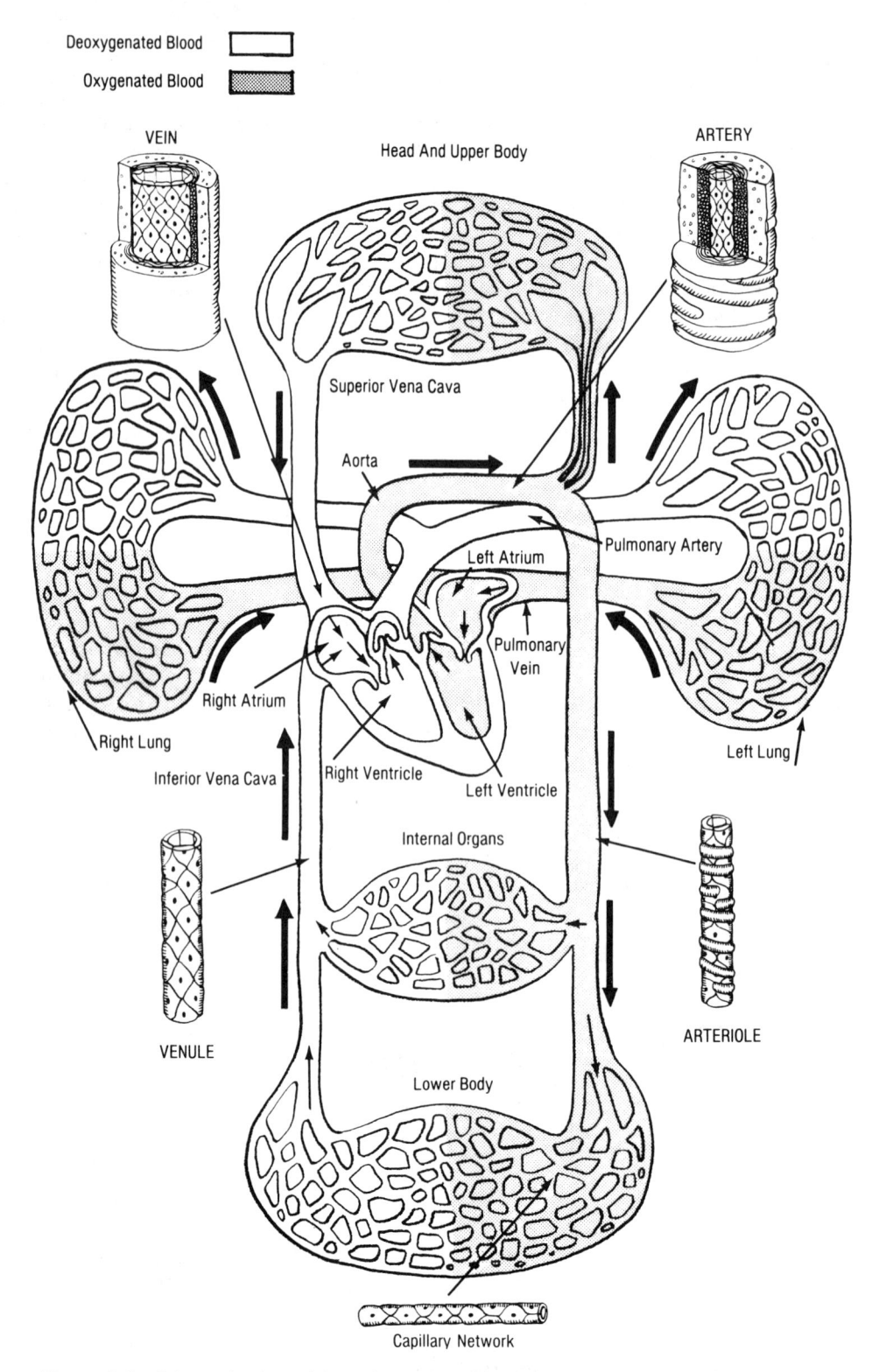

Figure 5-2 Schematic view of how the various blood vessels are arranged in the systemic circulatory system.

B. CAPILLARIES

Because the exchange of gases, water, electrolytes, etc. can only occur across the walls of the *capillaries,* their structure is vitally important. As can be seen in Figure 5-2, capillaries are located between the arterioles and the venules and they are considered to be the smallest of all vessels. The capillary walls are made up of very thin endothelial cell plates of protein and lipid. The length of a single capillary vessel is less than 1 mm. Because the capillaries inner diameter is sometimes hardly large enough for an erythrocyte (red blood cell) to pass through, it has been published that theoretically it would take 1 cc of blood between 5 and 7 hours to travel through a single capillary. However, because there are so many capillaries in the human body, this does not generally present a problem for sufficient blood flow. It has been stated that capillaries, when spread out, make up close to 60,000 miles. In fact, when considered as a whole, capillaries are said to be the largest organ in the body.

Figure 5-3 illustrates the microcirculation of a capillary bed. In the illustration, it can be seen that the blood reaches the capillaries from the arterioles by way of a series of *metarterioles,* and that some of the capillaries are larger (called *preferential channels*) than others (called *true capillaries*). Each of the large capillaries may branch off into many smaller ones. In Figure 5-3, it can also be noticed that at the capillary entry, a ring of smooth muscle surrounds the capillary vessel (referred to as *precapillary sphincter*). Because the walls of the capillaries have no muscle cells or

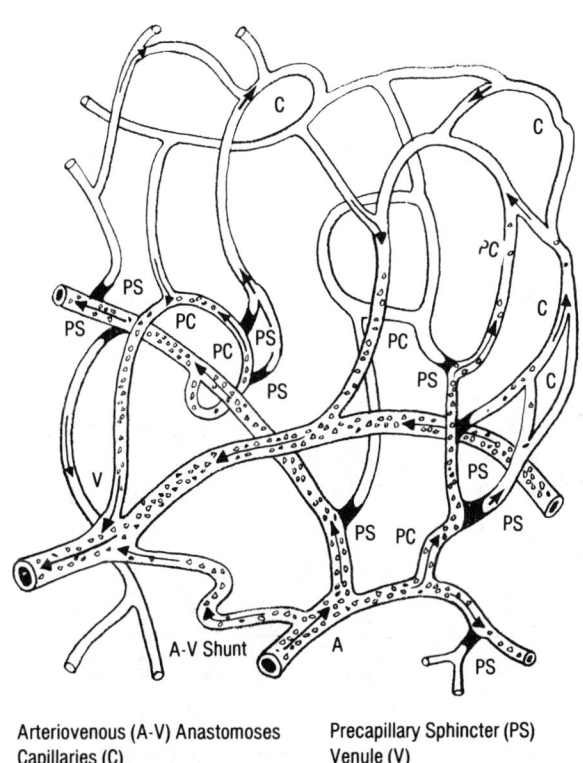

Arteriovenous (A-V) Anastomoses
Capillaries (C)
Preferential Channel (PC)
Precapillary Sphincter (PS)
Venule (V)
Arteriole (A)

Figure 5-3 Schematic illustration of the microcirculation of a capillary bed.

98 Essentials of Exercise Physiology

other contractable elements, this precapillary sphincter regulates the amount of blood flowing into the capillary bed. Channels for shunting arterial blood directly into the venous system when necessary without passing through the capillary bed are also present and can be seen in Figure 5-3. These channels are referred to as *arteriovenous* (A-V) *anastomoses* and are located primarily in the skin. Because the blood passing through the A-V anastomoses do not go through the normal blood route for exchanging oxygen and carbon dioxide and other nutrients at the tissue site, it is considered to be non-nutritive. However, it will have a warming effect on the skin since it results in an increased blood volume flowing into the veins.

It is acknowledged that when an individual is resting and not working, most of the true capillaries are closed and are not being used (normally, only the preferential channels are open during rest). When work commences, however, those capillaries in the working muscles become more functional. This obviously permits more blood to come into contact with a greater amount of muscle tissue, thereby allowing a greater exchange of gases to take place at this level. Also, during this period of time when body temperature may be going up as a result of work, blood flow may increase to the skin area in order to dissipate the increased core temperature.

C. VENULES AND VEINS

The venules are small veins which are found between the capillaries and the larger veins. The veins are the larger vessels which receives the blood (high in carbon dioxide and low in oxygen) from the venules and transports it to the heart. The veins increase in caliber as well as in wall thickness as they progress back towards the heart. Since the venules and veins are larger in size than the arteries and arterioles, and since there are more of them, it is quite obvious that more blood should be found in the venous systems. In fact, it has been calculated that the venous systems generally contain approximately 65 to 70 percent of the total blood volume during rest.

Figure 5-4 illustrates a unique feature of the veins. The illustration shows the presence of one-way valves which allow the blood to flow in one direction only (towards the heart), and also

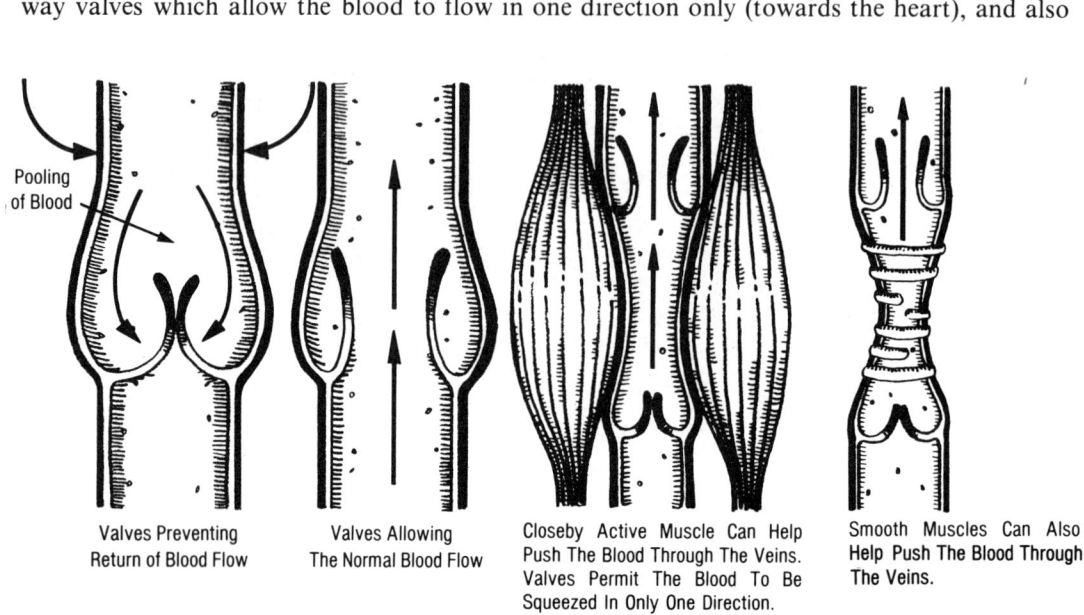

Figure 5-4 Illustration showing the presence of one-way valves in veins.

prevents the blood from draining back. As mentioned earlier, the size of the veins are much larger in total diameter than the arteries. This means that the blood moves back to the heart somewhat sluggishly compared with the surging force in the arteries. Figure 5-4 illustrates that when a vein within a skeletal muscle is actively compressed by nearby muscles during muscular contraction, its valves permit the blood to be squeezed only in one direction. Smooth muscles which encircles the veins are also able to push the blood back toward the heart. Thus, the return of venous blood, particularly from the feet and legs, is facilitated by this "muscle pump" of both the nearby active muscles and the smooth muscles.

II. HEMODYNAMICS: PHYSICAL LAWS GOVERNING BLOOD FLOW

There are three major hemodynamic factors which need to be considered in this section: (1) blood pressure, (2) velocity of blood flow, and (3) resistance to flow.

A. BLOOD PRESSURE

It is known that blood flows through the vessels of the circulatory system as a result of a *pressure gradient*. This means that blood flows from a point of high pressure to one of low pressure. For instance, in the systemic circulatory system, Figure 5-5 shows that the point of highest pressure occurs in the left ventricle (usually about 120 mmHg at body rest) during systole, and the difference between this point and the lowest pressure point in the right atrium is the driving force (along with the pumping action of the muscles just previously mentioned) that causes blood to flow throughout the entire systemic circulation. This situation is also true for pulmonary blood flow except the pressures are somewhat lower in magnitude.

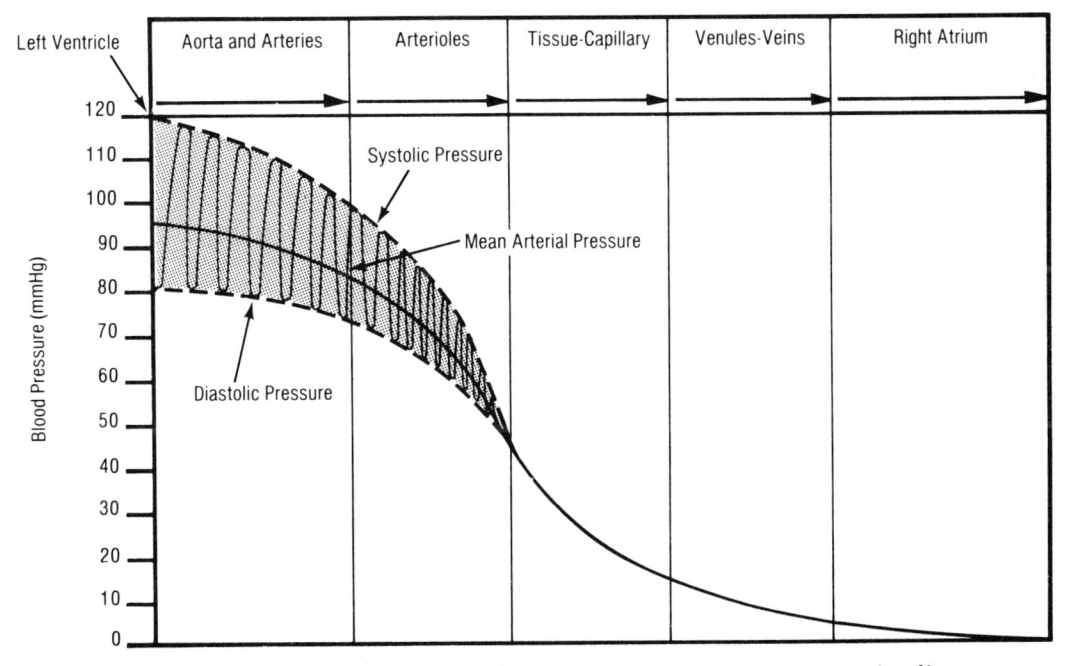

Figure 5-5 Schematic illustration of how blood flows from a point of high pressure to a point of low pressure in the body.

Figure 5-5 also illustrates that the pressure varies in the arteries. For example, the highest pressure recorded is called the systolic pressure, whereas the lowest is referred to as the diastolic pressure. The mean of these two pressures (systolic plus diastolic) during a complete cardiac cycle is referred to as the mean arterial pressure. Because the mean arterial pressure determines how fast the blood actually moves through the systemic circulatory system, it is generally considered to be one of our most important hemodynamic factors.

B. VELOCITY OF BLOOD FLOW

The velocity of blood flow past any given point depends upon the total cross-sectional area of the vascular system at that particular point, according to deVries. The following formula may be used to calculate the velocity of blood flow:

$$\text{Velocity of blood flow} = \frac{\text{blood flow}}{\text{diameter}^2}$$

Thus, if the same amount of blood must pass through a given area having half the diameter of another area, the velocity of flow must be four times as great.

Because the aorta in man has a total cross-sectional area of between 2.5 to 5.0 sq cm, and the quantity of blood flow from the heart into the aorta is about 5,000 ml per minute during rest, one can calculate from these figures (for example, using the 2.5 figure) using the above formula that blood passes through the aorta at a mean velocity of approximately 2,000 ml per minute or 33 ml per second. Since the combined cross-sectional areas of the arteries and arterioles do not differ greatly from that of the aorta, there is very little change in velocity. On the other hand, in the capillaries the rate of flow is decreased because of the increase in total cross-sectional area. For instance, each capillary is only about 1/100 mm in diameter; however, the combined cross-sectional area of all the capillaries is between 700 and 800 times that of the aorta. This indicates that the blood velocity is much slower in the capillary bed than in the aorta. Note that the velocity of flow in the capillary bed is about 1/700 to 1/800 that in the aorta or about 0.5 to 1.0 mm per second. This fact is extremely important to the system since we know that it is in the capillaries that the exchange of respiratory gases (oxygen and carbon dioxide) and other nutrients take place. At the same time, the total cross-sectional area of the veins at any given level is approximately double that of the corresponding arteries, which indicates that the velocity of the deoxygenated blood in the veins is only about one half that found in the oxygenated blood of the arteries.

C. RESISTANCE TO FLOW

The friction between the blood and walls of the vessels that the blood flows through determines the resistance to blood flow. For example, the closer the blood is clustered to the middle of the vessel, the less resistance it faces and thus the faster it flows. The resistance to blood flow is determined by three factors: (1) the diameter of the vessel, (2) the length of the vessel, and (3) viscosity or thickness of the blood, according to Mathews and Fox. This can be stated:

$$\text{Resistance} = \frac{\text{length} \times \text{viscosity}}{\text{diameter}^4}$$

Notice that in the above formula there is a direct opposite relationship between resistance and the blood vessels diameter to its fourth power. This is vitally important because it means that a slight change in the diameter of the vessel produces large changes in resistance. For example, as researchers have pointed out, if the vessel diameter is reduced to one-half its original size, resistance increases 16 times, or if the diameter doubles its original size, resistance decreases 16 times.

Poiseuille's law (a theoretically derived mathematical law) is often used by physiologists to express these relationships. It can be stated:

$$\text{Volume of blood flow} = \frac{\text{pressure} \times \text{diameter}^4}{\text{length} \times \text{viscosity}}$$

III. REGULATION OF BLOOD FLOW DURING REST AND EXERCISE

Regulation of the flow of blood to the different tissues of the systemic circulatory system is brought about by two mechanisms: (1) nervous, and (2) chemical.

A. NERVOUS REGULATION

Available evidence indicates that all of the nervous regulation of blood flow to the skeletal muscles is under the influence of the sympathetic nervous system. This system provides two types of nerve fibers to the smooth muscles of the blood vessels in the skeletal muscles: (1) cholinergic vasodilator fibers (releases acetylcholine at their endings) which play a role in increasing the active muscle blood flow in exercise through vasodilatation, and (2) adrenergic vasoconstrictor fibers (releases nor-adrenaline or norepinephrine at their endings) which restricts blood flow in inactive areas via vasoconstriction.

During rest, the blood flow through skeletal muscle is very small because the blood vessels that supply these muscles are in a state of vasoconstriction (intrinsic constriction which is largely independent of nervous control). It follows that increased blood flow in active muscles must be brought about by either an increased vasodilatation or a decreased vasoconstriction. Since vasodilatation apparently functions only in emotional situations or in the anticipation of exercise, the most important factor appears to be a decreased vasoconstriction in the active muscles (and an increase in vasodilatation) and an increased vasoconstriction in the less active tissues such as the skin and viscera. It should be mentioned that dilation of the vessels cannot be actively accomplished. Instead, when the smooth muscles in the blood vessels are relaxed, the internal pressure from the blood flow apparently brings about the dilation.

B. CHEMICAL REGULATION

Increased blood flow in muscles during exercise is also brought about by the chemical composition of the blood. As stated earlier, the smooth muscles in the blood vessels of the resting skeletal muscles (which are independent of nervous control) are in a state of vasoconstriction, and the increased blood flow through the active muscles is brought about by a decrease in this intrinsic constriction with an increase in vasodilatation. There is an abundance of information which indicates that this is due to the local action of chemical changes on the blood vessels. The following chemical agents have been suggested as responsible for this action: (1) a decrease in oxygen concentration, (2) an increase concentration of carbon dioxide and lactic acid with a decrease in pH (increase in acidity), (3) a release of intracellular potassium and histamine, (4) adenine phosphate compounds resulting from the breakdown of ATP (adenosine triphosphate), and (5) the vasodilator chemical compound called *bradykinin*. Potassium and low oxygen tension are considered to be the most important local vasodilator agents in active muscles.

Figure 5-6 illustrates the blood flow pattern for both rest and maximal exercise conditions. It is interesting to see how vasoconstriction and vasodilatation work together by restricting blood from one area and by delivering it to another part that needs it more during exercise. It is also interesting to notice how the various body parts differ in their need for blood during work. The brain, for example, maintains the same absolute amount during both rest and work, while the heart, with the increase in heart rate, increases its amount needed during work. The amount to the working skeletal muscles along with the skin for purpose of heat dissipation increases from rest to work. At the same time, the amount of blood to the other internal organs such as the kidneys, intestines, and stomach decrease with increases in work.

IV. BLOOD PRESSURE AND BLOOD FLOW RESISTANCE RESPONSES TO EXERCISE

A. MEASUREMENT OF BLOOD PRESSURE

Blood pressure may be determined either by *indirect (sphygmomanometer)* or *direct (catheter)* methods. The indirect method is the more common one used in physical education and exercise physiology. As illustrated in Figure 5-7, it involves a pressure cuff and a mercury or

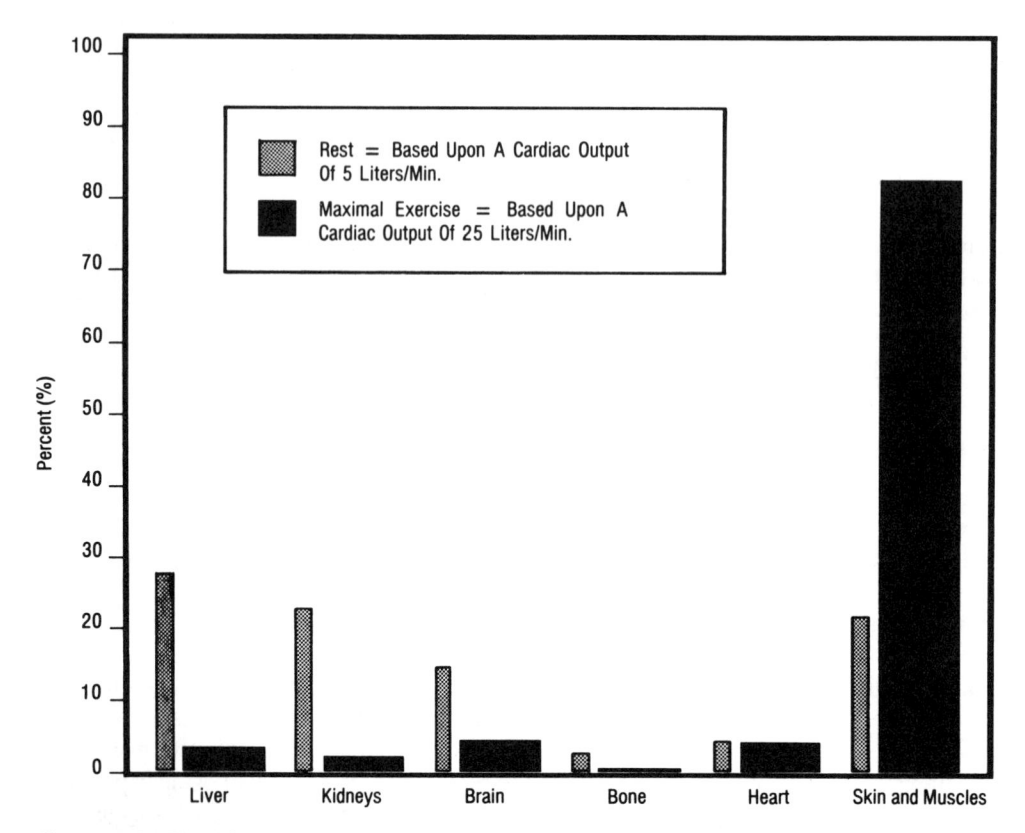

Figure 5-6 Blood flow pattern during rest and maximal exercise conditions.

Steps in Taking Blood Pressure

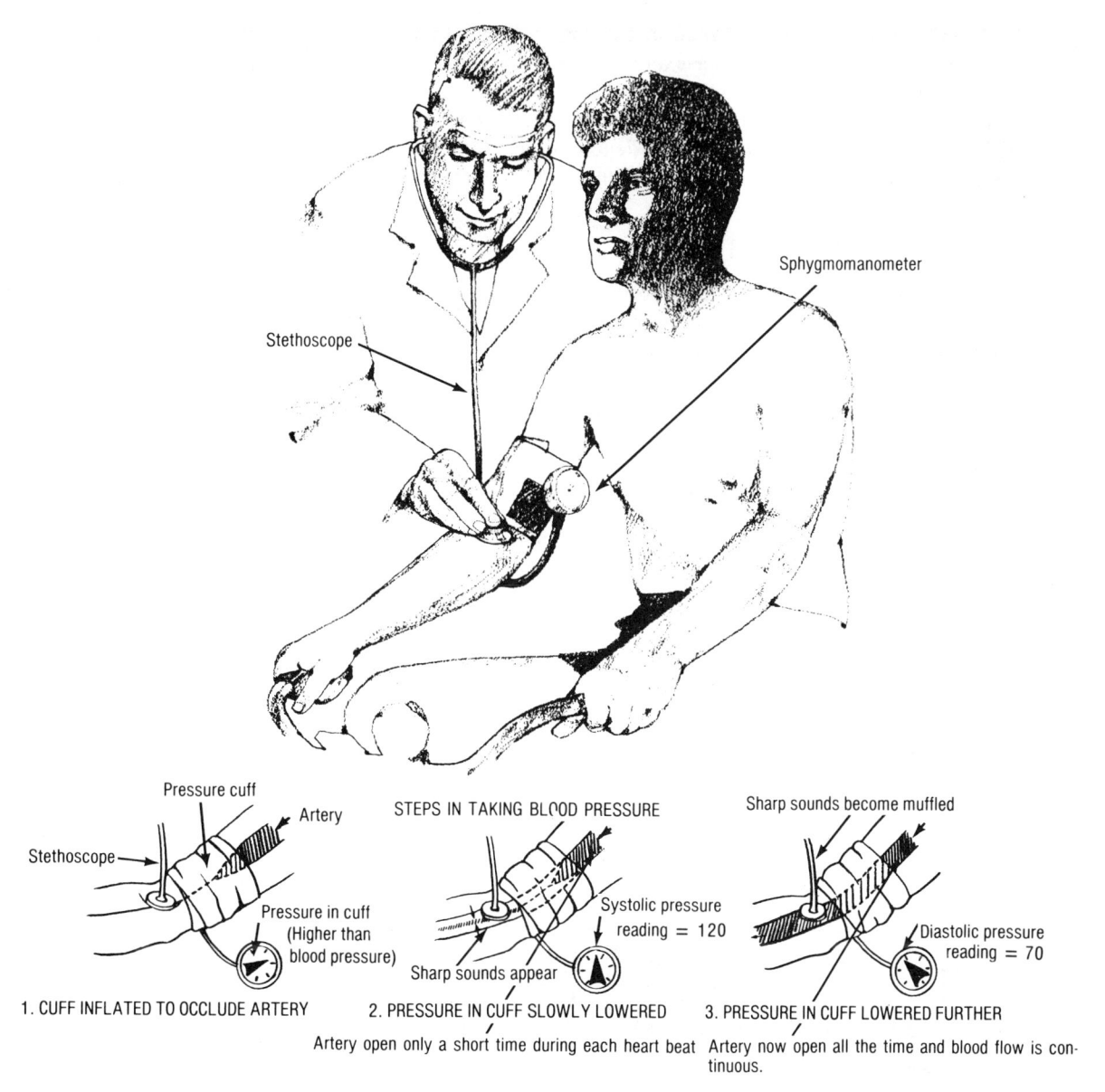

1. CUFF INFLATED TO OCCLUDE ARTERY
- Stethoscope
- Pressure cuff
- Artery
- Pressure in cuff (Higher than blood pressure)

2. PRESSURE IN CUFF SLOWLY LOWERED
- Sharp sounds appear
- Systolic pressure reading = 120
- Artery open only a short time during each heart beat

3. PRESSURE IN CUFF LOWERED FURTHER
- Sharp sounds become muffled
- Diastolic pressure reading = 70
- Artery now open all the time and blood flow is continuous.

Figure 5-7 Blood pressure determination by the indirect (sphygmomanometer) method.

aneroid manometer. The cuff is placed around the person's upper arm and should be approximately at heart level. *Systolic blood pressure* is the pressure needed to occlude the brachial artery, and it is found by listening (with a stethoscope) to the flow of blood just below the cuff. As the cuff pressure is gradually reduced, the pressure at which the sounds disappear or becomes muffled, is recorded as *diastolic blood pressure*. Mathematically, the difference between systolic and diastolic is referred to as the *pulse pressure*.

Caution should be taken when measuring exercise blood pressure by way of the indirect sphygmomanometer method since exercise comparisons between direct and indirect procedures have shown systolic pressure to be underestimated by mean values of somewhere around 8 to 15 mmHg. At the same time, recovery mean values have been reported of being overestimated by as much as 16 to 38 mmHg. Thus, if any degree of accuracy is to be obtained, the importance of practice in taking exercise blood pressure cannot be over emphasized by the physical educator and exercise physiologists.

B. EXERCISE RESPONSES

Figure 5-8 illustrates the typical, normal systemic blood pressure at rest and during maximal exercise. During exercise, blood pressure increases linearly as a result of an increase in cardiac output. These increases are brought about by both nervous and chemical influences, as was previously stated. It is clearly seen that exercise affects systolic pressure much more than diastolic or mean pressure. This is due to the fact that during exercise the resistance to blood flow is decreased, as illustrated in figure 5-9. The decreased resistance is the result of vasodilatation taking place in the arterioles or the working muscles. For example, resistance to blood flow can be determined in Figure 5-9 by use of the following formula:

$$\text{Resistance} = \frac{\text{mean arterial pressure}}{\text{cardiac output}}$$

Rest Conditions

Cardiac output = 4.5 liters/min
Mean arterial pressure = 93 mmHg
Resistance to blood flow = 20.67 mmHg/liter/min

Exercise Conditions

Cardiac output = 35 liters/min.
Mean arterial pressure = 126 mmHg
Resistance to blood flow = 3.60 mmHg/liter/min

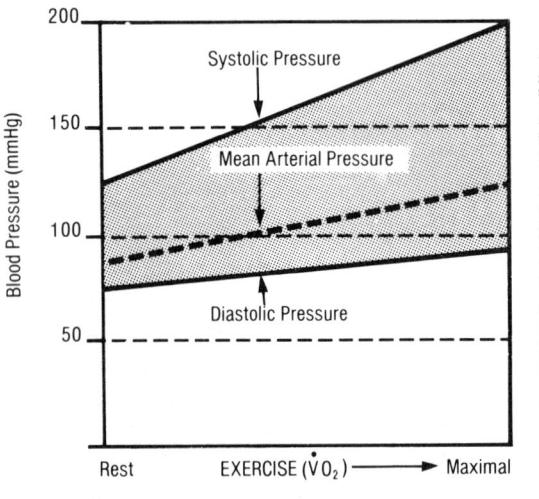

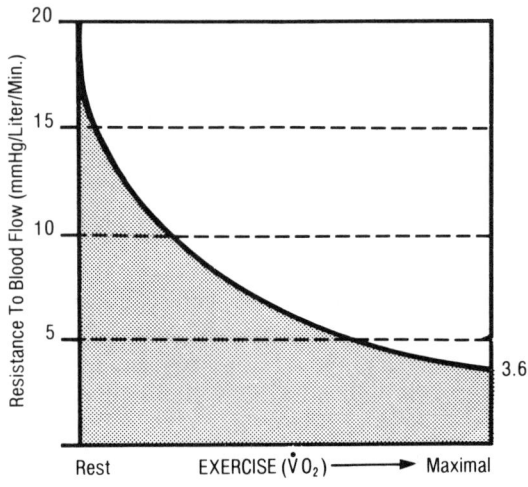

Figure 5-8 Illustration of blood pressure changes during maximal exercise.

Figure 5-9 Diagram of resistance to blood flow changes during maximal exercise.

This illustration obviously shows that more blood will be able to move from the arteries into the muscle capillaries with only slight changes in diastolic pressure. Notice in the illustration above that there is over a 5-fold decrease in resistance between rest and exercise. This is definitely an advantage during exercise. Changes in mean pressure will also be minimized since any mean arterial pressure increases (with increasing cardiac output) will be offset with the decreased resistance.

It should be pointed out that the type of exercise influences the increase in blood pressure. For example, Figure 5-10 illustrates typical changes during an isometric (static) handgrip contraction (where resistance is equal to 30 percent of the maximum voluntary force) and an exhausting progressive treadmill exercise (dynamic). Note the tremendous increase in blood pressure compared to heart rate response as well as the parallel increase in both systolic and diastolic pressures during isometric work. Some researchers have found small increases in heart rate, cardiac output, blood pressure, and muscle blood flow to a steady state when isometric contractions are less than 15 percent of the maximum force. Generally, exercises of this type can be maintained indefinitely. However, when isometric contractions are greater than 15 percent of

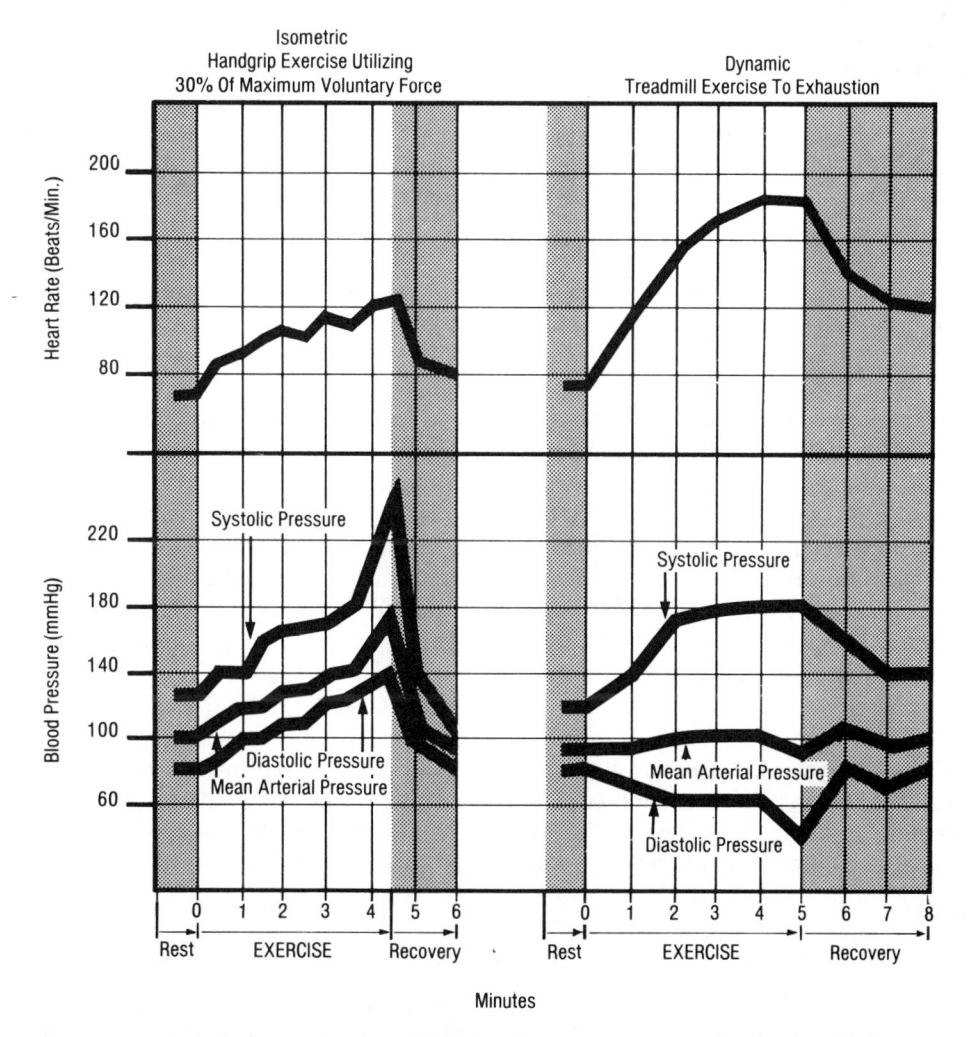

Figure 5-10 Effects of isometric and dynamic-type exercises on blood pressure.

maximum such as in Figure 5-10, all of these variables increase continuously until fatigue occurs. Figure 5-10 shows clearly that isometric exercise causes a much greater increase in blood pressure than did the dynamic exercise. Apparently, the body tolerates the increased blood flow of dynamic, rhythmic type activities such as running or jogging better than increased blood pressure. It is commonly believed among exercise physiologists that the increase in pressure from isometric type exercise is brought about, in part, by a nerve reflex originating in the exercising muscles and also by an increase in *intrathoracic* pressure (caused from making an expiratory effort against a closed glottis and thus restricting venous return to the heart). It is interesting to note that when one works dynamically with small muscles such as the arms instead of the legs, a greater than normal increase in blood pressure is also generally observed. This is especially true when one works with the arms such as in snow-shoveling or digging or in work above the waist such as in painting or doing carpenter-type work. Because of the uncommonly high blood pressure produced by isometric or dynamic arm work performed above the waist as in snow-shoveling or digging, this type of work is not recommended for older people and people with cardiovascular disease.

It should be mentioned that training also affects blood pressure. For example, prolonged work in the untrained subject leads to a progressive fall in systolic pressure which indicates nearing exhaustion. At the same time, training retards this phenomenon so that heavy work can be continued for a much longer period of time without a great deal of change in an individual's blood pressure. Training (endurance-type) also improves the blood pressure recovery process following exercise: the better trained the individual, the sooner blood pressure returns to the pre-exercise level. More about training will be said in a later chapter.

C. SELECTED FACTORS AFFECTING BLOOD PRESSURE

There are several factors that affect blood pressure besides exercise and training. Those covered in this chapter are: age, sex, emotion, and posture.

Age

The influence of age on the systolic and diastolic pressures is illustrated in Figure 5-11. It is clear from this illustration that blood pressure increases gradually throughout life. The normal systolic blood pressure for adults in western industrialized societies is around 140 mmHg, while the diastolic pressure is around 90 mmHg. The average blood pressure tends to be lower in underdeveloped countries than in western societies. On an individual basis, it should be pointed out that pressure values above 140 mmHg do not necessarily indicate an abnormal state of high blood pressure since the physiological range of normal for some individuals may occasionally reach into the range of abnormal for the total population. In fact, in older people, systolic values of 160 to 170 mmHg are accepted as normal.

Sex

Both the systolic and diastolic blood pressure values in women prior to menopause tends to be about 5 to 10 mmHg lower than that of the male. However, after menopause the female values are generally found to be slightly higher than their counterparts of similar age. A more detailed physiological comparison between men and women can be found in Chapter 11.

Emotion

It is well known that emotional states such as excitement, fear, and anxiety increase the

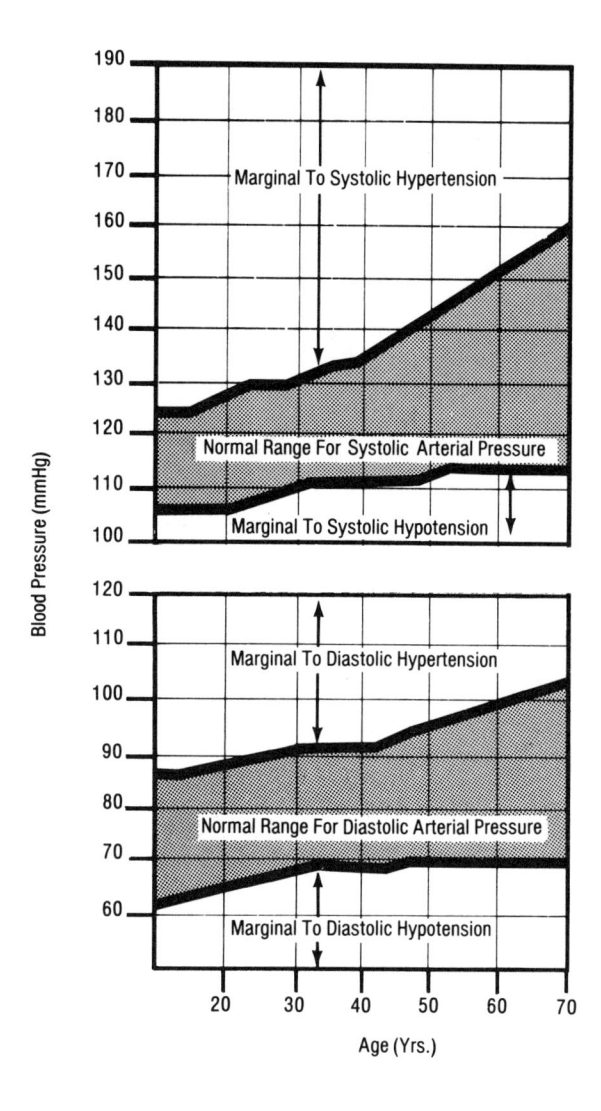

Figure 5-11 Normal resting blood pressure as a function of age.

arterial blood pressure. In fact, the slightest emotional involvement may cause falsely high results in blood pressure determinations. It is not clear as to what extent the effects of emotion are due to the liberation of adrenaline, however, it has been suggested among authorities that a flow of nerve impulses from the cerebral cortex to the medullary centers might also play an important part.

Posture

As is the case of the heart rate, the blood pressure is also affected by posture. When a reclining subject stands up, the hydrostatic pressure increase demands greater arterial pressure, and the response by the cardiovascular system generally overshoots the mark until the arterial pressure is usually 10 or 15 mmHg higher. It should be pointed out that in changing from supine to erect posture, there is a momentary fall in blood pressure (people may feel faint or dizzy) caused by the diminished venous return. However, this is normally overcome very quickly.

V. SUMMARY

(1) The blood vessels of the vascular system are classified as arteries, arterioles, capillaries, venules, and veins. The exchange of gases, water, electrolytes, etc. take place across the walls of the capillaries, while the other vessels function only as transport channels.

(2) Blood flowing through the microcirculation of a capillary bed may take one of three routes. They are:
    (a) *preferential channels* which are used to serve the metabolic needs of muscular tissue during rest:
    (b) *true capillaries* which open during exercise to serve the metabolic needs of muscular tissue; and
    (c) *arteriovenous anastomoses* which come into play to dissipate heat.

(3) Blood flows through the vessels of the circulatory system as a result of a *pressure gradient* (difference in pressure between two points).

(4) The velocity of blood flow past any given point depends upon the total cross-sectional area of the vascular system at that point. The velocity of blood flow may be calculated using the following formula:

$$\text{Velocity of blood flow} = \frac{\text{blood flow}}{\text{diameter}^2}$$

(5) The resistance to blood flow is determined by three factors:
    (a) the diameter of the blood vessel;
    (b) the length of the blood vessel; and
    (c) the viscosity (thickness) of the blood.
Resistance can be calculated from the following formula:

$$\text{Resistance} = \frac{\text{length} \times \text{viscosity}}{\text{diameter}^4}$$

(6) The resistance to blood flow can also be calculated from the following relationship provided cardiac output and mean arterial blood pressure are known:

$$\text{Resistance} = \frac{\text{mean pressure}}{\text{cardiac output}}$$

(7) Poiseuille's theoretically derived mathematical law is used to express the relationships of the various hemodynamic laws that govern the flow of blood. It is as follows:

$$\text{Volume of blood flow} = \frac{\text{pressure} \times \text{diameter}^4}{\text{length} \times \text{viscosity}}$$

(8) Regulation of blood flow is brought about by chemical activity and the sympathetic nervous system. Cholinergic fibers of the sympathetic system brings about an increase in blood flow in active tissue through vasodilatation, while sympathetic adrenergic fibers restricts blood flow in inactive areas via vasoconstriction. Once exercise is under way, the increased blood flow in the active tissues is augmented by chemical activity of the metabolites.

(9) Systolic blood pressure and mean values generally shows an increase during exercise, while diastolic pressure shows little or no increase. Isometric exercise generally causes a greater increase in blood pressure than dynamic exercise. Dynamic arm exercise generally causes a greater increase in blood pressure than dynamic leg exercise.

(10) Endurance training improves the exercise blood pressure process. In other words, training prolongs a drop (which indicates nearing exhaustion) in systolic pressure during heavy work in order that work can continue longer than it might normally would be able to. The blood pressure recovery process is also improved. That is, the better trained the person, the sooner blood pressure returns to the pre-exercise level.

(11) Besides exercise and training, several other variables such as age, sex, posture, and emotion affect blood pressure.

VI. REVIEW REFERENCES

(1) deVries, H. A. *Physiology of Exercise for Physical Education and Athletics,* 2nd edition, Wm. C. Brown Co., Dubuque, Iowa, 1974.
(2) Guyton, A. C. *Textbook of Medical Physiology,* 5th edition, W. B. Saunders Co., Philadelphia, 1976.
(3) Guyton, A. C., C. E. Jones, and T. G. Coleman, *Circulatory Physiology: Cardiac Output and Its Regulation,* 2nd edition, W. B. Saunders Co., Philadelphia, 1973.
(4) Guyton, A. C., and D. B. Young (editors). *Cardiovascular Physiology III,* University Park Press, Baltimore, 1979.
(5) Lamb, D. R. *Physiology of Exercise: Responses and Adaptations,* Macmillan Publishing Co., New York, 1978.
(6) Lind, A. R., and McNicol, G. W. "Muscular Factors Which Determines the Cardiovascular Responses to Sustained and Rhythmic Exercise," *Canadian Medical Association Journal,* 96:706-13, 1967.
(7) Mathews, D. K., and E. L. Fox. *The Physiological Basis of Physical Education and Athletics,* 2nd edition, W. B. Saunders Co., Philadelphia, 1976.
(8) Sawka, M. N., R. G. Knowlton, and J. B. Critz. "Thermal and Circulatory Responses to Repeated Bouts of Prolonged Running," *Medicine and Science in Sports,* 11:177-80, 1979.

6

NEURAL CONTROL OF SKELETAL MUSCLE ACTIVITY

KEY CONCEPTS TO BE GAINED FROM THIS CHAPTER

(1) The neuron is the structural unit of the nervous system. It initiates and directs all movements involving both voluntary and involuntary movements.

(2) The synapse, by way of its various functional characteristics, and the neuromuscular junction plays an important role in the neural control of skeletal muscular activity.

(3) The functional unit of skeletal muscular activity is the motor unit.

(4) While the cerebral cortex of the brain is the major overall center for voluntary control of muscular activity, the specific areas of the cortex involved are the sensory cortex, the motor cortex (pyramidal system), and the premotor cortex (extrapyramidal system).

(5) Skeletal muscle fibers follow the all-or-none law during muscle contraction.

(6) The cerebellum, thalamus, brain stem, basal ganglia and the reticular formation all play essential parts in the regulation of voluntary movement.

(7) The primary function of proprioceptors is to feed back information to the brain concerning the body and its parts in relation to time and space.

(8) Reflexes form the basis of all central nervous system activity.

(9) The reflex arc is the functional unit of the nervous system.

(10) Cross-education is greatest when work has been performed in overload.

(11) There is no relationship between reaction time and movement time.

The purpose of this chapter is not to give a complete anatomical and functional description of the nervous system, but instead, to describe how excitation of contraction takes place, and how the nervous system integrates all external as well as internal stimuli into smooth coordinated movements.

Neural Control of Skeletal Muscle Activity   **111**

The *central nervous system (CNS)* and the *peripheral nervous system (PNS)* acts as the controlling forces on muscle activity. The structural or fundamental unit of the nervous system is the *neuron* or *nerve cell* (Fig. 6-1). It is known that several billions of these cells are interconnected in different ways to form the central nervous system. The neuron contains a cell body which includes several processes called *dendrites,* an *axon,* and a *nucleus.* The dendrites conduct impulses toward the cell body and axons conduct them away. Each neuron has only one axon (also called a nerve fiber), but it may have many dendrites. Axons contain intracellular fluid, and they may make functional connections (synapses) with other dendrites or neurons, or they may terminate in effector organs such as muscles or glands. The axons of some neurons have a fatty material or covering called *myelin sheath* (these axons are referred to as myelinated axons). The myelin sheath is not always present (these axons are referred to as unmyelinated axons), but is characteristic of large, rapidly conducting fibers. The myelin sheath is interrupted at regular intervals by highly permeable structures called *nodes of Ranvier* (small uninsulated areas), which allow the axon to be in touch with the intercellular fluids. Because myelin is a good insulator, conduction of nerve impulses (with myelinated fibers) takes place at the nodes of Ranvier instead of continuously along the entire fiber. This ability to conduct from node to node is believed to be the major reason for the high transmission rate of myelinated fibers. Located outside the myelin

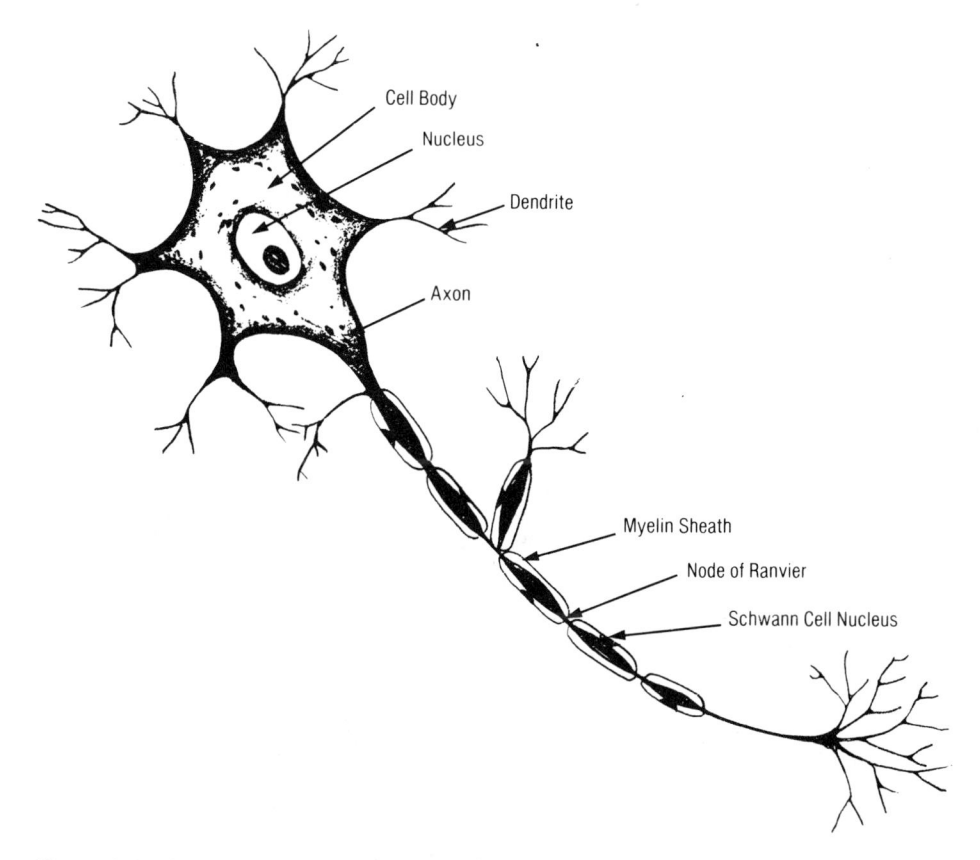

Figure 6-1 Structure of the neuron (nerve cell).

sheath is a nucleus called the *Schwann cell*. In addition to serving as insulation for the axon, Schwann cells play an important role in the regeneration of peripheral nerves that have been injured, as pointed out earlier by Clarke. This might explain, in part, why injury to the brain and spinal cord nerve tissue is more permanent than that of the peripheral nerve tissue since there are no Schwann cells in the brain and spinal cord.

Neurons are classified according to the way in which they transmit impulses. For example, neurons which receive stimuli from the environment such as odor, light, pressure, etc., and transmit them either to the brain or spinal cord via chemical-electrical signals are referred to as sensory or afferent neurons. On the other hand, neurons which transmit impulses from the central nervous system to muscles and glands causing them to contract are referred to as motor or efferent neurons.

I. EXCITATION OF CONTRACTION

Excitation is a self-propagating signal which flows rapidly from the motor end-plate through all parts of the muscle fiber and triggers the contractile mechanism, according to Loofbourrow. Excitation is a mechanism involving both physical and chemical changes as well as movements of electrically charged ions. During the resting state, positively and negatively charged ions (a mineral with an electrical charge) are located both inside and outside the membrane. However, as Figure 6-2 illustrates, the relative concentration of the ions is different on the inside and outside of the cell membrane. Figure 6-2 shows that the extracellular fluid or the outside of the cell is positively charged as compared with the intracellular fluid or inside of the cell. It is generally known that during rest, the membrane is polarized (the exterior being positively charged with respect to the interior) with a net resting potential of -85 millivolts. This indicates that the membrane on the inside is 85 millivolts more negative than the outside. Sodium (Na^+) and potassium (K^+) ions are primarily responsible for this situation. In fact, a *sodium pump* has been postulated as the mechanism responsible for actively transporting sodium ions from the cell in order that the resting membrane potential may be maintained. At the same time, a *potassium pump* has been postulated as the mechanism responsible for maintaining a high ratio of potassium

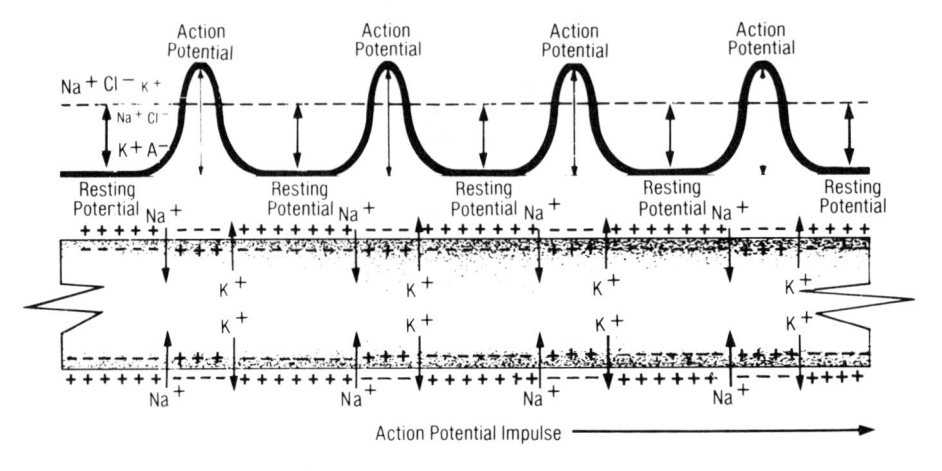

Figure 6-2 Schematic illustration of the resting and action membrane potential.

ions on the inside during rest. It should be pointed out that although Figure 6-2 shows there are large amounts of anions (negatively charged ions) found on the outside (chloride ions) as well as the inside (phosphate ions, sulfate ions, and protein ions), these anions are not freely diffusible through the cell membrane, and therefore, they all play a passive role in excitation of contraction.

When a fiber is stimulated, the membrane becomes highly permeable allowing sodium ions to flow inward thus reversing the membrane potential (Fig. 6-2). That is, the inside of the cell membrane becomes positive in relations to the outside. This process is referred to as *depolarization*. Hence, depolarization begins by passive inward diffusion of sodium ions and is then aided by active transfer of a *sodium carrier system,* as indicated by earlier researchers. It should be noted that the sodium pump is a mechanism for active *outward transport* and the sodium carrier is a system for active *inward transport*. As soon as the sodium ions begin flowing inward and disturbing the dynamic equilibrium, potassium outflow begins as passive diffusion and is then aided by active transfer of a *potassium carrier system*. Note also that the potassium pump is a mechanism for active *inward transport* of potassium ions, whereas the potassium carrier is a system for active *outward transport*. Depolarization is generally recorded as an action potential (electrical potential in millivolts) impulse. The action potential impulse moves the entire distance of the membrane in a self-propagating, wavelike pattern (Fig. 6-2).

Repolarization occurs as soon as the action potential returns to the resting potential. This is accomplished by passive diffusion and active transfer of potassium ions out of the cell. This is followed by a renewal of activity of the sodium and potassium pumps.

II. THE SYNAPSE

As stated earlier, the neuron is the structural unit of the nervous system. Between neurons there is an anatomical gap or junction which is called the *synapse,* a term meaning joining or a binding together. Figure 6-3 illustrates a typical neuron in synaptic relationship to another neuron.

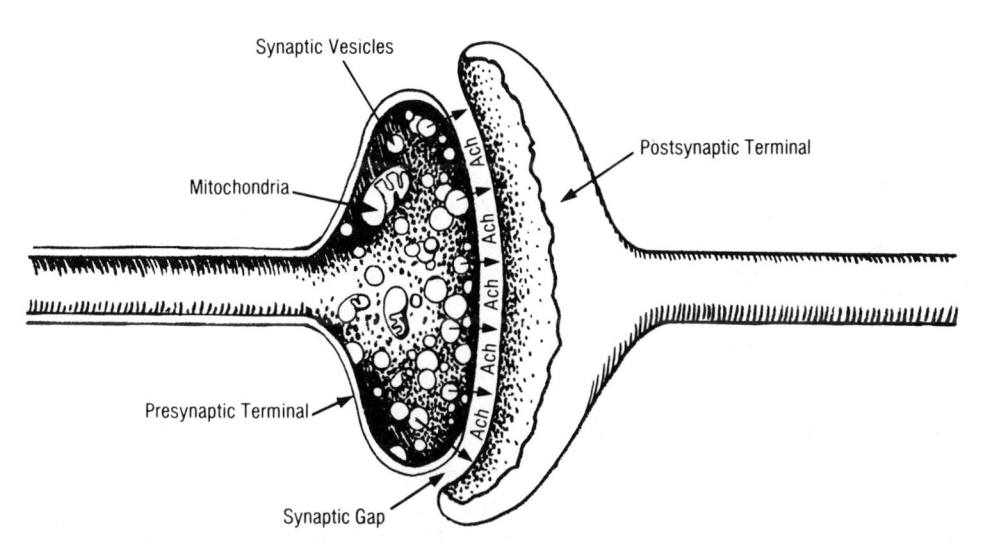

Figure 6-3 Structure of the synapse.

The electrical impulse that travels along the axon causes, in an unknown manner, the release of an *excitatory transmitter* substance called acetylcholine (ACh) from the synaptic vesicles at the end of the neuron. When a sufficient amount of the transmitter substance has diffused across the gap, receptor cells in the postsynaptic terminals are stimulated and the impulse is sent on setting up a muscle action potential, which in turn, leads to muscle contraction. Located on the postsynaptic membrane is the enzyme cholinesterase which is responsible for the inactivation of acetylcholine. This allows the membrane potential to be repolarized. More will be said about ACh and cholinesterase in a later section of this chapter.

The synapse has several important functional characteristics. They are:

A. TRANSMIT IMPULSES IN ONE DIRECTION ONLY

Impulses are transmitted through synapses only from the presynaptic terminals because the receptor cells are found only on the postsynaptic neuron. Obviously, for the impulses to be reversible, there would have to be receptor cells on both sides of the synaptic gap.

B. DELAY TRANSMISSION OF THE IMPULSE

In transmission of an impulse from a presynaptic terminal to a postsynaptic terminal, a certain amount of time is consumed for the chemical transmitter ACh to diffuse across the synaptic gap and thus stimulate the receptor cells. This results in a slight delay of the transmission of the impulse.

C. FATIGUE VERY EASILY

Although the presynaptic terminals are capable of being stimulated at high frequencies for long periods of time, eventually the number of discharges by the postsynaptic neuron will become progressively less and less due to fatigue. The mechanism of fatigue has been presumed to be simply exhaustion of the chemical transmitter ACh in the vesicles which is released under high-frequency stimulation faster than it can be resynthesized.

D. SUSCEPTIBLE TO DRUGS

Synapses are very vulnerable to the action of many drugs. For example, caffeine, theophylline, and theobromine, which are found in coffee, tea, and coccoa, respectively, all reduces the threshold for excitation of the neurons and thus increases neuronal responsiveness. However, strychnine does not reduce the threshold for excitation of the neurons, but instead, inhibits the action of the inhibitory transmitter on the neuron. This action increases the synapse responsiveness, according to researchers working in this area. On the other hand, hypnotics and anesthetics is believed to increase the threshold for excitation of the neurons and thereby decreases neuronal activity. Thus, some drugs do not allow the synapse to stop working when it is fatigued while other drugs inhibit the work of the synapse.

E. A RELATIVELY HIGH THRESHOLD

A high threshold generally means that it often takes more than one stimuli to excite and stimulate the chemical transmitter ACh sufficiently to cross over the synaptic gap and depolarize the postsynaptic terminal. The high threshold level of the synapse serves an important function in muscular activity. For example, if every stimuli was able to cross the synaptic gap, the body would be continually subjected to contractions of many muscle fibers. Thus, the high threshold of the synapse effectively functions to eliminate many stray impulses from traveling over the synaptic gap. However, when the stimulus is strong enough (approximately 11 millivolts above the resting potential of —85 millivolts) to comply with the appropriate threshold level, the impulse will cross over the gap and eventually cause muscle contraction. Note that this electrical increase in the resting potential of the neuron is referred to as an *excitatory postsynaptic potential (EPSP)*.

It is interesting to note that it is also possible for two or more weak stimuli's (below 11 millivolts) working together to be strong enough to depolarize the postsynaptic terminal, and thus bring about propagation of the nerve impulse. This adding together of stimuli is called *summation*. If several different presynaptic terminals are excited at the same time, this type of summation is termed *spatial summation*.

Note that if a single, weak stimulus does not excite the postsynaptic terminal, but it is strong enough to actually lower the membrane potential, and a second impulse arrives shortly afterwards (approximately 15 milliseconds), the postsynaptic terminal may, in some cases, become excited and activated. Because the impulses are separated by time, this type of summation is called *temporal summation*. Generally, there are many presynaptic terminals which are incapable of activating a postsynaptic terminal by themselves. Apparently, help is provided in terms of another presynaptic terminal which also does not activate the postsynaptic terminal but does lower the membrane potential, of which the first presynaptic terminal takes advantage. This assistance, according to authorities, is referred to as *facilitation*.

At this point, it should also be recognized that at the synaptic junction, an inhibitory transmitter substance (gamma-aminobutyric acid is one known inhibitory transmitter substance) may also be released from the synaptic vesicles of a neuron whose function is to actually raise the permeability of the postsynaptic membrane to potassium and chloride ions (not to sodium ions, however). This generates what is referred to as an *inhibitory postsynaptic potential (IPSP)* which results in the postsynaptic membrane becoming hyperpolarized rather than hypopolarized, as was pointed out previously by Edington and Edgerton. In order for IPSP to take place effectively in the nervous system, short internunical neurons are employed. These interneurons function more or less as the middleman between stimuli coming in and stimuli going out. When the short interneurons are employed, they permit us to overcome unwanted impulses, and at the same time, choose the ones that are the most important for us at that particular time. It is not hard to realize the confusion that would result if we were not able to screen out all the unwanted stimuli.

III. MOTOR UNITS

In the body, skeletal muscles normally contract in response to nerve impulses arriving over the motor nerve fibers. The motor nerve fibers terminate on muscle fibers in a framework known as *neuromuscular, myoneural junction,* or *motor end-plate* (Fig. 6-4). As the diagram in Figure 6-4 shows, a nerve fiber divides into several branches as it approaches a muscle and each motor end-plate aids many muscle fibers. A nerve fiber and its affiliated muscle fibers is referred to as a motor unit. Some motor nerves may serve hundreds of muscle fibers in muscles such as the leg muscles which do not demand a high degree of control and accuracy. On the other hand, muscles that are considered as fine control and delicate such as those controlling the eye may have as few as 5 to 15 fibers in each unit. It is interesting to note that the number of muscle fibers served by a single motor nerve is not necessarily determined by the overall size of the muscle. Instead, it is determined by the accuracy and delicacy of the movement.

A great deal of conversation has gone on in the past concerning the so-called *"all-or-none"* law as it relates to muscular contraction. It should be emphasized that this law of physiology is

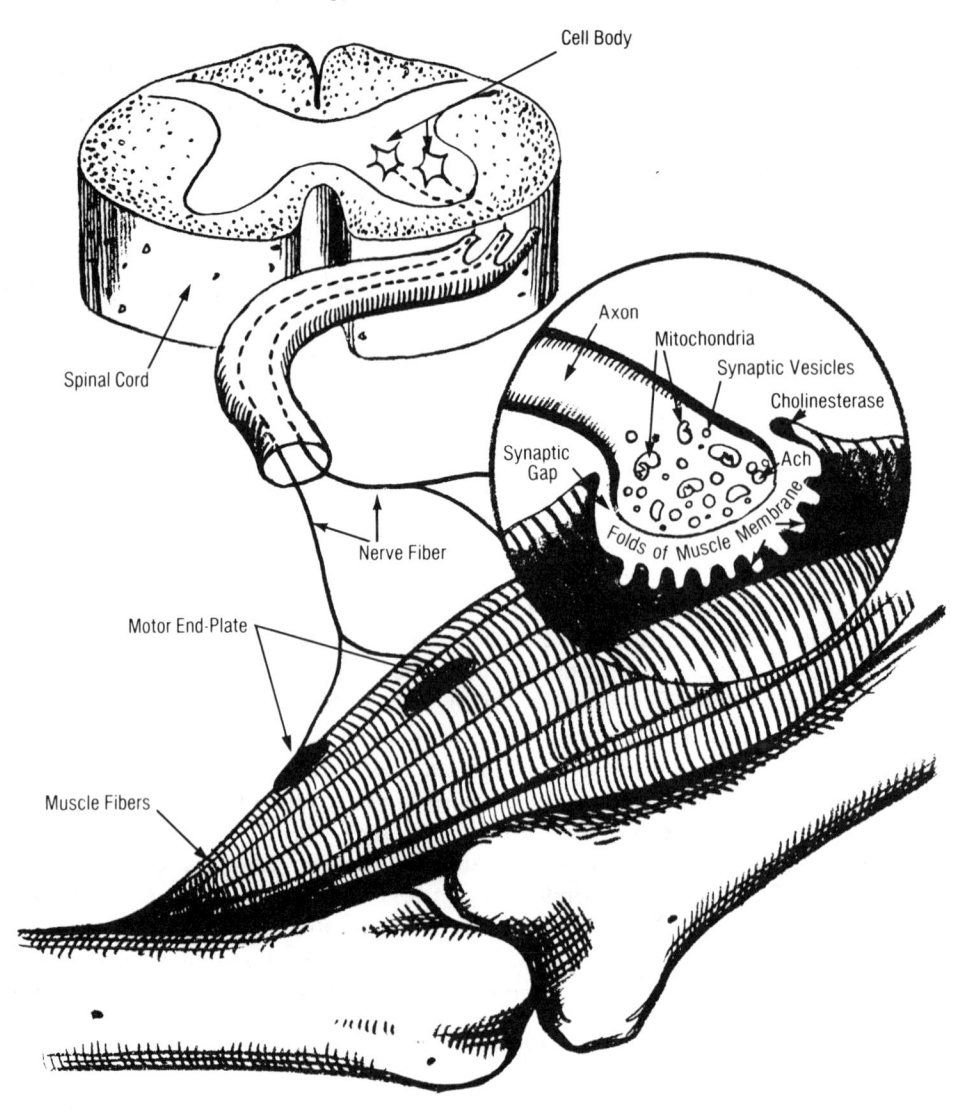

Figure 6-4 Structure of the neuromuscular (myoneural) junction.

applied to the individual muscle fibers of a given motor unit and not to a whole muscle. That is, a stimulus to a muscle fiber of a given motor unit causes an action potential to travel over the entire fiber or fails to stimulate it at all. A minimal stimulus will have the same effect as a strong stimulus on an individual muscle fiber. Thus, either all of the muscle fibers of a given motor unit contracts and relaxes or none of them contracts and relaxes. In other words, it is not possible for one or two of the muscle fibers of a given motor unit to relax and rest while the others contract. As was pointed out earlier, the all-or-none law does not apply to the whole muscle. Therefore, it is possible for a muscle such as the biceps to produce graded muscle contractions, ranging from a near non-noticeable contraction to a very strong highly-noticeable contraction. This, of course, depends upon how many motor units were actually called into action. All motor units do not come into play during submaximal work (such as recreational jogging), whereas during maximal contraction (such as in overload weight-lifting or all-out sprinting), most, if not all, do come into play. The more motor units brought into play and the quicker they are brought into play (by shorter rest periods), obviously, the greater the strength of contraction will be.

It is interesting to note that active and inactive motor units serving a particular muscle such as the biceps may exchange roles quite often in order that fatigue of any one motor unit may be prolonged or avoided. This is especially true in submaximal-type work such as in long-distance marathon running which takes several hours or in an 8-hour work day for a laborer. Note that this exchange would not necessarily help in maximal contraction such as in all-out sprinting where the firing of a given number of motor units is so fast that the rest period between contractions is nearly eliminated, if not completely, and thus, fatigue will set in quickly. This exchange in roles for motor units (called *asynchronous contraction*) is the key for the smooth, nonjerky skeletal muscle contractions that are typical of most everyday human movements.

IV. THE CHEMICAL TRANSMITTER

It is known that the arrival of nerve impulses at the motor end-plate triggers the release of a chemical transmitter called *acetylcholine (ACh)* from the synaptic vesicles on the presynaptic terminal. ACh then diffuses across the neuromuscular junction to the postsynaptic side. The arrival of ACh to the postsynaptic side changes the permeability of the muscle cell membrane (sarcolemma). This allows sodium ions to flow inward and potassium ions to flow outward, which in turn, brings about depolarization of the postsynaptic terminal. The wave of depolarization (action or electrical potentials) then spreads along the muscle in each direction from the motor end-plate, thus triggering the release of calcium from the sarcoplasmic reticulum, which in turn, puts the muscle contractile mechanism in motion. Upon arrival of ACh to the postsynaptic side, it is destroyed or broken down almost immediately (within approximately 2 milliseconds) into *acetate* and *choline* by an enzyme called *cholinesterase,* which is found on the postsynaptic membrane. In other words, cholinesterase, by breaking down ACh to acetate and choline, inactivates the depolarizing effect of ACh. Consequently, the muscle cell membrane is then repolarized and can respond shortly to another impulse.

V. VOLUNTARY CONTROL OF MUSCULAR ACTIVITY

It appears that the *cerebral cortex* is the center for voluntary skilled movements. The outside portion of the *cerebrum* is known as the cerebral cortex. Figure 6-5 illustrates the regions of the cerebral cortex that are primarily concerned with the motor movements. They are the *sensory cortex,* the *motor cortex,* and *premotor cortex.* The sensory cortex is the region that receives most of the afferent input from the various sensory receptors. This area is not only concerned with intergrating the incoming information, but it is also directly involved in initiating the appropriate actions. The motor cortex (*pyramidal system*), on the other hand, is concerned with small discrete movements by the contraction of specific and individual muscles such as the thumb and forefinger, toes, lips, etc. At the same time, the premotor cortex (*extrapyramidal system*), coordinates and controls complicated movement patterns involving groups of muscles.

The cerebellum's primary motor performance function is with the regulation, coordination, adjustment, and smoothing out of muscular movements. It does not initiate movement. It is generally known that it receives afferent impulses from the motor cortex, proprioceptors, cutaneous tactile receptors, auditory and visual receptors, and visceral receptors while sending out efferent impulses to the cerebral cortex and the lower motor neurons in the brain stem and spinal cord. Thus, some authorities believe that it performs its coordinating functions by continuously comparing the actual position of the body with the intended position indicated by impulses from the cerebral cortex. It has also been suggested in some circles that the cerebellum can perhaps predict from the present position of the muscles and joints what will actual take place as the movement is in progress, and hence give out signals which will prevent errors in the actual movement.

The *thalamus* makes up part of the *gray matter* called *nuclei*. The thalamus has been described by some researchers as the gateway or entrance to the cerebral cortex. Its major function is as a relay station for both sensory and motor signals.

The *brain stem* is an extension of the spinal cord. All incoming signals to the brain as well as outgoing signals travel through it. A primary function of the stem is the regulation of respiratory, cardiovascular, and gastrointestinal functions.

Figure 6-6 is a cross-section of the *cerebrum* showing the various motor and sensory sequences. The inside of the cerebrum is made up primarily of *white matter* which connects the cerebrum to the spinal cord. *Gray matter* is also found in smaller proportions. The white matter is composed of nerve fibers and these fibers form two types of nerve bundle tracts according to their

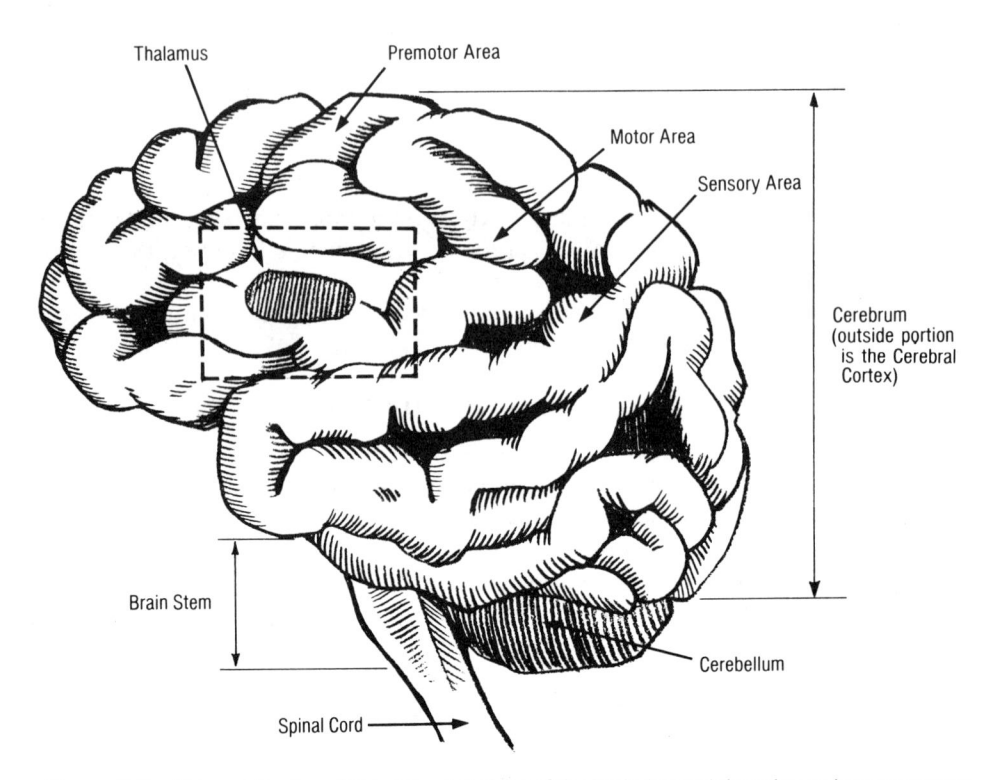

Figure 6-5 Schematic view of the various regions of the brain (cortex) that play an important part in the voluntary control of muscular activity.

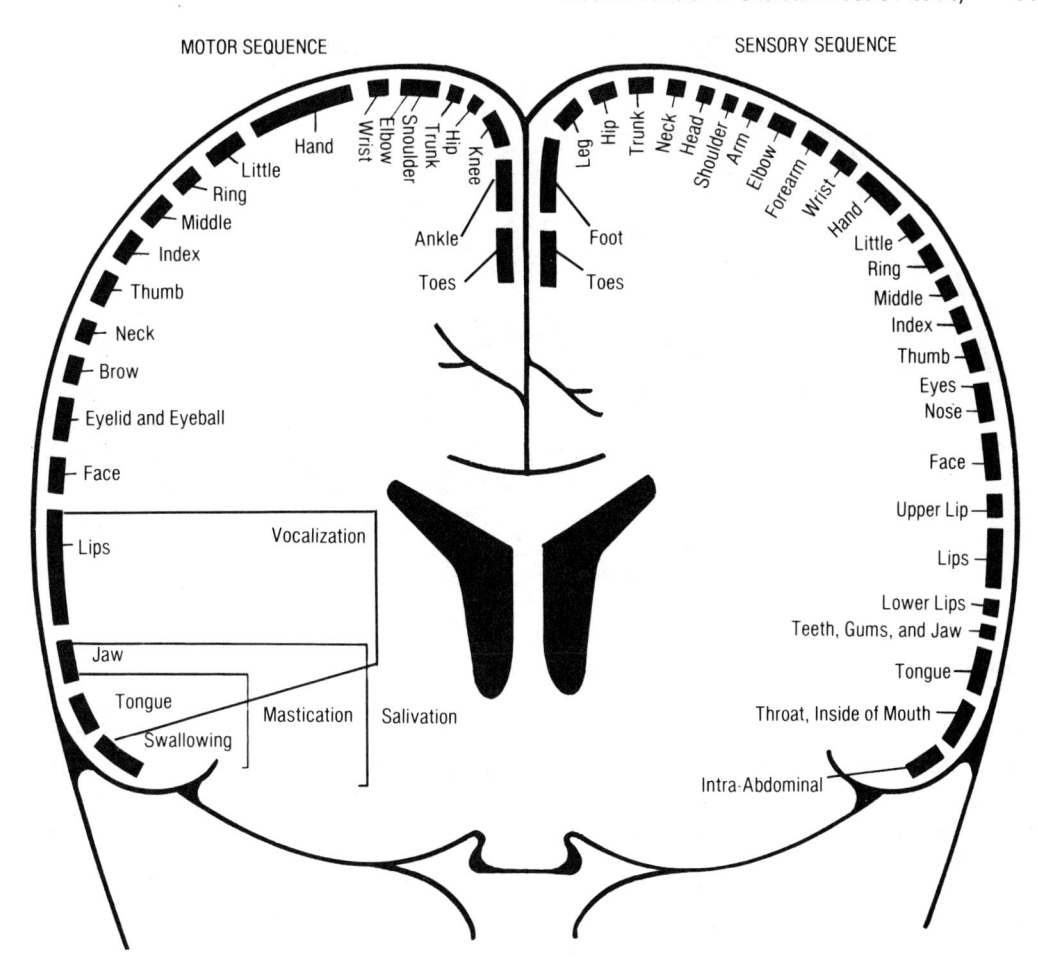

Neural Control of Skeletal Muscle Activity   119

Figure 6-6 Schematic illustration of the cross-section of the cerebrum.

functions. For example, the fibers that make up the afferent bundles are known as *ascending tracts* which carry afferent (sensory) signals to the sensory cortex. On the other hand, the fibers that make up the efferent bundles are referred to as *descending tracts* which transmit efferent (motor) signals from the various centers in the brain to the motor nerves. It is believed that the cerebrum and cerebellum work together very closely on all forms of coordinated motor acts.

Several other parts of the central nervous system are important in the coordination of muscular movement. Particularly important are the *basal ganglia* and the *reticular formation*. Briefly, the basal ganglia is found in close proximity to the thalamus. Figure 6-7 illustrates the three masses of nervous tissue that form the main part of the basal ganglia. They are the *caudate nucleus,* the *putamen,* and the *globus pallidus.* They are connected by afferent and efferent neurons to the cerebral cortex, to each other, to the reticular formation, to the substantia nigra, and to the thalamus. The basal ganglia's role in coordinating and controlling muscular movement is not well understood, however, observations of human disorders have shown that the basal ganglia are of

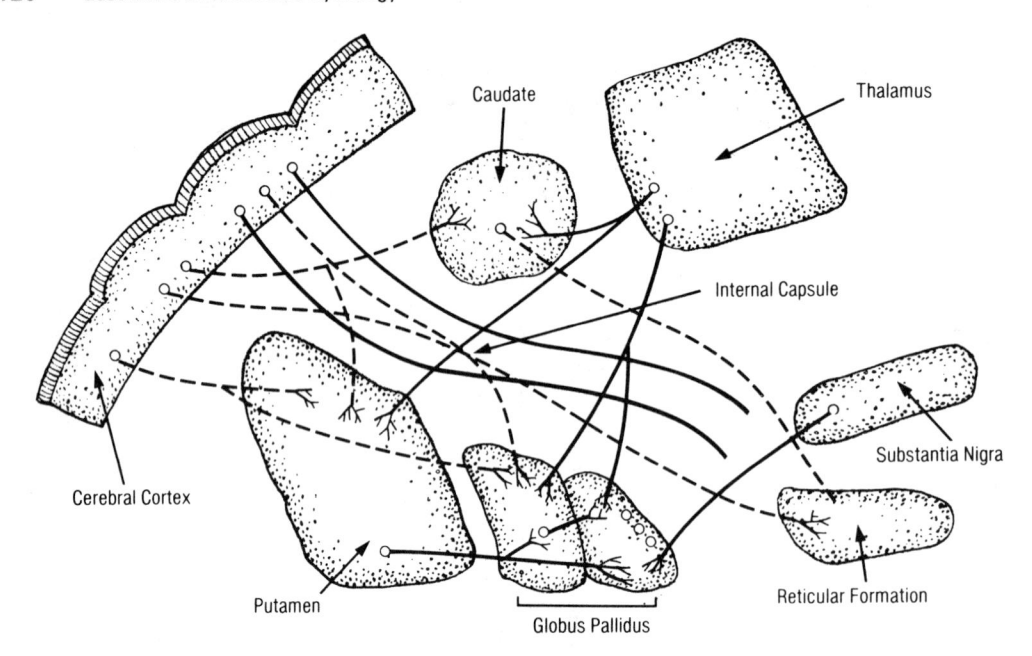

Figure 6-7 Schematic diagram of the basal ganglia.

great importance in the inhibitory functions of the extrapyramidal system. This phenomenon is tremendously important in controlling and coordinating motor actvity initiated by the motor cortex. Without this phenomenon existing with any degree of efficiency, an individual would experience unwanted muscular contractions which would certainly interfere with smooth coordinated muscular movements.

The *substantia nigra,* as illustrated in Figure 6-7, has been suggested as the major brain stem control for regulation of the gamma efferent nerve fibers. For example, authorities have found that destruction of this area causes almost complete loss of control of the gamma activating system of the muscle spindles. Furthermore, it has been suggested that when voluntary muscular functions are to be performed, activation of the substantia nigra by way of the basal ganglia, provides muscular tone and helps position various parts of the body so that discrete motor functions of the hands or feet can be carried out.

The *reticular formation,* as illustrated in Figure 6-7, is a mass of gray matter that stretches from the brain stem to the thalamus. The reticular formation sends to, and receives impulses from the cerebellum, spinal cord, the basal ganglia, thalamus and cerebral cortex. It regulates movement by exerting inhibitory effects on the antigravity (extensor) muscles as well as facilitatory effects on the lower flexor motor neurons in the spinal cord.

VI. INVOLUNTARY CONTROL OF MUSCULAR ACTIVITY

A. PROPRIOCEPTORS

The brain is fed-back the degree of contraction or relaxation of the skeletal muscles by impulses from sensory receptors within the muscles, tendons, and joints as well as from receptors located in the inner ear. These sensory receptors are called *proprioceptors,* and they permit us to perform smooth, coordinated movements such as diving or performing on a high beam without consciously thinking of the movement. They also play an important part in maintaining normal body posture. There are two types of proprioceptive feed-back functions for which we are concerned with in this chapter. They are *kinesthesis* or *kinesthetic muscle sense* whose sensory receptors are found within the muscle, tendons, and joints and the *vestibular apparatus* whose receptors are located in the inner ear.

Kinesthetic Functions

The muscle spindle, Golgi tendon organ, and pacinian corpuscle are the three types of sensory receptors most responsible for muscle, tendon, and joint sensation.

Muscle Spindles. The physiological structure of the muscle spindle is represented in Figure 6-8. The spindle receptor has a somewhat complex structure. Each spindle contains a connective-tissue sheath consisting of several *intrafusal* muscle fibers. As may be expected, stretch applied to the *extrafusal* fibers will also result in stretching the intrafusal fibers. Approximately half way down between the ends of the intrafusal fibers is the nuclear bag region. This is a heavily nucleated region that has lost all striations and cannot contract. Thus, when the spindle is stretched, the nuclear bag region also becomes stretched.

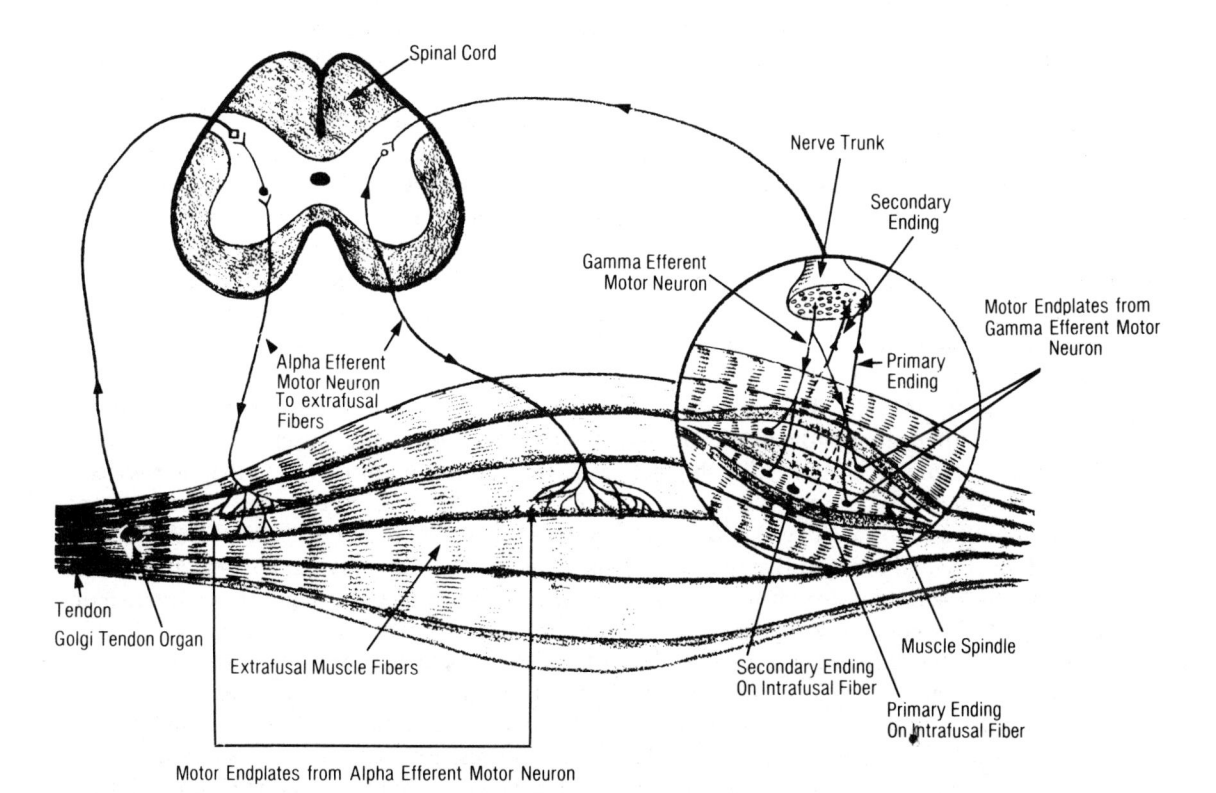

Figure 6-8 Structure of the muscle spindle and golgi tendon organ.

The spindle is supplied with two types of sensory end-organs: (1) the *primary ending* which is found wrapped around the central region of the spindle, and it evokes afferent impulses in its large, type Ia nerve (fast-conducting) fibers, and (2) the *secondary ending* which is located on each side of the primary ending receptor and it discharges afferent impulses in its small, type II nerve (slow-conducting) fibers. It is believed that the secondary ending receptor responds to stretch of the muscle spindle in the same manner as the primary ending receptor except that a far greater degree of stretch is needed to excite these receptors. This afferent impulse from the spindle is followed by a motor response such as contraction of the muscle that was stretched. This response is called the *stretch* (or *myotatic*) *reflex*. That is, the spindle actually facilitates the contraction of the muscle surrounding it.

The intrafusal muscle fibers of the spindle are innervated by small *gamma efferent* motor fibers, whereas the extrafusal fibers are innervated by the large *alpha efferent* motor fibers. The intrafusal fibers cannot contract in their center region where the primary and secondary ending receptors attach. On the other hand, their two end portions may contract. In fact, contraction of these end portions causes the central portion of the spindle to be stretched and thus excite the primary endings as well as perhaps the secondary ending.

Golgi Tendon Organs. The Golgi tendon organ is illustrated in Figure 6-8. It is found between the muscle tendon fibers and is stimulated by placing high tension on the tendons. Because the Golgi organ is located in series with the skeletal muscle fibers, it may respond to both passive stretching or active contraction of the muscle. On the other hand, the muscle spindle responds only when stretched (phasic and static). That is, because the spindle lies parallel with the extrafusal fibers, it stops firing and is thus unloaded as soon as the extrafusal fibers shorten in contraction. In addition, as stated earlier, the spindle may also facilitate contraction of the muscle surrounding it (stretch reflex), whereas the tendon organ appears to be a protective device for both the muscle and tendon from damage caused by excessive tension. Hence, the Golgi organ functions primarily to alert the central nervous system via a large type A fiber of overload on the muscle. This, in effect, causes an automatic reaction or tendon reflex to inhibit contraction of the muscle being stretched. This tendon reflex which prevents overstressing of the tissues is commonly referred to as the inverse myotatic reflex. Thus, the major difference in function between the spindle and the tendon organ is that the spindle detects changes in muscle length, whereas the Golgi organ detects change in muscle load.

Pacinian Corpuscle. The pacinian corpuscle is a large encapsulated end-organ found extensively in the region of the joints and in the sheaths of tendons and muscles. They are widely distributed and are also found in such places as in the periosteum of bones, in the interosseous membrane which connects the tibia and fibula in the lower leg, in joint capsules where synovial fluid is found, and in sensitive skin areas such as the finger tips. Because of their location, they respond quickly and are sensitive to deep pressure which allows an individual to detect passively where his body segments are without visual information. As illustrated in Figure 6-9, the pacinian corpuscles have a concentrically laminated capsule (appears to be the shape of an onion). Located in the center of the corpuscle is a non-myelinated nerve fiber whose axon, as it leaves the capsule, becomes myelinated with a node of Ranvier. When sustained pressure is exerted on the capsule, a single sensory stimulus is established and a generator potential (a local nonpropagated depolarizating potential) is developed. If the tension or pressure continues to be exerted and the electrical potential reaches a magnitude of approximately 10 millivolts, an action potential is then generated in the nerve. This means that the membrane of the axon has become highly permeable for sodium ions, thus allowing the spread of depolarization to take place in the terminals of the

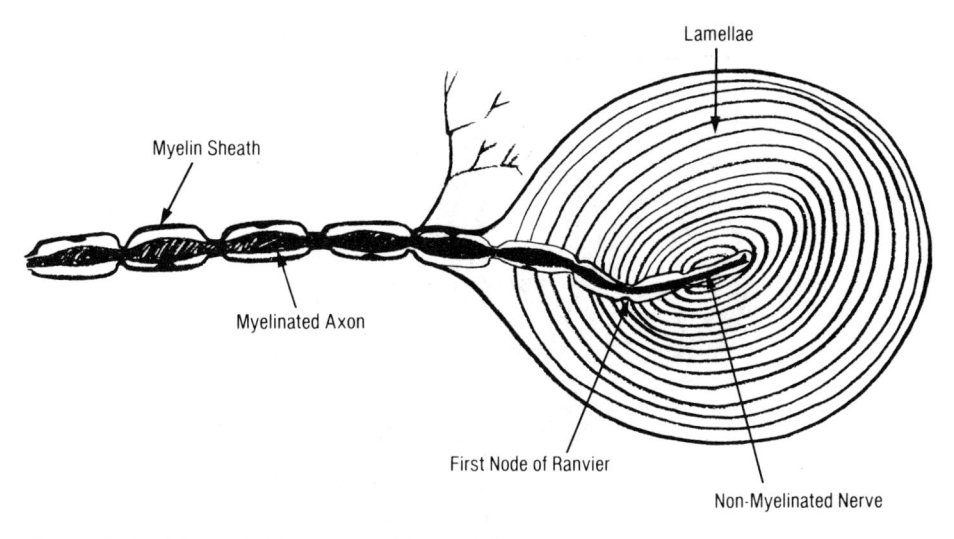

Neural Control of Skeletal Muscle Activity 123

Figure 6-9 Schematic illustration of the pacinian corpuscle.

neuron. The spreading currents set forth by the generator potential reaches the first node of Ranvier, as shown in Figure 6-9, and there it shifts the resting potential toward a self-propagating, wavelike action potential as was discussed earlier in this chapter. In essence, the function of the pacinian corpuscle appears to be that of keeping the central nervous system aware of the change in pressure rather than the amount of pressure.

Vestibular Function

Besides the three *muscle sense* receptors (muscle spindle, Golgi tendon organ, and pacinian corpuscle) already mentioned, the *vestibular apparatus* is also considered an important proprioceptive feed-back mechanism in the coordination of movement and body position. The vestibular sense receptors are located in the nonauditory labyrinths of the inner ear. The term layrinth refers to the intercommunication canals and cavities that make up the inner ear. It is called the *bony labyrinth system* because it is located within the temporal bone. Figure 6-10 illustrates the various parts that make up this system. They are the *cochlea cavity,* the *utricle, saccule,* and *semicircular canals.* The cochlea is concerned with audition, whereas the utricle, saccule, and semicircular canals are essential for equilibration. Figure 6-10 also illustrates that there are 3 semicircular canals (*superior, lateral,* and *posterior*), and they lie approximately at right angles to each other. Located at one end of the canals is a swelling known as the ampulla. Receptors sensitive to change in velocity are found in the *ampulla*. Sense organs are also found in the utricle and saccule structures.

The majority of the neurons which innervate the equilibratory receptors travel directly to the medulla while others go directly to the cerebellum. On the other hand, many secondary (collateral) fibers pass directly into the reticular activating system of the brain stem. This system sends impulses upward into the cerebral cortex and downward into the spinal cord, thereby completing the circuit for reflex movement in response to positional body change. Finally, a few fibers travel via the thalamus to the sensory cortex to get one aware of body position and changes in velocity.

124 Essentials of Exercise Physiology

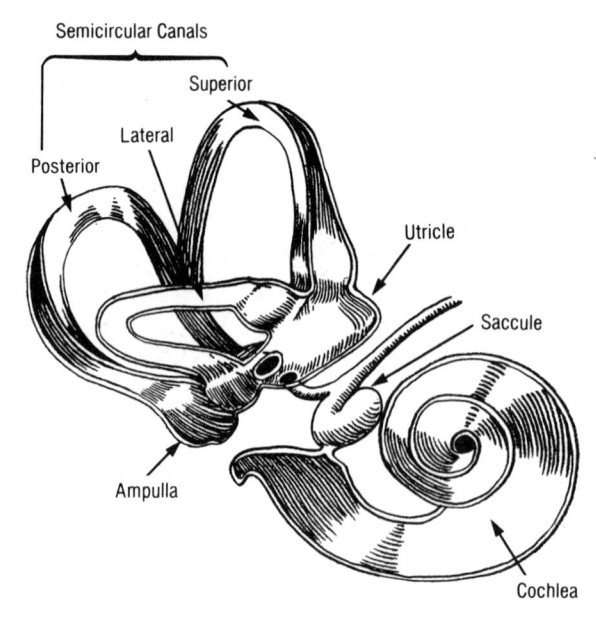

Figure 6-10 Structure of the bony labyrinth system.

The labyrinth system appears to play a dual role in coordination of movement; that is, to initiate appropriate reactions to movement, and to assist in maintaining the upright position. The semicircular canals are primarily concerned with responding to rotational acceleration and deceleration, while the utricle is mainly concerned with positional changes involving linear acceleration and deceleration. In man, the function of the saccule remains unclear, whereas in animals, authorities have fund that the saccule does respond to vibratory stimuli but not to positional changes.

B. RENSHAW CELLS

In addition to the aforementioned feed-back mechanisms for coordinating and controlling muscular activity, there is one other system that should be mentioned. This involves an internunical neuron in the spinal cord called a *Renshaw cell* which has the capability of synapsing with and inhibiting other motorneurons from coming into play (Fig. 6-11). For example, when the alpha efferent neuron sends out an electrical impulse, a recurrent axon collateral (which originates from the axons of the alpha motor neuron) is also innervated, which in turn, synapses directly with a Renshaw cell in the cord. The axons of the Renshaw cell circles back and synapses directly with the original alpha motor neuron as well as other motor neurons that go to synergistic muscles at the same segmental level, according to Clarke. The function of the Renshaw cell is to prevent other muscle fibers from coming into play and interferring with reflex and voluntary movement. This is apparently accomplished by the Renshaw cell being able to impart an inhibitory effect at the spinal cord level. Without this feed-back mechanism, fine coordinated movements would be difficult, if not nearly impossible.

C. REFLEXES

It is well known that *reflexes* form the basis of all central nervous system activity. Although reflexes take place at all levels of the brain and spinal cord, the majority of skeletal muscle reflexes

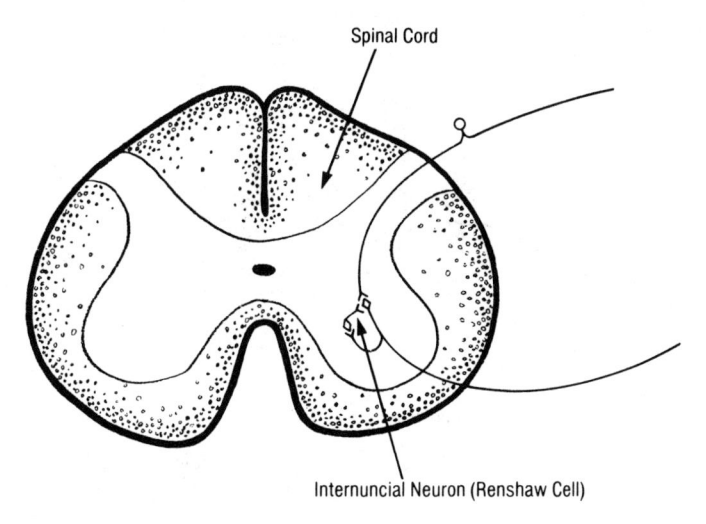

Neural Control of Skeletal Muscle Activity 125

Figure 6-11 Schematic view of the renshaw cell.

do not generally require the action of the higher brain cells. In some cases such as the classical knee jerk, we are made aware of reflex acts while others may actually occur without knowledge. For example, functions such as movements of respiration and digestion are also controlled through reflexes.

As stated earlier, the neuron is considered the structural unit of the nervous system. However, the simple *reflex arc,* as illustrated in Figure 6-12 is believed to be the functional unit of the nervous system. Generally, reflex arcs do not require the functioning of the higher centers of the nervous system. Reflex arcs involve a minimum of two neurons: the afferent (receptor) neuron and the efferent (effector) neuron.

More specifically, according to authorities, a reflex arc consist in each case of at least 5 parts: namely, (1) a *receptor* (specialized termination of a sensory nerve fiber with special sense organs), (2) *afferent neuron* (sensory transmitter of impulse from the receptor to the spinal cord), (3) *synapse* (a connection between the afferent and efferent neuron), (4) *efferent neuron* (motor transmitter of impulse from the spinal cord to the effector organ), and (5) *effector* (an organ which actually carries out the response such as a muscle or gland).

Reflexes may be arranged according to function such as postural reflexes, extensor reflexes, flexor reflexes, etc. Some of these reflexes may be denoted by a pathway of two neurons (the simplest type) while others require a more complex structure including more than two neurons. The *classical knee jerk,* as shown in Figure 6-12, as well as the *postural reflex* are examples of a two neuron reflex arc. They both are considered stretch or extensor reflexes.

The stimulus involved in the knee jerk reflex is the actual tapping of the patellar tendon of the quadriceps muscles. The quadriceps muscle is then stretched, thus causing the stimulation of the proprioceptive receptors in the muscle. The sensory impulses are then conducted in the spinal cord where a motor impulse results causing a contraction or shortening in the quadriceps muscle.

It is generally known that under most postural conditions there are many muscles that by their contractions serve to hold the body upright against the force of gravity. During postural control, the muscles antagonizing the pull of gravity are apparently stretched, thereby stretching the muscle spindles located in the muscles. The resulting afferent impulse is transmitted to the spinal cord by a sensory neuron, which synapses directly with a motor neuron. Efferent impulses

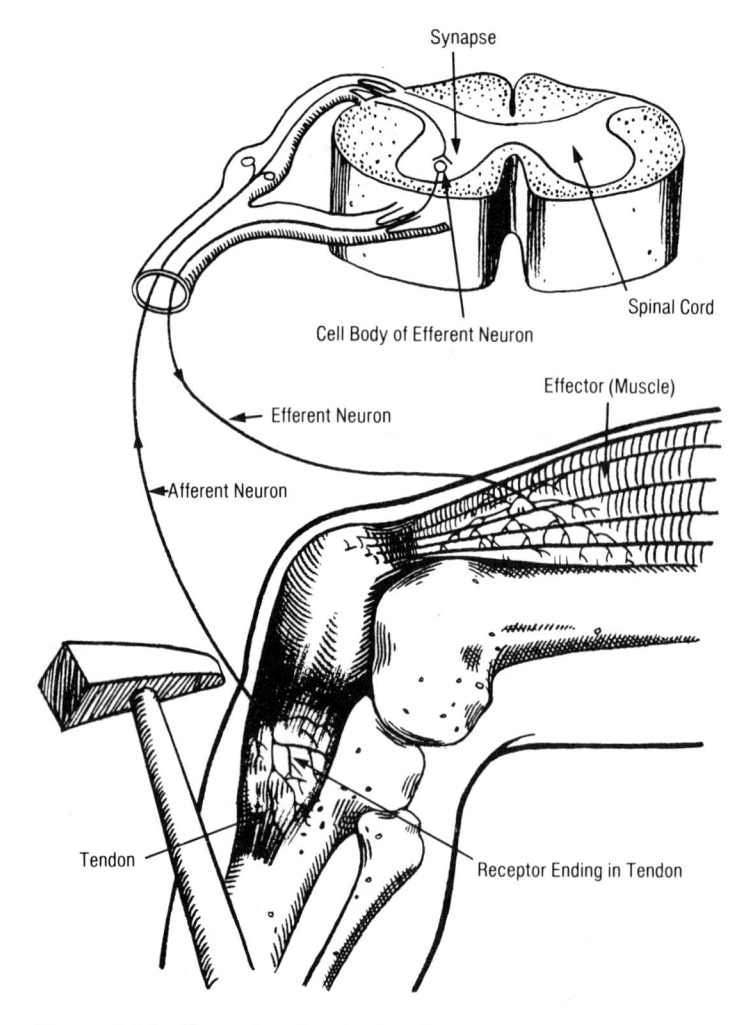

Figure 6-12 Illustration of a simple reflex arc.

are then evoked from the motor neuron, and the muscle contracts so that the pull of gravity is counterbalanced and thus body stability is maintained.

Flexor reflexes are those concerned with body protection via withdrawals. For example, the withdrawal of the hand from a hot object or the removal of the foot from contact with a sharp object such as illustrated in Figure 6-13. The impulses in these situations are transmitted over pathways which involves at least three neurons (sensory, internuncial, and motor) and two synapses. In fact, many of these types of reflexes generally include several interconnections with many association and motor neurons.

VII. REACTION TIME AND MOVEMENT TIME

The speed by which an individual can react in a given situation has been of great concern and interest to those in not only physical education and athletics, but also to those in business and

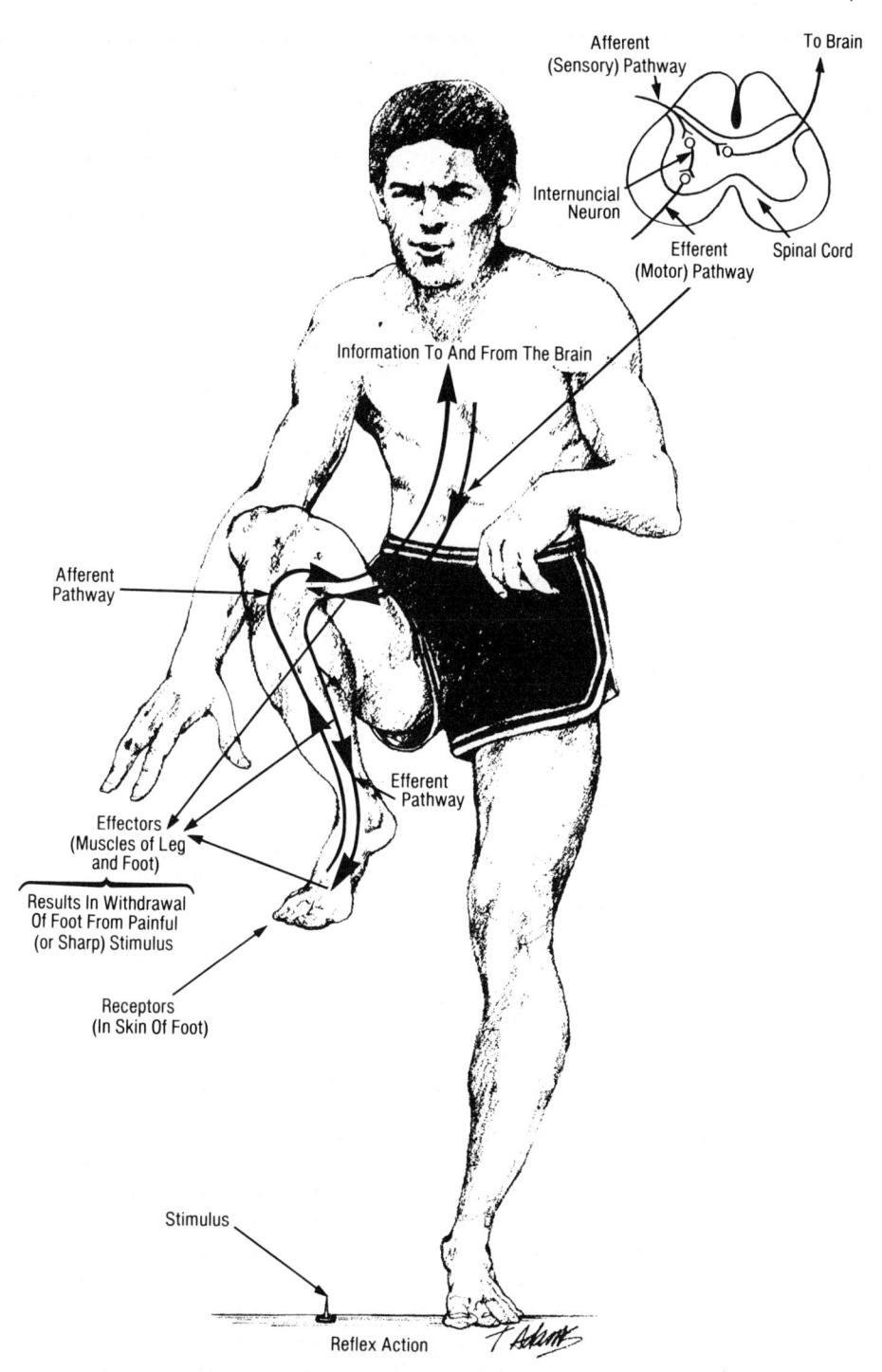

Figure 6-13 Schematic diagram of a flexor reflex.

industry. For example, in track and field, a difference in reaction to the starting signal for a short running event (such as the 100-yd dash) can result in either winning or losing by several feet or even inches. Or, on the other hand, the speed by which a person can react while working on an assembly line in a large factory may even mean the difference in keeping your job. Research of speed has generally focused on two aspects; namely, *reaction time* and *movement time.* Reaction time is defined as the length of time elapsed between the presentation of the simulus and the actual beginning of the movement. Movement time is defined as the length of time elapsed between the first sign of movement and the actual completion of the specific movement.

The measurement of reaction time is to present the subject with some type of stimulus, either visual, verbal, or tactile, which sets into motion an electric timer. The instant the subject moves to initiate some movement, the timer stops and the elapsed time is recorded as reaction time.

As mentioned previously for reaction time, the typical method of measuring movement time is to also present the object with some sort of stimulus, either visual, verbal, or tactile. Movement time can then be determined by having the subject react to the stimulus and move his or her entire body or specific body parts (arm or leg) a fixed distance and either contact an object or cross the path of a light beam or similar type device that permits follow-through, all of which stops the timer. Note that the instant the subject reacts to the stimulus to start the movement, the electric timer starts. At this point, it should be emphasized that since the measurements of reaction time and movement time are generally recorded to the hundredth or thousandth of a second, it is very important that the timer be extremely accurate.

An interesting question that has been debated and researched in recent years is the relationship between reaction time and movement time and whether one can be predicted from the other. The weight of evidence indicates that there is no significant relationship between them. In other words, the fact that a person tends to be a fast reactor does not necessarily mean that he will be a fast mover and vice versa.

The question of specificity as opposed to the generality of reaction time and movement time has also been brought up and debated in past years. In this area, considerable research has been done in attempting to determine whether an individual who has a fast reaction time for removing his legs from a microswitch in response to either a visual, verbal, or tactile stimulus, will he also be equally fast with his hand on the same task. The majority of the research agrees that there is a high degree of specificity by individual body segments (arms and legs) and movement. In other words, an individual who has a fast reaction time and movement time with an arm does not necessarily have a fast reaction time and movement time with the legs.

VIII. CROSS-EDUCATION

The fact that training and practice of the muscles of one limb (ipsilateral side) causes a significant improvement of strength and muscular endurance as well as the learning of motor skills in the contralateral (opposite side) extremity has interested researchers in the fields of physical education, physical medicine, therapeutics, and rehabilitation since the term "cross education" was introduced by Scripture and colleagues in 1894. Even today, however, the rationale for this cross transfer is still not completely understood. Many experimenters studying the theoretical basis are of the opinion that the explanation for this transfer lies in the area of neurology. For example, it has been suggested that this phenomenon is brought about by a diffusion of motor impulses from the 70 to 85 percent of contralaterally descending nerve fibers of the pyramidal system to the remaining 15 to 30 percent of ipsilaterally descending nerve fibers.

While some controversy still exists concerning the most effective means of developing cross transfer of strength, endurance, and skill, most researchers agree that, in general, sufficient overflow is greatest when work has been performed in overload. In some studies, however, it appears that during the training of the ipsilateral side, the contralateral extremity (in some cases), may have been undergoing some sort of an isometric-type contraction without being aware of it. Thus, the untrained limb (in these cases) was not theoretically unexerised.

From the available information, it would appear that in order for cross transfer effects to be achieved, intact motor innervation is apparently needed. In summary, while the clinical importance of cross education in the treatment of immobilized and nonfunctioning innervated muscles cannot be over emphasized (for maintenance of muscle tone and prevention of atrophy), it is unfortunate that most of its application thus far has been in its use in gathering experimental data and not in its therapeutic application.

IX. SUMMARY

(1) The structured unit of the nervous system is the nerve cell or neuron. The dendrites conduct nerve impulses toward the cell body while the axons take them away.

(2) Neurons are bound together by an anatomical gap called the synapse. A synapse has 5 fundamental characteristics:
   (a) they transmit impulses in one direction only;
   (b) they delay the transmission of the impulse;
   (c) they fatigue very easily;
   (d) they are very susceptible to drugs, and
   (e) they have a relatively high threshold.

(3) The membrane of a resting axon is polarized, that is, the exterior being positively charged with respect to the interior. Large amounts of sodium and potassium ions are found on the outside and inside, respectively. When the cell membrane is stimulated, depolarization occurs. That is, sodium ions flowing inward during the rising portion of the action or spike potential, and thus causing the inside of the cell to become positive in relation to the outside. Potassium outflow begins immediately, hence restoring the resting state of the cell membrane and bringing about repolarization. The action potential impulse travels the entire distance of the membrane in a self-propagating, wavelike pattern.

(4) The arrival of nerve impulses at the neuromuscular or myoneural junction triggers the production of an excitatory transmitter called acetycholine (ACh) and depolarization of the postsynaptic membrane occurs. The wave of action potentials then spreads along the muscle in each direction from the motor end-plate, thus triggering the release of calcium from the sarcoplasmic reticulum which in essence puts the muscle contractile process in motion. Upon arrival of ACh to the postsynaptic side, it is destroyed or broken down almost immediately into acetate and choline by an enzyme called cholinesterase which is found on the post-synaptic membrane. This inactivates the depolarizing effect of ACh.

(5) The cerebral cortex is the center for voluntary control of skilled movement.
   (a) The sensory cortex is responsible for intergrating and initiating the appropriate action.
   (b) The motor cortex (pyramidal system) is concerned with the coordination of small discrete individual muscle movements.
   (c) The premotor cortex (extrapyramidal system) controls complicated movement patterns involving groups of muscles.

(6) The cerebellum is concerned with the regulation, coordination, and adjustment of muscular movements. It receives afferent impulses from the motor cortex and various sensory receptors, while it transmits efferent impules to the cerebral cortex as well as to motor neurons in the brain stem and spinal cord.

(7) The basal ganglia coordinates and controls muscular movement by exerting an inhibitory effect on the extrapyramidal system.

(8) The substantia nigra provides muscular tone and helps position various parts of the body so that discrete motor functions of the hand and foot can be performed.

(9) The reticular formation regulates muscular movement by exerting inhibitory effects on the extensor muscles as well as facilitatory effects on the lower flexor motor neurons in the spinal cord.

(10) The feedback to the brain of what the muscles are doing in order that coordination of movement can take place is known as proprioception and involves two types of information: namely, (a) kinesthetic, from sensory receptors in the muscles, tendons, and joints, and (b) vestibular, from receptors of the nonauditory labyrinths found in the inner ear.

(11) Reflexes play an important part in involuntary control of muscular movement. While reflexes take place at all levels of the brain and spinal cord, most of the skeletal muscles reflexes do not require action of the higher brain cells.

(12) The simple reflex arc involves the following:
   (a) a sensory receptor which receives the stimuli;
   (b) an afferent neuron to transmit the stimuli to the spinal cord;
   (c) a synapse in the spinal cord to bound the afferent neurons to the efferent neuron;
   (d) an efferent neuron to transmit the stimuli to a muscle or gland;
   (e) an effector organ such as a muscle or gland to receive the stimuli.

(13) There is no significant relationship between reaction time and movement time. In other words, the fact that a person may be a fast reactor does not necessarily mean that he will be a fast mover and vice versa.

(14) Investigators generally agree that there is a high degree of specificity by individual limbs and movement. That is, an individual who has a fast reaction time and movement time with an arm does not necessarily have a fast reaction time and movement time with the legs.

(15) The cross-transfer effects of strength, muscular endurance, and skill are well documented. Intact motor innervation is required and overloading of the trained extremity results in the best transfer effects.

X. REVIEW REFERENCES

(1) Astrand, P. O., and K. Rodahl. *Textbook of Work Physiology,* 2nd edition, McGraw-Hill Book Co., New York, 1977.
(2) Clarke, D. H. *Exercise Physiology,* Prentice-Hall, Inc., Englewood Cliffs, New Jersey, 1975.
(3) Edington, D. W., and V. R. Edgerton. *The Biology of Physical Activity,* Houghton Mifflin Co., Boston, 1976.
(4) Eyzaguirre, C., and S. J. Fidone. *Physiology of the Nervous System: An Introductory Text,* 2nd edition, Year Book Medical Publishers, Chicago, 1975.
(5) Guyton, A. C. *Textbook of Medical Physiology,* 5th edition, W. B. Saunders Co., Philadelphia, 1976.
(6) Hunt, C. C. (editor). *Neurophysiology,* University Park Press, Baltimore, 1975.
(7) Lamb, D. R. *Physiology of Exercise: Responses and Adaptations,* Macmillan Publishing Co., New York, 1978.
(8) Langley, L. L. *Physiology of Man,* 4th edition, Van Nostrand Reinhold Co., New York, 1971.

(9) Loofbourrow, G. N. "Neuromuscular Integration," in *Science and Medicine of Exercise and Sport,* 2nd Edition, (W. R. Johnson and E. R. Buskirk, editors), Harper and Row, Publishers, New York, 1974.
(10) Singer, R. N. *Motor Learning and Human Performance,* Macmillan Publishing Co., New York, 1975.

7

EXERCISE AND TEMPERATURE REGULATIONS IN HOT AND COLD CLIMATES

KEY CONCEPTS TO BE GAINED FROM THIS CHAPTER

(1) Thermal balance in the human body is maintained by keeping a balance between heat loss and heat gain.

(2) Temperature of the human body is maintained within a very small range with the outer shell temperature being about three degrees lower (depending on the external temperature as well as the amount of clothing being worn) than the inner core temperature.

(3) The hypothalamus along with the adrenal medulla and the thyroid endocrine glands play an essential role in the regulation of temperature in the body.

(4) Temperature regulation during exercise in a hot climate involves vasodilatation and sweating, whereas regulation in cold weather involves vasoconstriction and shivering.

(5) Exercising in hot-humid climates pose different physiological problems on the human body than when working in hot-dry weather.

(6) Heat disorders can be reduced and work performance maintained by: (a) adequate water and salt replacements; (b) adequate period of acclimatization to heat; (c) sufficient rest periods and water breaks during practice; and (d) knowledge of the limitations placed on the human body involving work, clothing attire, and ambient conditions.

(7) The practice of "making weight" by wrestlers by way of crash diets and dehydration is highly condemned and not recommended by the medical profession as well as the American College of Sports Medicine Association.

(8) Although adaptation to cold is probably a combination of both physiological and psychological factors, the most important physiological factors appear to be metabolic insulation, hypothermic and peripheral circulation.

It is a well-known fact that under normal conditions, the internal temperature of the human body generally remains at a constant level of 37°C (98.6°F). Yet several factors such as exercise, illness, and external temperature may upset this constancy by either increasing or decreasing the body temperature. For instance, on some occasions the temperature of the environment is much higher than that of the human body, and thus under these conditions the body tends to gain in heat (upper level of Fig. 7-1). On the other hand, if the outside temperature is lower than that of the human body, then the body loses heat (lower level of Fig. 7-1). In addition, approximately 80 percent of the energy expended during exercise is actually transformed into wasted heat. If this wasted heat is not dissipated, then body temperature will generally rise. There are occasions (especially during strenuous work) under extreme environmental conditions where the human body may not be able to regulate its temperature satisfactorily. If this happens, illness (such as dehydration and heat cramps, heat exhaustion, and heat stroke) can result, or in severe cases, death can ensue (Fig. 7-1). If the temperature of the body is to remain at or near 37°C, heat production and heat gain must equal heat loss and vice versa.

I. BALANCE BETWEEN HEAT LOSS AND HEAT PRODUCTION

There are three ways by which heat is lost from the body: the *skin, lungs,* and *excretions.* Skin is the most important of the three. Approximately 85 percent of heat is lost via this organ, although this depends on external and internal conditions. Heat is lost from the skin by the following four means: radiation, convection, evaporation, and conduction. Each will be discussed separately.

A. RADIATION

Heat is lost from the skin by *radiation* when the body temperature is higher than the surrounding object such as walls and furniture. On the other hand, we gain heat by way of radiation when the external objects are warmer than the human body. Radiation is based on the principle that molecules within the body are constantly vibrating, and as a result, heat is being given off in the forms of electromagnetic waves.

B. CONVECTION

When the body temperature is higher than the surrounding air or water (such as in swimming), heat is lost from the skin by way of *convection.* Thus, the surrounding air is warmed by air currents from the body. The convection currents replace warmed air with cold air, and they also replace moist air with relatively dry air. The amount of heat loss from convection depends on the temperature as well as the speed by which the air flows over the surface of the body. We gain heat by convection when the surrounding air is warmer than the body.

C. EVAPORATION

Heat is lost from the skin by *evaporation* (diffusion of water molecules from body surface to air) of sweat from the body surface since the evaporation of any given fluid utilizes and hence removes heat from the surrounding objects and air. In order for evaporation to be an effective mechanism for cooling the body, the sweat from our body must be changed into a gaseous water vapor at the body surface. Energy, in the form of heat, is needed for this change and it is absorbed from the area body surface. This absorbing of heat energy results in cooling. In fact, for every liter

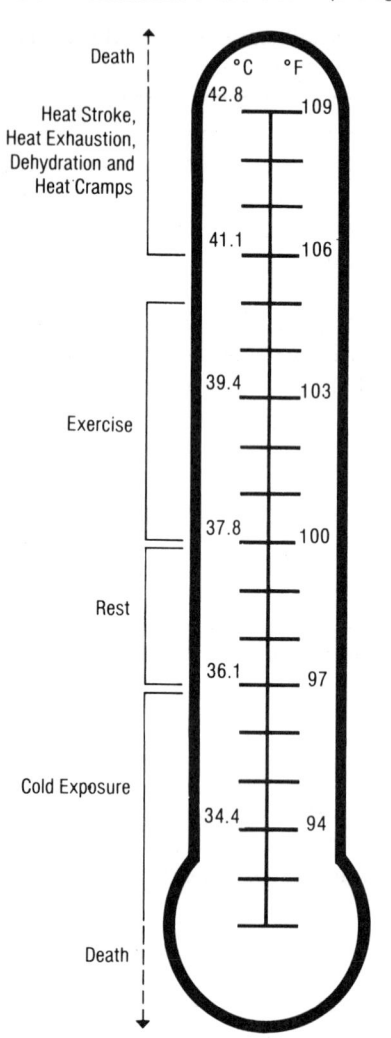

Figure 7-1 Schematic illustration showing the effects of various factors on body temperature.

of sweat evaporated, the body dissipates approximately 580 kilocalories of heat energy. It should be noted that if the sweat from the body cannot be evaporated and does nothing more than fall to the ground, cooling of the body by way of evaporation cannot take place.

During exercise, the major portion of heat loss is through evaporation of sweat from the body surface. In addition, when air temperature is higher than that of the human body, the majority of heat is lost by evaporation. The amount and rate of heat lost by evaporation depends upon the movement of air across the surface of the body as well as the relative humidity (RH) of the air. The lower the humidity, the greater the heat loss via evaporation; whereas the higher the humidity (air highly saturated with water vapor) the smaller the heat loss. During vigorous exercise, especially in a hot and humid environment, perspiration can exceed as much as 4 liters per hour. Although the rate of perspiration changes with the temperature, there is some perspiration even at low temperatures. Perspiration of this nature is referred to as *insensible water loss.* Insensible water loss leaves the body at all times unless the ambient humidity is 100 percent RH. This moisture or extracellular fluid diffuses through the skin, through the pores of the sweat glands, and from the lungs.

D. CONDUCTION

Heat may also be lost from the skin by *conduction*, as in coming in direct contact with an object possessing a colder temperature. Heat is always conducted from the warmer to the colder object. If the outside object is warmer than the human body, then heat is gained by conduction.

II. HEAT GAIN

Heat is gained by the human body primarily as a result of all the internal metabolic processes. However, there may be a small gain by radiation and convection from the external environment, such as the sun, a newly resurfaced black-top road, desert sand and rock, etc., if they are at a higher temperature than the body. A small gain may also be obtained through conduction if the body is exposed to a source having a high temperature such as hot water. The amount taken in with hot food and drink is almost negligible. Heat production from metabolism takes place in the tissues. Although every tissue contributes to this, the skeletal muscles furnish the largest amount. Therefore, increasing heat production is obtained primarily by increasing muscular activity. In strenuous activity, heat production from metabolism has been known to increase by as much as 30 times its normal. In bitter cold weather, the metabolic heat production is achieved by an involuntary response known as shivering, which may in fact, increase the metabolic processes by as much as 400 percent. The human body generally starts to shiver when the skin temperature has dropped to approximately 19°C (66°F).

III. REGULATION OF BODY TEMPERATURE

How is the temperature balance between heat production and heat loss maintained? There are several neural centers in the spinal cord and the brain which control such activities as vasoconstriction, vasodilatation, sweating, muscle tone, and shivering. In order for body temperature to remain at or near a constant level, the integration of these various activities is essential. This is the function of the *thermoregulatory system* located in the hypothalamus. The role of the thermoregulatory system in regulating body temperature is accomplished by two centers: (a) anterior hypothalamus center and (b) posterior hypothalamus center.

A. ANTERIOR HYPOTHALAMUS CENTER

This center controls heat dissipating events. For instance, if this center is stimulated, the blood vessels of the skin are dilated, thus resulting in a greater flow of blood to the surface. Also, impulses are transmitted to the sweat glands, increasing perspiration, and to the respiratory center, causing panting. All these physiological responses act to increase the rate of heat loss from the body, and thereby prevent overheating of the body. Destruction of this center causes a person to react normal in a cold environment, but in hot climates the common methods of losing heat (conduction, radiation, convection, and evaporation) are inoperative and hence the body temperature rises.

B. POSTERIOR HYPOTHALAMUS CENTER

The posterior hypothalamus center calls on heat conservation events, and thereby prevents chilling of the body. For example, if the center is stimulated, the blood vessels of the skin are constricted, thus reducing the blood flow to the surface. In addition, it is well known that the surface hairs on the body are also stimulated to become erect, and thus they come into play to reinforce the insulating layer of air surrounding the skin. At the same time, shivering is brought about through the same mechanism to increase heat production. As a result of this centers destruction, exposure of the person to cold climate does not increase metabolism or heart rate; therefore, heat production lags, and the body temperature drops.

The hypothalamus responds reflexly to afferent impulses initiated by the thermoreceptors in the skin, and to changes in the temperature of the arterial blood that flows through it. The skin receptors react to changes in the environmental temperature, whereas the hypothalamus receptors respond to small temperature changes (as little as 0.2 to 0.5°F) of the arterial blood flowing through them.

C. ADRENAL MEDULLA AND THYROID ENDOCRINE GLANDS

The adrenal medulla and the thyroid endocrine glands also take part in the regulation of either heat production or heat loss. When the adrenal medulla is stimulated, large amounts of *epinephrine* and *norepinephrine* hormones are released into the blood. These two hormones have the ability to increase the basal metabolic rate and therefore increase heat production. The exact means by which this is accomplished is not clear, however, according to some authorities researching in this area, epinephrine and norepinephrine enhance the breakdown of glycogen into glucose as well as increase the rate of some of the enzymatic reactions that promote oxidation of foods. Since these two hormones may cause constriction of the cutaneous blood vessels, they are also of value in conservation of body heat.

When the thyroid gland is stimulated, large quantities of the hormone called thyroid is released into the blood. The action of this hormone is similar to that of norepinephrine, however, the thyroid hormone continues to be active for as long as 4 to 8 weeks after its release into the blood. Norepinephrine, on the other hand, remains active for only a few minutes. Large secretions of the thyroid hormone can cause the metabolic rate to increase as much as 200 percent of normal. Again, the exact mechanism by which the thyroid hormone affects the cells of the body is not known, but it is generally known to increase the quantities of most of the cellular enzymes. Hence, this may explain its metabolic effects.

IV. TEMPERATURE MEASUREMENT

A. CORE AND SKIN

The human body may be regarded as having an *inner core* (deep central areas including heart, lungs, abdominal organs, and brain as well as deep regions of the muscle masses of the extremities) at a temperature around 37°C and an *outer shell* (includes the skin, subcutaneous tissues, and the shallow areas of the muscle masses) of variable temperature. Generally, the outer shell temperature is somewhere between 23°C and 34°C (depending upon the ambient temperature, the amount of clothing being worn, etc.). Although it appears that external temperature does not affect core temperature within a given range at rest or during work, skin temperature is affected by the external environment. In addition, exercise may cause the core temperature to be as much as 20°C higher than that of the skin. It is generally believed that at rest the ideal difference between the inner core and the outer shell is about 4°C.

Most authorities generally consider that approximately two-thirds of the body mass is at the core or rectal temperature, while one-third of the body mass is at the shell or mean skin temperature. This relationship may be expressed by the following equation:

$$\text{Mean body temperature} = 0.33 \times \text{skin temperature} + 0.67 \times \text{core temperature}$$

The mean skin temperature is normally found by taking measurements with either thermocouplers or thermistors at various sites on the body surface. The classical site of core temperature measurements is the rectum. It is usually accomplished with the aid of mercury thermometers, thermocouplers, or thermistors. This relationship between the core and skin temperature is important since it is used in estimating the actual amount of heat that is gained or lost over a given period of time. The *kilocalorie (kcal)* is generally used as the unit of heat energy. Recall from Chapter 2 that a kcal represents the amount of heat needed to increase the temperature of 1 kg of water 1°C. Therefore, if 1 kcal is added to 1 kg of water, the temperature will increase 1°C. Thus, the specific heat of water (defined as the number of kcal needed to change the temperature of 1 kg of water 1°C) is equal to 1.0 or 1 kcal/kg of water/°C. At the same time, the human body, as a whole, has a mean specific heat of 0.83. This is slightly below the 1.0 for water because the human body not only contains water, (approximately 80% of body is water) but also proteins and lipids of lower specific heat. This means that for every 0.83 kcal added per kg of body tissue a 1°C increase in temperature will take place (0.83 kcal/kg of body tissue/°C). For example, in order to increase the temperature of the body by 1°C, an individual weighing 145 pounds (66 kg) would have to add or store 55 kcal of heat (0.83 × 66 kg).

Below is a simplified illustration of how body temperature would increase during both rest and exercise conditions if we were not able to maintain heat balance by radiation, convection, conduction, and evaporation.

Rest Illustration

Recall from Chapter 2 on energy and metabolism that during rest, the normal person takes in about 250 ml (or .25 liters) of oxygen per minute. Also recall that the caloric equivalent of one liter of oxygen depends upon the food that is being metabolized for the body's source of energy. Remember from Chapter 2 that during rest, the normal respiratory quotient (R.Q.) or respiratory-exchange ratio (R) is 0.82. This means that for each liter of oxygen taken in during metabolism, 4.83 kcal of heat will be produced, or in this illustration 1.21 kcal (.25 liter × 4.83 kcal per liter) per minute. This results in 72.6 kcal per hour. Again, recall from previous discussion that specific heat of the human body is 0.83 kcal/kg/°C. This means, therefore, that if the person weighed 145 pounds (66 kg), he or she would have to add or store 55 kcal of heat (0.83 kcal/kg/°C × 66 kg) in order to increase the temperature by 1°C. In this illustration, the person produced 72.6 kcal in 1 hour. Thus, if no heat were lost, the body temperature for this individual would increase around 1.3°C in 1 hour (72.6 ÷ 55).

Exercise Illustration

In this example, assume that a jogger running for 1 hour averages taking in 1.5 liters of oxygen per minute (1.5 liters × 60 minutes = 90 liters). During this period, the R.Q. is again assumed to be equal to 0.82. This means that a total of 435 kcal of heat will be produced (90 liters × 4.83 kcal per liter) in the 1 hour of jogging. Using the same body weight (66 kg) and specific heat of body tissue (0.83 kcal/kg/°C) for this illustration as was used in the rest illustration, if no heat were lost, the body temperature for this same individual would increase around 7.9°C in 1 hour (435 ÷ 55).

It should be clear to the reader from this simplified illustration the importance of radiation convection, conduction, and evaporation in maintaining heat balance during physical activity.

V. AGE

It is generally believed that regulation of body temperature in the premature and newborn baby is quite different from that found in adults. Briefly, these differences are related to the lack of control exercised by the infants nervous system over the blood vessels and other organs involved in temperature regulation. Temperature variations due to emotion, crying, or activity are usually greater during the first year of life than in the adult.

Elderly people regulate body temperature at approximately the same level as the younger adult, however, they are less able to adjust to cold or extreme heat. It appears that this fragility is not caused by any one factor but rather to overall changes in nutrition, health and exposure.

VI. SEX

It is common knowledge that preovulatory women generally have approximately the same oral temperature as men. On the other hand, during ovulation body temperature usually rises 0.2° to 0.5°C and remains slightly higher throughout the remainder of the cycle. The exact cause for this increase is not clear. However, it has been reported in various studies that certain hormones, including *pregnenolone* and *pregnanediol,* cause fever when injected in man, and hence may be a partial explanation.

Men and women respond differently to thermal stress. In addition, it appears that females may have a slightly higher sweating threshold (2° to 3°F) than males. For examples, evidence is available to indicate that the female sweats less than the male because she does not apparently start sweating until the environmental temperature is about 2°F above the male's sweating threshold. This may be due, in part, to the female's sex hormone, estrogen, which inhibits sweating to some degree. Since the temperature gradient from the inner core to the outer shell is smaller for women, the physiological cost of maintaining heat balance in hot weather is greater and hence seems to be more limiting in terms of physical performance.

The outer shell temperature of women is generally higher in warm weather than that of the male. This may be due, in part, to the greater acclimatization or training of the male. Also, in cold weather, women have a lower outer shell temperature than men and a heat loss of approximately 10 percent less. According to authorities studying heat and cold tolerance of different sexes, this may be partially due to a more effective vasoconstriction in women as well as to a greater amount of adipose tissue (about 10%) in women.

VII. DIURNAL CHANGES

Body temperature is usually at its lowest (about 36.1°C) in the early morning hours, and at its highest (about 37.4°C) in the late afternoon or early evening. These variations can be reversed by merely changing one's daily living habits such as eating and sleeping. According to experts, this variation is credited to the circadion rhythm seen in other areas of physiology and is affected by daily routines such as sleeping, eating, light, and time. It also appears that long periods of travel will cause cycle changes. For instance, evidence is available to indicate that when a person travels in an airplane for 8 to 10 hours, it may take the cycle 3 or 4 days to actually readjust to the new time. An adjustment also takes place when night workers go on day shifts and vice versa. Fasting has also shown to reduce the amount of these variations.

VIII. INDIVIDUAL DIFFERENCES

It is well known in the exercise physiology circles that the fat and overweight, endomorph person is at a somewhat disadvantage in the heat, but has some advantage in the cold. For instance, the fat person not only has more insulation (subcutaneous fat) as a barrier to conductive heat loss, but he also has a smaller body surface area for the evaporation of sweat per unit mass of tissue than the skinny, thin ectomorph person. Consequently, heat loss in a fat person occurs at a much slower rate than in a thin individual. At the same time, however, the fatter the individual, the lower his resistance to heat. Thus, it is obvious that a fat person is better able to tolerate cold while the thin person is better able to dissipate heat in a hot climate.

IX. EXERCISE AND TEMPERATURE REGULATIONS IN HOT CLIMATES

As mentioned earlier, temperature regulation during exercise in a hot climate involves vasodilatation and sweating as a function of the anterior hypothalamus of the brain. Vasodilation (expansion of a blood vessel) increases skin blood flow, and thus enhances the transfer of metabolic heat from the deep core to the skin surface. Secretion of sweat, on the other hand, provides water for evaporative cooling.

A general increase in blood flow from the deep core to the skin and limbs by the circulatory system allows for a greater amount of heat to be lost by conduction, convection, radiation, and evaporation. As the cooled blood returns to the deep core area, it once again picks up the heat and transports it to skin where it is dissipated in the manner previously mentioned.

Figure 7-2 illustrates the effect of exercise on body temperature. It can be seen that exercising at a work load of about 75 percent of maximum oxygen uptake values in a comfortable room temperature environment increases core temperatures to about 38 to 39°C during the early part of the exercise and then it remains steady at this new level until the exercise is completed. Skin temperature, on the other hand, is reduced mainly because of evaporative heat loss through the sweating mechanism. Thus, as can be noticed in Figure 7-2, the result of these temperature changes between the core and skin is an apparent increase in the thermal gradient between the core

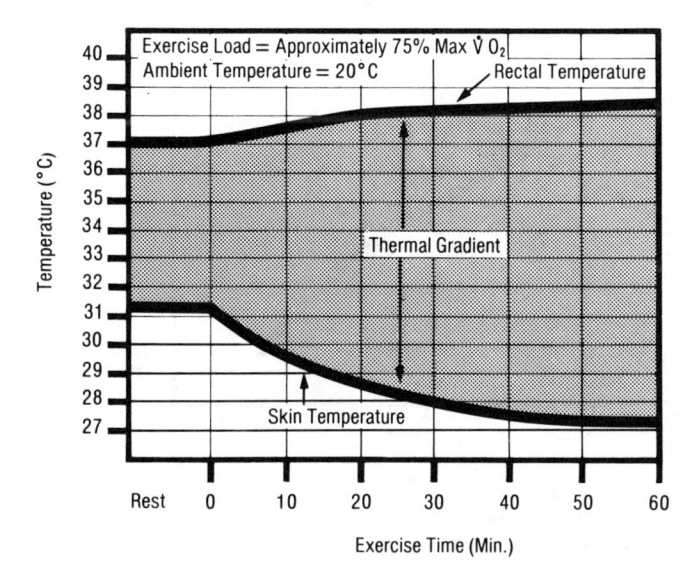

Figure 7-2 The effects of exercise on body temperature.

140   Essentials of Exercise Physiology

and skin. This increase in the thermal gradient obviously helps in getting rid of the heat by way of the four previously mentioned mechanisms.

A. SWEATING

When environmental temperatures rise above the skin temperature (normally around 34°C), the circulatory adjustments are not sufficient for heat dissipation by convection and radiation because of the reduced gradient or negative gradient between the skin and environment. In fact, when external temperatures are greater than the skin temperature and a negative gradient appears, the body is actually gaining heat by radiation and convection. Thus, the only means for heat loss at temperatures above skin temperature is by evaporative *sweating*. At the same time, however, if the rate of metabolism is increased by exercise, sweating must be called upon at lower temperatures. This is illustrated in Figure 7-3 where a subject worked at a work load of approximately 900 Kpm/min. at various environmental temperatures ranging between 5°C and 36°C. It can be seen that when the subject exercised at the lower environmental temperatures, radiation and convection accounted for approximately 70 percent of the heat loss. The subject's skin temperature was recorded to be 21°C. When the exercise was performed at the highest environmental temperature (36°C), the skin temperature was 35°C, and thus the subject actually gained heat from the outside environment. The subject in this illustration apparently counteracted this gain by increasing his evaporative sweating loss. For instance, when the subject exercised in the cold, he was known to have evaporated 150 grams of sweat, whereas in the hot climate, he evaporated 700 grams.

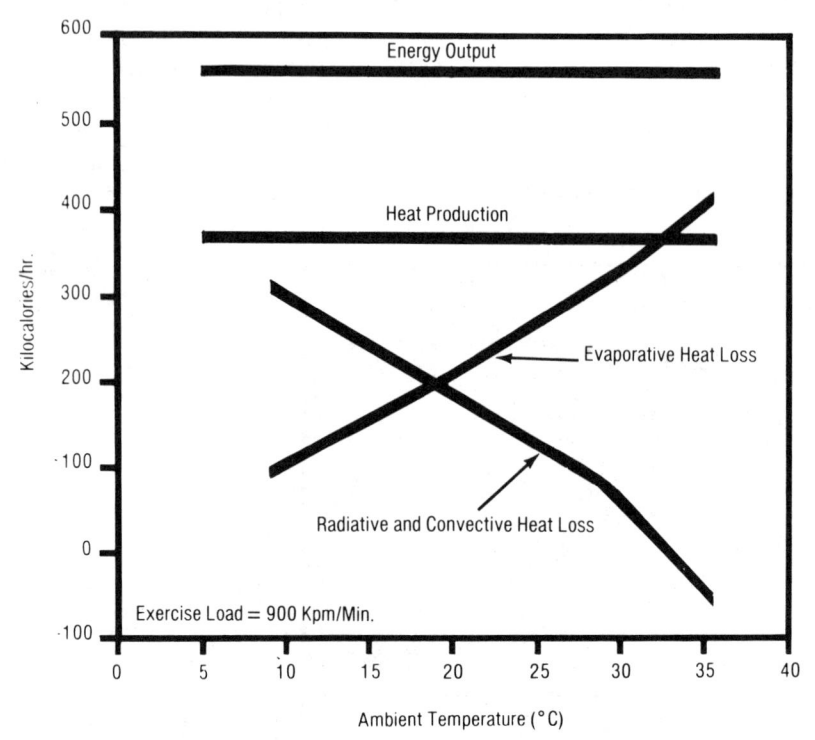

Figure 7-3   Schematic illustration of heat loss by way of evaporative sweating, radiation and convection when exercising in various environmental temperatures.

It is common knowledge that sweating is an effective cooling mechanism. It has been calculated that there are about 2.5 million sweat glands in the skin. It appears that the sweating rate is increased not only by increasing the number of active glands, but also by increasing the rate of output of each gland as heat exposure is made more severe. The capacity for sweating varies considerably among people. For example, it is common information that some people have no sweat glands at all. As an individual becomes acclimatized to heat, the amount of sweat given off in relation to a standard heat stress will increase.

As was pointed out earlier in this chapter, in order for thermal sweat to be effective, it must evaporate from the skin surface. The rate of evaporation depends on the difference between the vapor tension of water at the skin surface and in the environmental air (note that the wearing of clothes will retard evaporation from the skin). When environmental air is warm and relative humidity is high, the vapor tension of air and water is high and thus thermal sweating is not effective. This generally accounts for the discomfort that people usually witness when exercising on warm, humid days.

Since exercising in hot-humid climates can pose different problems than when working in hot-dry weather, the author has chosen to discuss each separate.

B. HOT-HUMID CLIMATES

Information is available to indicate that workers who are exposed to severe heat and high relative humidity can sweat at rates as high as 4 liters per hour over short periods of time. In fact, it is known that some people working in intense heat can maintain a sweat output of approximately 2 liters per hour for periods of 5 hours or longer.

Because of the reduced thermal and vapor pressure gradients brought on by climates that are hot and humid, tremendous demands are asked of both the cardiovascular system and the evaporative sweating mechanism. This is especially noticeable during work in hot, humid weather as compared to work in hot, dry surroundings. For example, for the same intensity of work, the heart rate and sweat rate are both higher in hot, humid conditions as compared to the hot, dry weather.

In weather that is hot and humid, it is common knowledge that the heart has to work much harder than normal because the amount of blood flowing through the skin is generally increased (due to vasodilatation of the skin blood vessels) and highly saturated with oxygen. Under these conditions, less oxygen is available to the working muscles, and hence lactic acid starts to accumulate in the blood at a much lower intensity of work. It should be pointed out that the humidity imposes an additional heat dissipation problem. Recall from earlier discussion that in order for thermal sweat to be effective, it must evaporate from the skin surface, and that the rate of evaporation is depended upon the difference between the vapor tension of water at the skin surface and in the environmental air. When the atmospheric air is hot and relative humidity is high the vapor tension of air and water is high, and as a result, the vapor pressure gradient between the skin and air is reduced. This means, unfortunately, that the evaporative mechanism for heat dissipation is generally not as effective during work in hot, humid weather as compared to a more normal climate.

Because of the added strain on the circulatory system to provide sufficient blood to the working muscles and to the skin for heat dissipation, it is quite obvious that exercise in environmental surroundings of high temperature and high relative humidity can place severe strains upon the cardiovascular system.

Figure 7-4 illustrates the combined effect of high temperature and high humidity upon heart rate for both trained and untrained subjects. It is seen that heart rate during rest, exercise, and

142 Essentials of Exercise Physiology

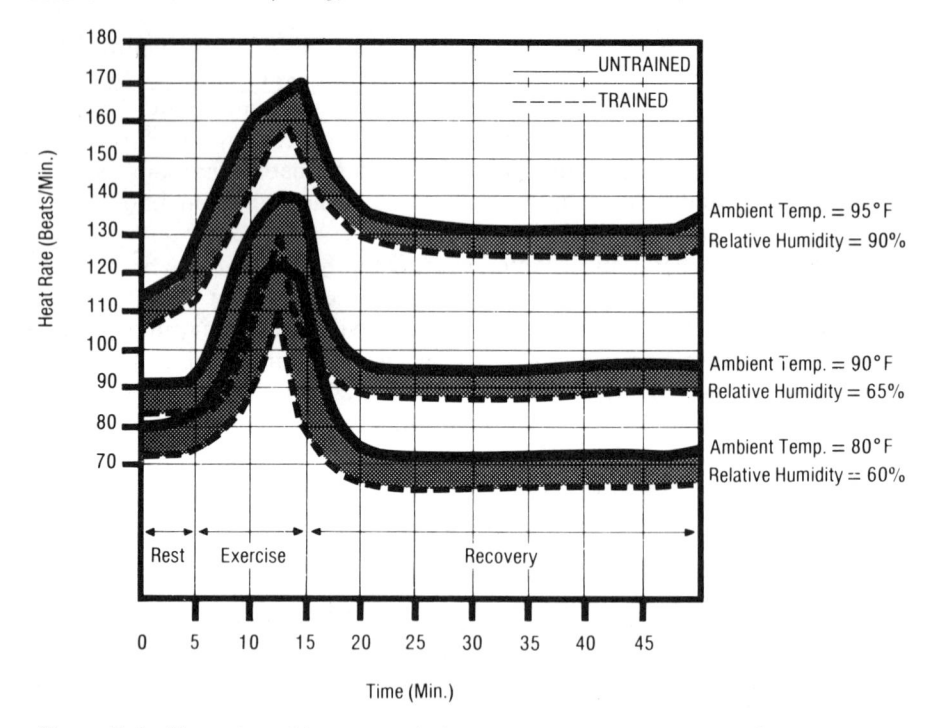

Figure 7-4 Illustration of heart rate during rest, exercise, and recovery for trained and untrained subjects in various high temperatures and high humidities.

recovery is consistently higher as temperature and humidity rise. In fact, following 15 minutes of work in temperatures of 90° to 95° F, and relative humidity between 65 and 90 percent, heart rate does not completely recover to normal even after 45 minutes. Evidence has also been published showing that when subjects exercise at the same intensity, pulmonary ventilation and oxygen consumption are generally higher at hot (90° F) and humid environments, but are lower at hot (108° F) and dry environments than at room temperatures.

At this point, it should be emphasized that although it is common knowledge that environmental conditions of high heat and high relative humidity pose a strain on the circulatory and sweating mechanism, and therefore, can have adverse effects on athletic performance in some events, it appears from the available evidence that the events that are the most effected are those lasting more than 15 minutes in duration. Also, it appears that certain activities where repeated short, quick work-bouts over an extended period of time are carried out in heat and humid conditions are also adversely effected and may not be performed at optimal levels. Without doubt, some of this adverse heat effect on performance is psychological and not physiological. That is, some people are less motivated to work and perform in heat than others, and therefore, they fail to perform up to their maximum capacity.

C. HOT-DRY CLIMATES

The ability of an individual to perform prolonged moderate work in a hot and dry climate apparently is not limited by the evaporative processes as he or she is in hot, humid conditions. In a hot and dry environment the ambient air can absorb large amounts of moisture before becoming saturated. When working in this kind of climate, however, heat must still be taken from the core to the skin for heat dissipation in order to maintain normal body temperature. Like work in hot, humid conditions, this requires adjustments on the circulatory system from its normal state. Since the volume of oxygenated blood flowing through the skin is normally increased (for heat dissipation) as a result of vasodilatation in the skin blood vessels, the heart has to work much harder. Again, because less oxygen is readily accessible to the working muscles under these conditions, lactic acid (the fatigue product) starts to accumulate in the blood at a somewhat lower intensity level of work. As a result of the increased strain on the circulatory system to furnish sufficient blood to the active muscles and to the skin for heat dissipation, it can be seen that work in climates close to or above skin temperature can place severe strains on the cardiovascular system, even when the external air is relatively dry. Because of the fact that the entire process of heat dissipation relies upon the elimination of water in sweating, it is rather clear that when exercising in hot climates (especially with high relative humidity), dehydration is a strong possibility and preventive measures should be taken to avoid it. More will be said about dehydration and other effects of extreme heat in the following section.

X. EFFECTS OF EXTREME HEAT

The human body is made up of a total of approximately 40 liters of intracellular and extracellular fluid. Of this total, the blood in the form of plasma (3 liters) and blood cells (2 liters) take up approximately 5 liters. Because, as was pointed out earlier, some people working in intense heat can lose 2 or more liters of body fluid per hour for periods of 5 hours or longer, the loss of body fluid (especially from the blood) is the most serious problem of sweating and it can lead to *dehydration.*

Dehydration is common in workers in hot climates. It is due to excessive amounts of water being lost in sweat without an adequate replacement. A drop in body fluid during prolonged exercise is not only accompanied by an increase in body temperature, but also a reduction in cardiac output, stroke volume, blood volume, velocity of blood flow and a fall in blood pressure. All of these can and will adversely effect performance unless body fluids are replenished to facilitate the sweating mechanism and to help keep the body temperature at a lower level. If coaches and trainers would see that their players consumed as much as one quart of water before practice or competition in hot, humid weather, and if they would insist on every player consuming as much as one cup of water every 10 to 15 minutes during practice breaks, many of the problems associated with heat stress could probably be eliminated.

The loss of fluid during excessive sweating not only results in dehydration, but also in salt imbalances (namely, sodium, potassium, and chloride) within the body and if not replenished by either additional salt in the daily diet or perhaps a daily salt tablet, it may lead to fatigue, nausea, and *heat cramps.* When working in extreme heat (such as during early season physical conditioning or a lumber jack working an 8-hour day shift), it is possible to lose as much as 10 to 30 grams of salt per day. Since a normal, healthy person generally consumes between 7 and 15 grams of salt in their daily diet, it is apparent that an extra supply of salt may be necessary for those people working in extreme heat. While it may be beneficial for some laborers who work in the heat 8 to 10 hours per day to consume extra salt each day in the form of salt tablets, most experts agree that the 7 to 15 grams of salt that a person normally consumes in their diet each day is more than adequate for most working people. Most authorities also agree that athletes only need to add 2 to 4 extra teaspoons of salt to their food each day or perhaps ingest several glasses of water each day with a half of teaspoon of dissolved salt in each glass.

Because a trained athlete generally looses less salt in their sweat than a non-trained person (due to heat acclimatization), ingestion of large quantities of salt for trained athletes is not required nor recommended. In fact, too much salt can be more detrimental to the athlete and lead to serious medical problems than too little salt. Caution should be taken when consuming large quantities of salt without sufficient water during practices and game situations in the hope that it will improve your performance. *Note that experts recommend a minimum of 1 pint of water with each 7-grain salt tablet.*

A substantial amount of evidence has been published showing that if an over abundance of salt is ingested into the stomach, dehydration may, in fact, be facilitated because of body fluids being drawn by osmosis from the cells into the stomach. Not only will the athlete experience discomfort with a stomach filled with fluid, but his performance may in deed be adversely effected.

In addition to dehydration and heat cramps, exercising in extreme heat may also lead to heat exhaustion and heat stroke unless preventive measures are taken. Each will be discussed separately.

A. HEAT EXHAUSTION

In this condition the cardiovascular system is at fault, as is indicated by a low blood pressure and a rapid, yet weak and soft pulse. These symptoms may eventually lead to dizziness or syncope (fainting). Heat exhaustion is generally not a question of temperature regulation since the body temperature may be normal or even a little below normal. In contrast to heat stroke, the skin is usually cool and moist (clammy). Elderly people and those in questionable health as well as those individuals who are not acclimatized to extreme heat are more likely to suffer heat exhaustion. Complete rest and adequate fluid intake is usually sufficient for recovery.

B. HEAT STROKE

This condition is the most severe form of heat damage since it results from brain damage. It is a failure of the heat-regulating system. This condition is generally more common in hot climates with high humidity since temperature regulation by either radiation or vaporization is limited. The symptoms are cessation of sweating (dry, hot skin) and a sharp rise in body temperature. In addition, pulse rate and blood pressure are generally above normal. A person in this condition may be unconscious, in convulsions, or possibly in a state of delirium. It is common for the body temperature in this condition to rise to 110° to 114°F. Unless the temperature is quickly reduced by ice packs or cold baths, the brain cells are affected and eventually destroyed.

Because of the seriousness involved in heat illness with athletes (particularly with football players and wrestlers) and older people now becoming more actively involved in recreational jogging, a great deal has been written by the medical profession as well as various other sports-related groups concerning ways to prevent heat illness. Table 7-1 is a summary of the recommendations made by various experts in the field for preventing heat illnesses.

XI. HEAT ACCLIMATIZATION

Continuous exposure to heat causes a gradual adjustment or *acclimatization* of the human body resulting in a higher capacity for exercise and less discomfort of heat exposure. *Heat*

Table 7-1. Summary of Recommendations for Preventing Heat Illnesses

1. Encourage a pre-season training program. In other words, a period of heat acclimatization should be carried out before working in the heat.
2. Practice in lightweight uniforms. Long-sleeved jerseys and stockings (such as in football) should not be worn until the weather turns cool.
3. Players should be weighed before and after workouts. An individual who has lost over 5 lb (2.3 kg) should be observed very carefully. Individuals who lose over 10 lbs. (4.5 kg) in a practice should be considered in the danger zone.
4. Provide for adequate salt and water replacement. Water, in some form, should be allowed during all practices and games.
5. Allow for sufficient rest periods during practice.
6. Workouts and/or distance runs should be conducted during the cool-part of the day (generally early mornings and late evenings) on hot days.
7. Conduct daily dry- and wet-bulb* temperature readings. The relative humidity should also be recorded daily. When the wet-bulb temperature is over 50°F, all members of the team should be alerted (especially those teams that have to have their bodies covered with uniforms such as football players). Many water and rest breaks should be allowed. When wet-bulb temperatures are above 75°F, practices should be conducted in shorts or they should be cancelled. Note that the American College of Sports Medicine has issued a position statement concerning distance running in heat and their position is that distance races (16 kilometers or 10 miles) should not be conducted when the wet-bulb temperature exceeds 82.4°F or 28.0°C. It is also important to remember that whenever relative humidity is around 95% or higher, precautions should be taken at all temperature levels.

*This instrument is suspended outside in the air where it is away from trees, buildings, etc. that might cast a shadow or interfere with air movement. This instrument takes into account humidity, air velocity, degree of cloud coverage, and temperature. In other words, it accounts for conduction, radiation, convection, and evaporation in determining temperature. The instrument should be suspended for a period of 30 minutes before taking a reading from it. The instrument may be purchased from the Howard Engineering Co., P.O. Box 3164, Bethlehem, Pa. 18017.

acclimatization (in the outdoor environment) or *acclimation* (in environmental chamber) results in lower exercise-pulse rates, incresed stroke volume, increased sweat production (the rate and onset of sweating is increased), less amount of salt is lost in the sweat, greater blood flow to liver and kidneys, increased plasma volume, and a lowered skin and internal body temperature.

Also, blood pressure following heat acclimatization appears to be more stable and adequately regulated during exercise. The reduction in the salt content of the sweat is believed to be due to an increased amount of aldosterone hormones released into the blood stream during heat exposure. Without this decline in salt concentration, the human body (in most cases) would suffer a salt deficit.

The increase in sweat production is more common in hot and humid climates than in dry. For instance, this increase generally amounts to about 15 percent in a hot dry environment, whereas in cooler but more humid climates the increase may vary from as much as 60 to 100 percent over the original levels. The increased sweat production is brought about by a greater number of sweat glands being actively involved in the sweating mechanism following heat acclimatization. In spite of this increased number of functioning sweat glands, less sweat is lost from the body in the form of water droplets because of the fact that sweat is now more evently dispersed over the entire body surface, thus allowing for a greater amount of heat to be lost by way of water evaporation.

The drop in skin temperature provides for a better cooling of the blood flowing through the skin. Thus, the body can afford to cut down on the skin blood flow. It also means that an equivalent rate of sweating is obtained at a lower body surface temperature following heat acclimatization. The improved distribution of sweat over the surface of the skin is an advantage in hot and humid environments. The lower pulse rates appear to be a reflex action to the lower skin and internal body temperature. The reason for the increased stroke volume is not fully known. However, since cardiac output does not change as a result of heat acclimatization, it may be responding and adjusting to the lowered pulse rate and unchanged cardiac output. An increased venous blood flow to the right atrium does not appear to be adequate for the stroke volume changes. The improved liver and kidney blood flow is the result of the decreased blood flow to the skin. A large skin blood flow does not appear to be needed for the acclimatized person since heat dissipation is primarily provided by evaporation of sweat. Some researchers working in the area of heat acclimatization have also found a slight increase in plasma volume (about 5%), although this increase appears to be transitory and not permanent.

Finally, as heat acclimatization proceeds, subjective symptoms such as nausea, dizziness, and syncope (fainting) which are associated with heat exposure are progressively reduced until people are able to work without discomfort.

Although the rate of development of heat acclimatization is still debated among some investigations, most experts agree that even though few changes take place within the first 4 to 14 days, the best improvements in heat tolerance is generally brought about between 8 and 12 weeks of intensive interval or continuous endurance training. For best results, the training intensity should be greater than 50 percent of an individual's maximum oxygen uptake. Available evidence indicates that heat acclimatization is usually retained for several weeks following heat exposure.

At this point it should be emphasized that although physical training in a cool climate will improve the tolerance of an athlete to exercise in the heat as well as increase the rate of heat acclimatization, it still does not necessarily mean that he or she will be totally acclimatized to compete in the heat. In fact, unless time is devoted for exercising and training in the heat, performance for the athlete may be disappointing. In other words, physical conditioning can not take the place of acclimatization. If physical work is to be performed in the exposure to hot weather, then muscular work should be incorporated in the acclimatization period.

Heat acclimatization is apparently related directly to the conditions of exposure. For instance, investigators have found that people who live in hot climates are only partially acclimatized (about 50%) when compared with individuals who have been exercised and trained under controlled hot-room conditions. Also, if heat acclimatization has been carried out for a particular level of work for a given environment, then a person will not necessarily be acclimatized for a higher level of work even in the same identical environment. In addition, the person will not be prepared physiologically for a more severe climate. Further acclimatization takes place only if a person is exposed to a higher heat level. Finally, it is important to remember that during the period of acclimatization and heat exposure, it is vitally important that water and salt losses be replaced in order to maintain optimum health and performance.

XII. MAKING WEIGHT FOR WRESTLERS

One of the major complaints of amateur wrestling is the practice of rapid and extreme weight reduction. "Making weight" for wrestlers generally involves a combination of food restriction, fluid deprivation and dehydration. Physicians, athletic trainers, coaches, and professional groups are all in complete agreement in condemning the practice. In fact, most wrestlers dislike the crash methods, but they are apparently willing to utilize it in order to gain the advantages which it may give them (by being able to compete in weight classes below their normal body weight) or to protect themselves against opponents who also seek such advantages.

It is not unusual for wrestlers to lose up to 7 percent or more of their normal body weight within a period of one week in order to qualify for lower weight classes. Although several articles have been written by physicians as well as other professional groups warning against the possible health hazards that are associated with crash diets and dehydration, no conclusive pattern in the human research has been experimentally established to provide an objective evaluation of the practice from a health as well as physical performance viewpoint. While the research is somewhat inconclusive concerning the effect of rapid weight loss and dehydration on physical performance, athletes and responsible officials should be aware of the single or combined physiological effects that making weight by means of crash diets (such as food restriction) and dehydration (such as fluid deprivation) has on the human body. Physiological changes that are generally associated with these diet practices are:

(1) a decrease in muscular strength,
(2) a reduction in work performance time,
(3) a decrease in plasma and blood volume,
(4) a decrease in cardiac output,
(5) a decrease in oxygen consumption,
(6) a decrease in renal blood flow,
(7) a drop in liver glycogen stores,
(8) an increased amount of electrolytes being lost from the body,
(9) a decrease in the amount of fluid being filtered by the kidney,
(10) higher heart rates during submaximal work, and
(11) impairment of thermoregulatory processes.

Because it is possible for the above changes to hinder growth and development, there would appear to be no sound justification (physiological or medical) for use of the potential health hazard diets that are being presently followed by many wrestlers. The American College of Sports Medicine takes the position that these potential health hazards can be eliminated if state and national organizations will:

(1) Determine each wrestlers body composition several weeks prior to the competitive season and those whose fat content is less than 5 percent of their certified body weight should obtain medical clearance before being permitted to compete.

(2) Discourage wrestlers from consuming less than their minimal daily caloric needs without prior medical approval. The caloric needs should be determined on the basis of age, body surface area, growth and physical activity levels and obtained from a balanced diet. The minimal needs for high school and college wrestlers range from 1200 to 2400 kcal/day.

(3) Discourage the habit of fluid deprivation and dehydration by (a) educating the coaches and wrestlers on the physiological and medical consequences that can result, (b) prohibiting the use of rubber suits, steam rooms, hot boxes, saunas, laxatives, and diuretics to "make weight," (c) arranging for weigh-ins just before competition, and (d) arranging for more official weigh-ins between team matches.

(4) Allow for more participants per team to take part in those weight classes which have the highest number of wrestlers actually certified for competition.

(5) Standardize rules and regulations involving the wrestlers eligibility for the Championship tournaments. In other words, the wrestlers should only be allowed to compete in those weight classes in which they had the highest number of matches throughout the regular season.

(6) Encourage organizations at the local and county level to collect data on a regular basis involving the hydration state of wrestlers and its relationship to growth and development.

XIII. EXERCISE AND TEMPERATURE REGULATIONS IN COLD CLIMATES

Temperature regulation during work in a cold climate involve *vasoconstriction* and *shivering*. Vasoconstriction (narrowing of a blood vessel) of the skin blood vessels reduces heat loss by as much as 1/6 to 1/3 by reducing heat transfer from the deep core to the skin surface. Shivering, on the other hand, increases heat production. As a result of vasoconstriction, the effective thickness of the skin surface is enlarged and this lowers thermal conductivity from the interior. This is accomplished primarily by a reduction in blood flow, and partly because the blood in the veins of the limbs is shifted from the surface veins (that is so prominent in heat exposure) to the deep veins (Fig. 7-5). Since the routes of venous blood returning from the extremities may be shifted, a *countercurrent heat exchange* is set up. For example, it is generally known that arterial blood is cooled as it approaches the extremities, and venous blood is warmed as it returns to the deep core. This is clearly illustrated in Figure 7-5. Notice that when a subject is exposed to a cold external temperature of 10°C, the arterial blood leaving the chest will have a temperature of about 37°C. By the time the blood reaches the area of the wrist, it may be as low as 25°C. It is also important to notice in Figure 7-5 that as the venous blood approaches the area of the chest, it reaches a temperature of nearly 37°C. Because of the close proximity of the deep veins (or so-called *venae comitantes*) to the arteries, the venous blood absorbs a large portion of the heat as the arterial blood flows through the arm. According to some authorities, since cooling of arterial blood in the limbs is dependent upon the rewarming of cold blood returning in adjoining veins from more distal areas, cooling of the body core is prevented. This allows the deep core temperature to remain near the normal 37°C. Figure 7-5 also illustrates that when a subject is exposed to a hot environment of 30°C, the blood from the arm returns primarily through surface veins, which facilitates further cooling of the blood.

Upon exposure to cold temperatures, vasoconstriction and blood flow shifts are so efficient that they may actually cause the deep core temperature to increase as much as 0.5°C. In fact, in a cool environment, it has been estimated that because of vasoconstriction and blood flow shifts, heat loss from the hands and feet may be reduced to values as low as 2 percent of the total heat loss. On the other hand, in cold temperatures peripheral vasoconstriction also has a disadvantage. For instance, during vasoconstriction the temperature in the skin may approach that of the outside environment. If this occurs, one is likely to suffer cold fingers and toes.

Changes in the size of blood vessels and the vascular bed have only limited protective capacity against cold temperatures. When external temperatures are below 25°C the peripheral circulation of a nude man is maximally vasoconstricted, and therefore, he cannot maintain heat balance by additional vasomotor activity. Thus, with sufficient cold stimulus, another protective mechanism to maintain heat balance is an increase in metabolism brought on by either skeletal muscle activity or shivering.

A. SHIVERING

Shivering represents involuntary muscular activity and consists of synchronous activation of

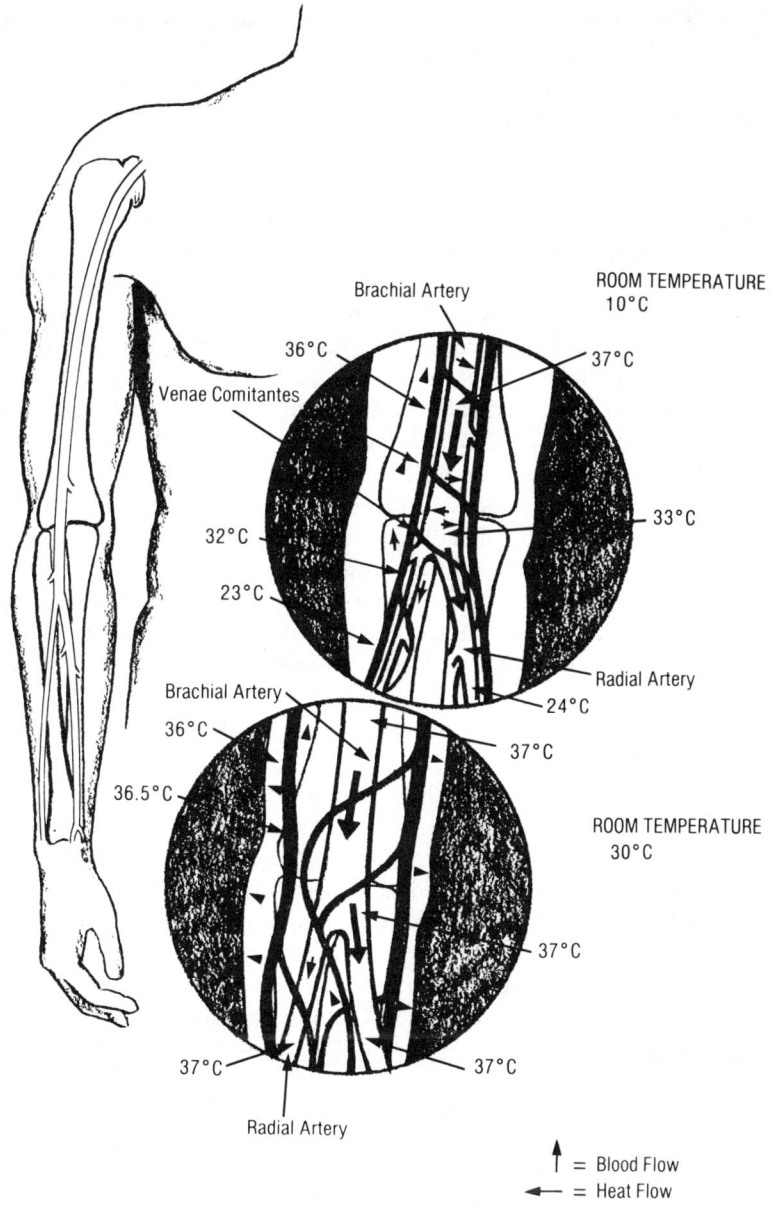

Figure 7-5 Schematic illustration of the countercurrent heat exchange in the human extremity.

nearly all muscle groups. In other words, the antagonists muscles of the body are actually contracting against each other. Shivering may be manifested as slight tensing of muscles with light chilling or, in the case of extremely cold weather, as uncontrollable whole body spasms or shakes. Shivering is commonly known to be an effective heat production mechanism in that all of the chemical energy released is converted to heat with no energy going toward work. Heat production from shivering is relatively high. In fact, evidence shows that shivering may produce as much as somewhere around 42.5 cal/hr, almost 7 times greater than man's normal resting metabolism at room temperature. A seminude man left in temperatures of 5°C for a period of 60 minutes will more than double his heat production by shivering. Naturally, with physical work the metabolic rate may be further increased in cold environments.

B. CLOTHING

Although clothing is important in terms of insulation for the inactive person in cold weather, an individual engaged in a strenuous winter sport such as skiing or speed skating needs little clothing because of his high heat production. Since vigorous activity may cause the metabolic rate to increase by as much as 25 to 30 times basal values, and since clothing may act as a partial water vapor barrier, it is obvious that clothes worn during muscular activity in cold weather can become a hinderance in the temperature regulation process. For instance, it is known that most active people generally sweat profusely even in cold environments, and if the clothing worn is heavy and allows for no ventilation, then the sweat is condensed in the clothing and hence does not achieve skin cooling. Eventually, however, during periods between work, the sweat evaporates and thus takes away from the body heat that it cannot afford to lose at that time. Therefore, an important consideration for individuals working in cold weather is that the clothing worn should allow for considerable ventilation as well as vapor permeability. While some people wear protective scarves or clothing over their faces to protect themselves against the possibility of chapped lips or a dry mouth and throat due to the low humidity in the cold air, it should be pointed out that there is no evidence at this time to indicate any lung tissue damage as a result of exercising in cold weather.

C. COLD ACCLIMATIZATION

It is generally known that repeated exposure to cold temperatures results in greater ability to tolerate cold. However, no definite pattern of acclimatization to cold environments has been reported for humans, and some investigators question the occurrence of such a pattern. On the other hand, animals kept at 5°C definitely indicate an acclimatization. This includes an increased metabolism of 50 to 100 percent, which is linked with a decrease of shivering activity (so-called *nonshivering thermogenesis*). It appears that this nonshivering thermogenesis may originate in the muscle tissue, but not from muscle contraction. The chemical mechanism of this extra metabolism has not yet been reported, however, it is possible that the hormones, *norepinephrine* and *thyroxine* play a major role in the elevation of the metabolic rate. Norepinephrine, injected into the acclimatized rat, may cause about a threefold increase in metabolism. Following a period of 3 to 4 weeks of human as well as animal cold acclimatization, the thyroid gland gradually enlarges, and thus increases the rate of thyroxine secretion. Apparently, this mechanism increases the basal metabolic rate by as much as 15 to 25 percent.

Although local skin cold acclimatization for the human is well defined, attempts to demonstrate whole body cold acclimatization in human populations have resulted in some contradictory as well as in unresolved problems of racial, ethnic, and dietary involvements. Nonetheless, the general trend of human cold acclimatization is hinted to be related to the following: (1) metabolic, (2) insulation, (3) hypothermic, and (4) peripheral circulation.

Some experiments in which human subjects have been chronically exposed to cold strongly suggest that increased heat production without shivering can be developed the same as it can in animals. In a study comparing thermoregulation in Eskimos and European (control) subjects, the non-shivering *metabolism* of the Eskimo natives was found to be abut 30 to 40 percent greater than that of the European controls. While it was suggested that this difference might have been due to the Eskimo's diet, another carefully controlled study with Alaskan natives showed that the higher non-shivering metabolism of the natives as compared to controls was not due to diet.

Environmental physiologists working with Korean and Japanese female divers found an increased basal metabolic rate (BMR) of 35 percent in winter water (air temperatures around 0°C and water temperatures around 10°C) as compared to a constant BMR for a group of non-diving control natives. Internal temperature for the divers was found to drop from 37°C to 33°C or less. It appears that these female divers are perhaps better insulated for winter temperatures than non-divers who are not acclimatized to be able to tolerate such low core temperatures. The better divers were also able to stay at the greatest depths for longer periods of time than the other divers.

On the other hand, when subjects were exposed for 8 hours per day at temperatures of 12.5°C over a 14 to 32-day period, a rapid fall in total metabolic heat production has been reported in some circles.

One of the few remaining groups of people that are consistently exposed to cold are the Australian Aborigines (stone-age people), who customarily sleep unclothed on the ground at night in near freezing temperatures. Information is available from this group of people to indicate that the cold conditions of which these people are exposed to have no effect on their metabolism. Evidence also is available to show that the *insulation* of the Australian Aborigines body shell was somewhat increased by vasoconstriction, and that the natives were able to tolerate moderate amounts of *hypothermia* (rectal temperature was reduced to 35°C). It appears that the Australian Aborigines have an inborn ability to tolerate greater body cooling without necessarily increasing metabolism. Most investigators have shown that internal body temperature is generally lower in the cold-acclimatized person than in the non-acclimatized person during standardized cold tests.

Peripheral adaptation to cold has been observed in Gaspe' Northern Norwegian fishermen. With this group of subjects, researchers have found evidence for local acclimatization to cold by having warmer finger temperatures in ice water than was found for a group of controls. With the immersion of both hands and feet in ice water, the fishermen gave lower pressor responses than did the controls. Eskimo natives have also shown to be able to maintain a higher rate of blood flow to their fingers during various cooling tests than a group of controls. Thus, it would appear that when a person allows his hand to be repeatedly exposed to cold for a period of time, this cold stress will eventually cause an increased blood flow through the hands. Although this will result in a greater amount of heat lost from the hands, it will improve the ability of them to perform hand and finger dexterity in the cold.

In summary, it is rather obvious that there is a need for more research in the area of whole body cold acclimatization in humans. These studies are needed for not only athletes competing in cold weather, but for those people who take part in recreational activities in cold climates as well as those who have to work 8 to 10 hours per day in this type of environment.

XIV. SUMMARY

(1) Heat loss occurs from the body by way of the skin, lungs, and excretions with the skin being the most important depending upon external and internal conditions (about 85% of heat is lost via the skin).

(2) Heat is lost from the skin by radiation, convection, evaporation, and conduction while heat gain is due primarily to metabolism that takes place in the tissues. Some heat gain may also result from radiation, convection, and conduction when the external temperature is higher than the body temperature.

(3) Body temperature is regulated mainly by the anterior and posterior hypothalamus centers. The anterior center controls heat dissipation events by causing vasodilatation in the blood vessels of the skin, while at the same time, stimulating activities of the respiratory center (causing panting) and the sweat glands. The posterior center controls heat conservation events by causing not only vasoconstriction in the skin blood vessels, but shivering activities as well as the erection of skin hairs (for purpose of increasing the insulating of the skin).

(4) The adrenal medulla, by releasing epinephrine and norepinephrine hormones into the blood, also play a part in the regulation of body temperature by both heat loss and heat conservation events. Note that these two hormones have the ability to not only increase the metabolic rate, but they may also cause vasoconstriction in the skin blood vessels.

(5) The thyroid endocrine glands aids in the regulation of body temperature by releasing the hormone called thyroid into the blood. The action of this hormone is to increase the metabolic rate and therefore increase heat production.

(6) The human body temperature is generally maintained within a relatively small range with the outer shell skin temperature being kept somewhere between 23°C and 34°C (depending on the external temperature as well as the amount of clothing being worn) and the inner core around 37°C.

(7) Human body temperature variations are functions of age, sex, diurnal changes, and individual differences.

(8) When exercising in hot weather, temperature regulation involves vasodilatation and sweating whereas work in cold weather includes vasoconstriction and shivering.

(9) Work performance in hot, humid weather is somewhat limited because of the rising body core temperature and strain that is placed on the cardiovascular system due to the ineffectiveness of the evaporative mechanisms for heat dissipation.

(10) Exercise performed in hot, dry conditions is rather limited because of the rising body core temperature and strain placed on the cardiovascular system due to dehydration.

(11) Effects of extreme heat can lead to the following heat disorders: (a) dehydration, (b) heat cramps, (c) heat exhaustion, and (d) heat stroke.

(12) The medical profession and other experts in the area of environmental physiology recommend the following for preventing heat illnesses:

    (a) encourage a pre-season training program,
    (b) practice in lightweight uniforms,
    (c) players should be weighed before and after workouts,
    (d) provide for adequate salt and water replacement,
    (e) allow for sufficient rest periods during practice,
    (f) workouts should be held in early mornings and late evenings, and
    (g) conduct daily dry-bulb and wet-bulb temperature readings.

(13) The following physiological adjustments are noticed while working in the heat following a period of acclimatization:

    (a) lower exercise pulse rate,
    (b) increased stroke volume,
    (c) increased sweat production
    (d) less amount of salt is lost in the sweat,
    (e) greater blood flow to liver and kidneys,
    (f) increased plasma volume,
    (g) lower skin and internal body temperature,

(h) better regulation of blood pressure, and

(i) improved distribution of sweat over surface of skin.

(14) Although the rate of development of heat acclimatization is still debated, it is generally agreed that some changes occur in about 4 to 14 days. However, the best improvements are believed to be brought about between 8 and 12 weeks of intensive interval or continuous endurance training. For best results, the training intensity should be greater than 50 percent of an individual's maximum oxygen uptake. These changes are generally retained for several weeks following heat exposure.

(15) When exercising in heat, the loss of body water is the most serious problem of sweating since it reduces the blood volume, cardiac output, stroke volume, and velocity of blood flow as well as leading to dehydration and a progressively increase in core temperature. Many problems associated with heat stress could be perhaps eliminated if the coach or trainer would see that the athlete consumed as much as one quart of water before practice or competition and every 10 to 15 minutes during practice, have water breaks for the players.

(16) Too much salt can be more detrimental and lead to serious medical problems for the athlete than too little salt. Caution should be taken when consuming large quantities of salt without sufficient water during practices and game situations. Experts agree that a minimum of 1 pint of water should be taken with each 7-grain salt tablet.

(17) Physicians, trainers, coaches, and the American College of Sports Medicine as well as other professional groups are all in complete agreement in condemning the practice of "making weight" for wrestlers by way of crash diets and dehydration because of the potential health hazards.

(18) It appears that the most serious problem that an athlete has during competition in cold weather is finding proper clothing that allows for maneuverability as well as adequate ventilation (for heat dissipation) and vapor permeability.

(19) Both physiological and psychological factors are probably involved in cold acclimatization with the following being the most important physiological factors: (a) metabolic (b) insulation, (c) hypothermic, and (d) peripheral circulation.

XV. REVIEW REFERENCES

(1) American College of Sports Medicine. "Position stand on weight loss in wrestlers," *Medicine and Science in Sports,* 8:xi-xiii, 1976.

(2) Bullard, R. W. "Temperature Regulation," in *Physiology,* 4th edition, (E. E. Selkurt, editor), Little, Brown, and Co., Boston, 1976.

(3) Downey, J. A. "Physiology of Temperature Regulation in Man," in *Physiological Basis of Rehabilitation Medicine,* (J. A. Downey and R. C. Darling, editors), W. B. Saunders Co., Philadelphia, 1971.

(4) Drinkwater, B. L., and S. M. Horvath. "Heat Tolerance and Aging," *Medicine and Science in Sports,* 11:49-55, 1979.

(5) Edington, D. W., and V. R. Edgerton. *The Biology of Physical Activity,* Houghton Mifflin Co., Boston, 1976.

(6) Folk, G. E., Jr. *Textbook of Environmental Physilogy,* 2nd edition, Lea & Febiger, Philadelphia, 1974.

(7) Gisolfi, C. V., and J. S. Cohen. "Relationships Among Training, Heat Acclimation, and Heat Tolerance in Men and Women: The Controversy Revisited," *Medicine and Science in Sports,* 11:56-59, 1979.

(8) Guyton, A. C. *Textbook of Medical Physiology,* 5th edition, W. B. Saunders Co., Philadelphia, 1976.

(9) Hubbard, R. W. "Effects of Exercise in the Heat on Predisposition to Heatstroke," *Medicine and Science in Sports,* 11:66-72, 1979.

(10) Lamb, D. R. *Physiology of Exercise: Responses and Adaptations,* Macmillan Publishing Co., New York, 1978.

(11) Mathews, D. K., and E. L. Fox. *The Physiological Basis of Physical Education and Athletics,* W. B. Saunders Co., Philadelphia, 2nd edition, 1976.
(12) Nadel, E. R. "Control of Sweating Rate While Exercising in the Heat," *Medicine and Science in Sports,* 11:31-35, 1979.
(13) Pandolf, K. B. "Effects of Physical Training and Cardiorespiratory Physical Fitness on Exercise-Heat Tolerance: Recent Observations;" *Medicine and Science in Sports,* 11:60-65, 1979.
(14) Roberts, M. F., and C. B. Wenger. "Control of Skin Circulation During Exercise and Heat Stress," *Medicine and Science in Sports,* 11:36-41, 1979.
(15) Roberts, M. F., C. B. Wenger, J. A. J. Stolwijk, and E. R. Nadel. "Skin Blood Flow and Sweating Changes Following Exercise Training and Heat Acclimation," *Journal of Applied Physiology,* 43:133-37, 1977.
(16) Rowell, L. B. "Human Cardiovascular Adjustments to Exercise and Thermal Stress," *Physiological Review,* 54:75-159, 1974.
(17) Senay, L. C., Jr. "Early Response of Plasma Contents on Exposure of Working Men to Heat," *Journal Applied Physiology,* 44:166-70, 1978.
(18) Senay, L. C., Jr. "Effects of Exercise in the Heat on Body Fluid Distribution," *Medicine and Science in Sports,* 11:42-48, 1979.

8

EXERCISE AND ALTITUDE

KEY CONCEPTS TO BE GAINED FROM THIS CHAPTER

(1) Physiologically, the most critical factor affecting physical performance at high altitude is the decreased partial pressure of oxygen which, in effect, decreases the arterial oxygen saturation of the blood.

(2) There are specific performance-related tasks in which a period of acclimatization to altitude is required.

(3) Several physiological adaptations take place during acclimatization to altitude that is conducive to increased efficiency.

(4) The specific training and conditioning effects at altitude depend largely upon not only the individual, but also the type of exercise as well as the previous level of training.

(5) Exposure to altitude may result in a functional disorder known as mountain or altitude sickness.

Prior to the 1968 Olympic Games in Mexico City (altitude of approximately 7,300 feet or about 2,300 meters), scientific studies of work performance at high altitudes had been concerned primarily with problems of military significance or of mountaineering expeditions. Now, however, there is a tremendous interest in the effects of altitude on athletic performance. In fact, every large country and several of the smaller ones have undertaken investigations both at home and abroad to determine the specific effects of high altitude on sports performance. Several international symposia have recently been conducted to discuss problems related to work performance at high altitude. Thus, it is quite obvious that the interest in the effect of altitude on human performance is considerable. The purpose of this chapter is to discuss the limitations imposed on physical performance by high altitude.

I. EFFECTS OF HIGH ALTITUDE ON PHYSICAL PERFORMANCE

A. DECREASE IN TOTAL BAROMETRIC PRESSURE

It is well known that as we ascend to higher and higher altitudes, the total barometric pressure* decreases because of the decreased weight of the atmosphere (Table 8-1). Since the force of gravity is somewhat smaller at high altitude than at sea level, the energy required to lift the body as in the pole vault and high jump would be theoretically decreased. As most authorities recognize, however, the practical effect on physical performance is probably quite small.

B. DECREASE IN PARTIAL PRESSURE OF OXYGEN

Although the percentage of oxygen in the atmosphere (20.93%) remains the same regardless of altitude (the number of oxygen molecules per unit volume decreases, however, which means that in order to receive the same number of molecules in a given breath of air at high altitude that we receive at sea level, we must take in more air), the decreased barometric pressure causes the partial pressure of oxygen (P_{O_2}) to be decreased (Table 8-1). The decreased oxygen pressure at high altitude decreases the arterial oxygen saturation of blood (Table 8-1) which, in turn, decreases the amount of oxygen available to the working tissues. Physiologically, the decreased P_{O_2} is the most critical factor of high altitude because the individual's work capacity depends largely upon his ability to take in and utilize oxygen rapidly.*

C. DECREASE IN DENSITY OF AIR

In addition to the diminished pressure of oxygen in the atmosphere, there are additional features of the high altitude environment that should be mentioned. For example, the decreased density of the air reduces the resistance of the airways to the flow of air into and out of the lungs. This permits greater volumes of air to be taken in during work with no significant increase in ventilation cost. The reduced density of the air acts in favor of those performances in which air resistance is a factor (sprint-type activities, jumping, pole vaulting, weight throwing, and other high-velocity events which are powered largely by anaerobic metabolism). In the 1968 Olympic games in Mexico City, it was determined by the United States Ballistic Research Laboratory that the four weight throwing events had theoretical advantages of: 6 cm for the shot put; 53 cm for the hammer throw; 69 cm for the javelin; and 162 cm for the discus.

Table 8-1. Effect of Altitude on Barometric Pressure, Atmospheric and Alveolar Oxygen Concentrations, and Arterial Oxygen Saturation

Altitude (ft)	Barometric Pressure (mm Hg)	Atmospheric P_{O_2} (mm Hg)	Alveolar P_{O_2} (mm Hg)	Arterial Oxygen Saturation (%)
0	760	159	104	97
10,000	523	110	67	90
20,000	349	73	40	70
30,000	226	47	21	20
40,000	141	29	8	5

*Note that barometric pressure reflects the force of earth's gravity acting on the atmosphere; therefore the atmospheric pressure is greatest at the surface of the earth and gradually gets smaller as one moves to higher altitudes.

*When the arterial oxygen saturation of the blood drops to somewhere between 25 and 50%, unconsciousness generally occurs. Because of this, pilots and mountain climbers are required to use oxygen at altitudes over 20,000 feet (Table 8-1).

D. COOLER AND DRYER AIR

The air is generally cooler and dryer at high altitude. Although the cooler temperature makes work more pleasant, and in fact, can help performances involving prolonged exertion, the dryer air can also increase the water loss from the respiratory tract which may contribute to the dehydration of exercise. Also, dryness of the throat is often experienced by athletes as a result of the dry air.

E. SUNBURN AND SNOW BLINDNESS

It is not uncommon for skiers and mountaineers to experience sunburns and snow blindness at high altitude. The reasons for this is because solar radiation is much more intense at high altitude than at sea level and because the skin tends to be dryer (due to the fact that the winds generally blow harder at higher elevations) at high altitudes. Skin burns at high altitude are also related to the decreased density of the air.

There is no doubt that in all events (aerobic-type) in which prolonged exertion is involved there is a decrement in performance at high altitude. In swimming, this means that a decrease in performance takes place at any event over 200 meters, and in running, at any distance of 800 meters or more. This was clearly shown in the Pan-American Games at Mexico City in 1955 and in the pre-Olympics in 1965 and 1966. For example, in free style swimming, although the best time for 100 meters was only 3.2 seconds over the world record, at 400 meters it was 11.2 seconds and at 1,500 meters was 15 seconds greater, and 3,000 meters was 32.15 seconds greater. These findings are logical in terms of our understanding of the ATP and CP system and the aerobic and anaerobic energy pathways discussed in Chapter 2. Recall that the body is able to provide energy via the ATP and CP and anaerobic systems for short periods of time without large quantities of oxygen. Thus, any activity that can be performed before the depletion of readily available energy stores in the body will not be affected by the decreased P_{O_2} at high altitude, whereas those activities requiring energy from the aerobic (with oxygen) pathways are affected significantly.

II. PHYSIOLOGICAL ADAPTATIONS TO ALTITUDE

What are the physiological adjustments of which an individual is capable to help him to perform work more efficiently at high altitude? These are extremely complex and still only partially understood. However, the primary problems that the body encounters is to adjust for the decrease in pressure gradients of oxygen, which takes place between: (a) tracheal air and alveolar air, (b) alveolar air and arterial oxygen, (c) arterial oxygen and capillary oxygen, and (d) capillary oxygen and venous oxygen. These are illustrated in Figure 3-9 in Chapter 3.

The human body adjust for this decrease in pressure gradients of oxygen by altering its respiratory and cardiovascular responses to exercise and work in several ways. They are: (a) an augmented pulmonary ventilation, (b) an enlarged hemoglobin concentration in the blood, (c) a greater diffusing capacity of the lungs, (d) an increased vascularity of the tissues, (e) an increased myoglobin content of the muscles, and (f) a greater ability of the cells to adjust to the low partial pressure of oxygen and make use of the available oxygen.

A. AN AUGMENTED PULMONARY VENTILATION

Initially, the rate and depth of pulmonary ventilation increases to a maximum of about 65 percent. Although this is an immediate compensation for the high altitude, if the individual remains at high altitude for several days, his ventilation may eventually increase to as much as 5 to 7 times normal. The principal cause of this increase is as follows:

158 Essentials of Exercise Physiology

The initial increase of 65 percent in pulmonary ventilation not only provides more oxygen, but at the same time, the increased ventilation tends to "blow off" large quantities of carbon dioxide (at the same time, the hydrogen ion concentration is reduced), which results in a lowered partial pressure of carbon dioxide (P_{CO_2}). This, in turn, brings about a respiratory alkalosis (increased pH of body fluids) and a shift in the oxygen dissociation curve to the left. (Note that a complete discussion of the oxygen dissociation curve may be found in Chapter 3). At altitude, both of these changes inhibit rather than aid the stimulus for increased ventilation from the lowered oxygen pressure (hypoxia). However, two important effects occur during the following days to nullify this inhibition. First, the inhibitory effect (on the respiratory center) caused by the low P_{CO_2} slowly fades away so that this is no longer a handicap to increased ventilation. Second, by reducing the blood bicarbonate level, the kidneys gradually restores the acid-base balance (the high pH) back to normal.

It should be pointed out that the lowered blood bicarbonate level not only reduces the buffer capacity of the blood, but with it, the ability to tolerate high blood lactic acid levels. This means that anaerobic capacity, which is normal on the immediate arrival at high altitude, is gradually lowered during continued stay. On the other hand, however, as a result of these changes, the respiratory center now responds with full force to the chemoreceptor stimuli resulting from low oxygen pressure, and the ventilation increases to approximately 5 to 7 times normal. This slow process of developing more and more ventilation is referred to as *acclimatization* to high altitude.

Figure 8-1 illustrates the typical breathing response at different altitudes during exercises of comparable work loads. It is quite clear that the overall trend is similar at sea level and higher altitudes, in that at all levels there is nearly a linear relationship between ventilation and oxygen consumption until maximum oxygen uptake values are obtained. Once maximum oxygen uptake values have been reached, the greater disproportionately increases in ventilation is obviously due to the build-up of lactic acid (end product of anaerobic metabolism) and the role that the respiratory system plays in buffering the lactic acid. Thus, traveling to high altitudes apparently has very little effect on maximal ventilation even though investigators have found both increases and decreases.

B. AN ENLARGED HEMOGLOBIN CONCENTRATION IN THE BLOOD

Another adjustment in which the body makes that favors acclimatization is an increase in the number of red blood cells, for hypoxia causes rapid production of these cells by the bone marrow. Usually, in full acclimatization to low oxygen the hematocrit (the percentage, by volume, of the red blood cells in the whole blood) increases from a normal value of 40 (women) to 45 (men) percent to an average of about 59 percent which, in turn, increases the blood viscosity. At the same time, the hemoglobin concentration increases from the normal 15 grams percent to an average of approximately 20 grams percent. The increases in hematocrit and hemoglobin concentrations are probably due to the overall decreases in plasma volume.

In addition, the blood volume generally increases by as much as 20 to 30 percent. This results in a 50 to 90 percent total increase in circulating hemoglobin. What is the effect of the increase in red cells and hemoglobin on cardiac function? Experimentally, it has been found that an increase in blood hematocrit above the normal level of 40 to 45 percent reduces the cardiac output because of increased blood viscosity; as a result, at altitude, this means that the heart must do more work in order to compensate for the increased blood viscosity. In fact, if it were not for a capacity for adjusting the number of open capillaries (note that this will be discussed later) the work of the heart at altitude would be greatly increased.

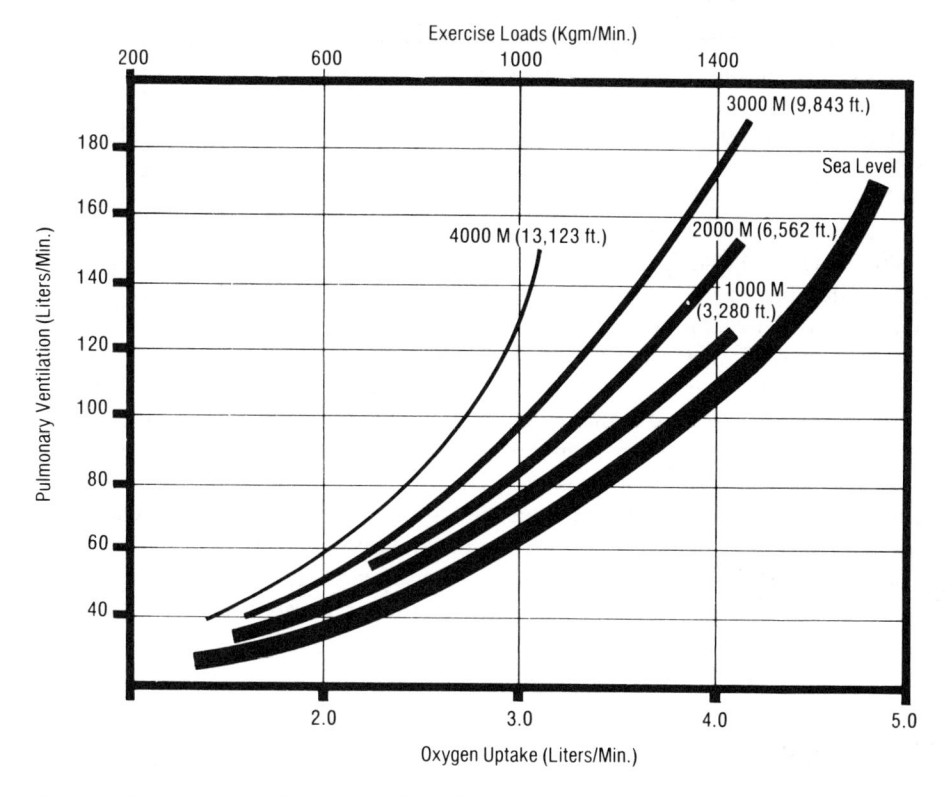

Figure 8-1 Schematic illustration of the breathing response at various altitudes during exercises of comparable work loads.

At this point, it should be mentioned, however, that the formation of many new cells is a rather slow process requiring at least several weeks to help acclimate a person to high altitudes. Prolonged residence at altitudes as low as 12,000 feet often develop red blood cell counts as high as 7 to 8 million per cu. mm as compared with the normal count of 5 million.

C. GREATER DIFFUSING CAPACITY OF THE LUNGS

Another acclimatization modification of the respiratory system at altitude is a greater diffusing capacity of the lungs. The normal diffusing capacity for oxygen through the pulmonary membrane is around 20 ml per mm Hg pressure gradient per second. During exercise at sea level or at high altitude, this diffusing capacity can increase as much as 3 times its normal figure. Two reasons are generally given for this increase: (1) an augmented pulmonary capillary blood volume, which expands the capillaries and increases the surface through which oxygen can diffuse into the blood, and (2) an augmented lung volume, which presumably expands the surface area of the alveolar membrane.

D. AN INCREASED VASCULARITY OF THE TISSUES

When a person moves from sea level to high altitudes, there is an immediate increase in heart rate and in cardiac output during rest (often as much as 10 to 20 percent) and submaximal exercise (as much as 20 to 30 percent). As acclimation proceeds, heart rate usually falls back to normal sea level rates. Cardiac output generally follows the same pattern as heart rate, however, it has been shown by several researchers that even after an adjustment period of some 10 weeks, sea level values for cardiac output are usually not obtained. This initial increase in cardiac output is apparently primarily dependent on the increased heart rate and not the stroke volume. For example, higher heart rates have been reported by several researchers for submaximal exercises at higher altitudes than for corresponding work at sea level. Since altitude investigators on stroke volume have shown either a decrease or a slight increase for submaximal exercise of such small magnitude, it definitely could not account for the major portion of the increased output. At the same time, however, stroke volume apparently takes on a greater proportion of the cardiac output as the intensity of work increases.

While maximum exercise cardiac output is affected very little at intermediate altitudes (13,000 feet), it may be reduced significantly at extremely high altitudes with the decrease due primarily to a reduced maximum exercise heart rate. For instance, normal exercise cardiac outputs of 22 to 25 liters per minute at sea level have been shown to drop as low as 16 to 17 liters per minute at 19,000 feet with a simultaneous reduction in maximum exercise heart rate from 192 (at sea level) to 135 (at 19,000 feet) beats per minute and only a slight reduction in stroke volume. The explanation for the reduction in maximum exercise heart rate at high altitude has been linked to not only the increased blood volume and blood viscosity, but also to hypoxia's (lowered oxygen pressure) direct effect on the heart.

During the course of exercise at moderate altitude, maximum oxygen uptake decreases. Since the maximal values for heart rate, stroke volume, and cardiac output are affected very little during acute exposure to altitudes up to around 13,000 to 14,000 feet, the reduction in maximum oxygen uptake must be due entirely to the decrease in the oxygen content of the arterial blood (Table 8-1). For example, it has been illustrated quite clearly that when subjects perform all-out work at a simulated altitude of 13,200 feet (4,000 meters), they are only able to obtain maximum oxygen uptake values of around 72 percent of their sea-level values. At the same time, their arterial oxygen content values reach only about 74 percent of their sea-level values. Maximum cardiac output, on the contrary, reaches values as high as 100 percent of the sea-level values.

Another adjustment in which the body makes that favors acclimatization is an apparent increase in the number of capillaries along with a better distribution of blood to the areas (such as the muscles, heart, brain, and other organs that normally require large amounts of oxygen increases) where gas exchange is needed for optimal performance. This means that the hemoglobin molecule comes into much closer contact with the active tissue cells than normally and, as a result, provides a supply of oxygen to each cell even with a somewhat lower oxygen tension. Evidence of a slight increase in arterial blood pressure has been found along with a drop in total peripheral resistance as a result of vasodilatation. This obviously indicates a better overall distribution of blood to the tissues and is brought about by the opening up of new capillaries in the small blood vessels in order to suit the character of the blood flowing through them.

E. AN INCREASED MYOGLOBIN CONTENT OF THE MUSCLES

In addition to the above mentioned favorable altitude adjustments, there also is an increase in myoglobin, the oxygen carrying pigment in the muscle. Information is available to indicate that with prolonged stay at altitude, the myoglobin concentration in both the heart and the skeletal muscles increases, which obviously favors acclimatization to high altitude.

F. A GREATER ABILITY OF THE CELLS TO ADJUST TO THE LOW PARTIAL PRESSURE OF OXYGEN AND MAKE USE OF THE AVAILABLE OXYGEN

It is generally known that human beings that are native to high altitudes of 13,000 to 17,000 feet have a greater number of certain cellular oxidative enzyme systems than those individuals who live at sea level. It is apparent that these human beings can utilize oxygen that is available much more effectively than the sea level inhibitants.

It is interesting to note, however, that non-native human beings who have been exposed to high altitudes for as long as a year do not encounter similar increases in oxidative enzymes. Thus, it is likely that the increased oxidative enzyme systems experienced by native human beings ("naturally acclimatized" persons) results from either (1) many years of existance at high altitudes, or (2) from genetic differences that have come about through generations of selection at these altitudes.

It is of further interest to note that naturally acclimatized individuals can survive for several hours at altitudes of approximately 30,000 feet without needing supplemental oxygen. Needless to say, this would be lethal to even the best acclimatized non-native.

At this point in our discussion, it should be pointed out that once a person returns to sea level following several weeks of stay at high altitude, all of the physiological changes brought about by acclimatization will be lost within a period of about 2 weeks. However, continued training at sea level will apparently delay these losses. More will be said about training at high altitude and returning to sea level later in this chapter.

III. ALTITUDE TRAINING AND CONDITIONING

A. EVENT TO BE PERFORMED

It is generally agreed among researchers in the area of altitude that any event (performed at altitude) lasting more than 2 minutes will require a period of training at altitude in order to obtain optimal performance. At the same time, it should be pointed out that although athletes performing in competitive events of a few seconds to 2 minutes duration (anaerobic-type activities which include sudden bursts of muscular strength such as jumping and throwing or speed events such as sprinting) are unaffected at altitude because they do not require optimal circulatory and respiratory adaptations, complete recovery from this type of work will require a longer period of time (in order to pay off the oxygen debt) than at sea level.

B. TIME REQUIRED FOR ACCLIMATIZATION

As Figure 8-2 illustrates, although the time necessary to acclimatize to altitude is directly related to the preceding training state of the individual athlete (for example, a well-trained individual will acclimatize more rapidly than an untrained person), it is generally agreed among altitude experts that a minimum period of 3 weeks is needed for acclimatization to take place at altitudes of 2,000 meters or higher involving aerobic-type activities. At lower elevations, the period required is probably less. It is interesting to note that at Mexico City (elevation of approximately 7,300 feet or about 2,300 meters) during the 1968 Olympics most physiological adaptations were accomplished within 2 to 3 weeks. While it is interesting to note that age is apparently not a hindrance to acclimatization, it should also be remembered that no matter how well acclimatized an individual becomes, performance or aerobic activities will always suffer to a certain degree at high altitude.

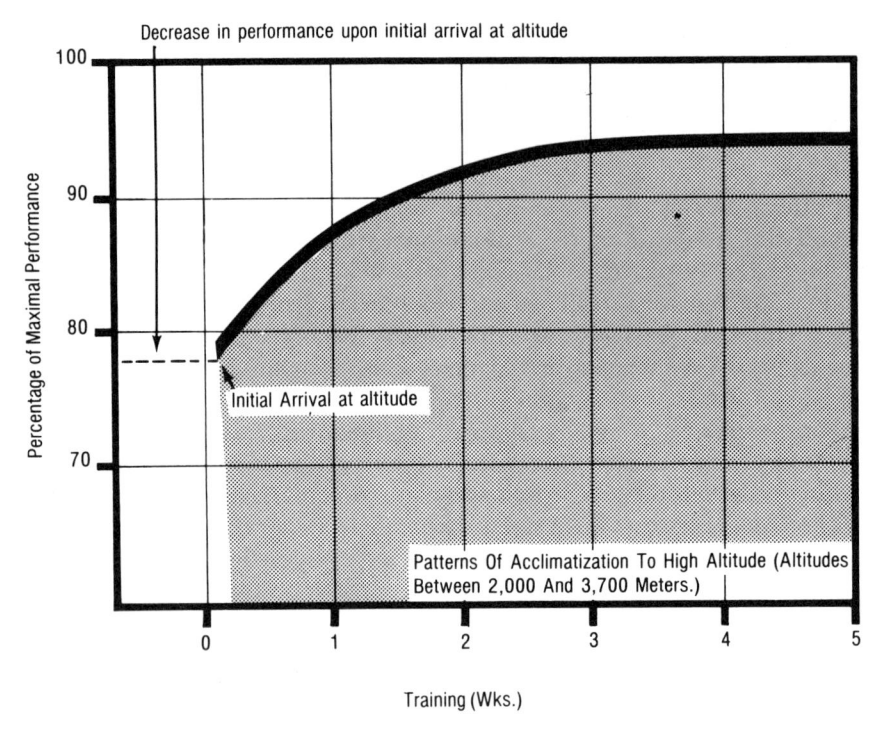

Figure 8-2 Schematic illustration of time needed for acclimatization to take place at high altitudes.

C. INTENSITY REQUIRED FOR TRAINING

With regard to the intensity of training at altitude, some exercise physiologists recommend that during the first week at altitude the work intensities should be rather light, followed by a gradual increase to the maximum. For athletes, some authorities recommend starting immediately, at a high intensity, in order that they quickly become accustomed to the changed conditions. While this procedure apparently presents no danger to the health of the athlete, it is obviously not recommended for the sedentary person who is going from sea level to high altitude. Other experts in this area have pointed out that the exercise intensity should be as high as possible in order to minimize the detraining effects that normally come about from the fact that maximal training intensity at altitude is usually lower than that at sea level.

Although training programs similar to those used at sea level can apparently be incorporated at high altitude, one should be aware of the fact that muscular fatigue will generally set in earlier. This means that during training at high altitude, one is forced to accept a slower tempo as well as a reduced intensity and duration. It also appears that intermittent training at sea level and moderate altitude may be beneficial in improving performance at altitude. As one might expect, this type of program would permit the individual to maintain his or her muscle power status during sea level competition and also adjust to the thinner atmosphere during high altitude competition. One variation of this type of training that has shown to be successful at an altitude of 2,300 meters is training for a period of 9 days at altitude and 5 days at sea level. This is followed by 9 more days at altitude and 7 more days at sea level, and finally 16 days at altitude with a final return to sea level.

Since detraining effect increases with altitude, there appears to be no evidence that performance is improved by training at a higher altitude than for performance at a lower altitude. In fact, according to some experts, a longer period of altitude training than necessary may even be detrimental to performance, because of a detraining effect on the muscles.

D. TRAINING AT ALTITUDE AND RETURNING TO SEA LEVEL

Although training at altitude improves performance at altitude, there is little evidence to suggest that it improves performance of highly trained athletes after returning to sea level (more than sea level training would). This is illustrated quite clearly in Figure 8-3. In this illustration, the subjects were college runners who trained for approximately 4 weeks at each altitude before returning to sea level. The training intensity for each altitude is shown in the illustration.

While there is little evidence to indicate that training at altitude improves the performance of highly trained athletes after returning to sea level, one possible exception is that the anaerobic capacity of the body may be increased slightly by high altitude training. It has been suggested that this increase in anaerobic capacity might be due, in part, to the increased myoglobin content, or to an augumented buffering capacity. Another suggestion has been that it might be due to an increase in the pain threshold.

It has been indicated by some that one of the major reasons for not finding any improvement in highly trained athletes once they return to sea level is because the training intensity and duration that is required for these athletes (to reach peak performance) cannot be achieved at

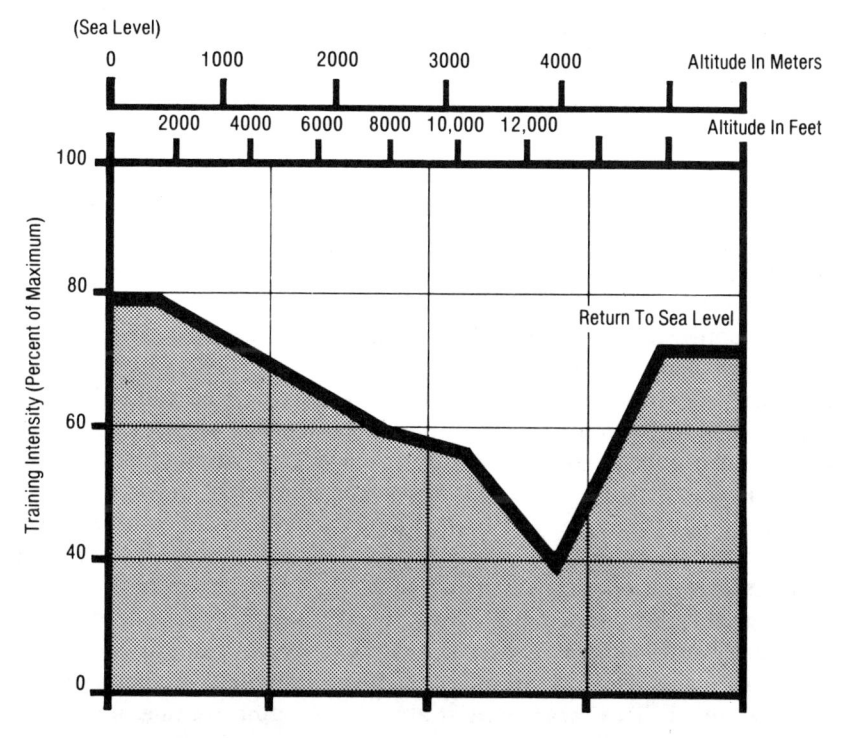

Figure 8-3 Schematic illustration of training at high altitude and returning to sea level.

altitude the same as it can at sea level. Figure 8-3 is a typical illustration of how altitude reduces the training intensity or efforts of trained athletes at various altitudes.

It is interesting to note that some investigators have shown that training at altitude may improve performance in unconditioned, nonathletic individuals once they return to sea level. However, it should be pointed out that in these particular reports the improved sea level performances were not determined if they were due solely to the altitude training or to just the altitude exposure itself. In other words, the unconditioned individuals (with probably having a lot of room for improvement) could possibly have improved their performance with additional training even at sea level.

At this point, it should be mentioned that some of the physiological changes (for instance, the reduction in blood bicarbonate that takes place at altitude which results in a reduced buffer capacity for lactic acid) resulting from altitude training may actually hinder performance at sea level.

It appears that athletes who reside and train at high altitude do not perform significantly better than athletes who train at sea level and then become acclimatized to the high altitude. A substantial amount of evidence has shown that athletes who train at high altitude do not necessarily perform better at sea level than athletes who train at sea level.

E. INDIVIDUAL DIFFERENCES

In addition, it should be remembered that because of individual differences in ability to acclimatize, some individuals will require longer periods of time to adjust to high altitude than others, while at the same time, some may never acclimatize In fact, there are examples of long-distance athletes who perform outstanding at sea level, but consistently fail at high altitude.

IV. MOUNTAIN (OR ALTITUDE) SICKNESS

The decrease in the oxygenation of the blood brought on by low atmospheric oxygen pressure, induces a functional disorder known as *mountain or altitude sickness*. Individuals who have trouble becoming acclimatized to high altitude will generally suffer from mountain sickness. The symptoms include nausea, vomiting, headache, insomnia, acceleration of heart rate, cyanosis, gastrointestinal disturbances, lack of appetite, apathy, euphoria, deterioration of neuro-muscular coordination, diminution of visual acuity, decrease in auditory perception, fatigue, and lowered stamina.

It appears that the greatest incidence of symptoms are noticed within 2 to 12 hours after arrival at altitude, and most people apparently become symptom-free within 5 to 7 days. Both the trained and untrained athlete may experience various degrees of mountain sickness. Reduced work efficiency is apparent (for both the trained and untrained) during this period of time. However, due to the fact that the well-trained athlete is able to tolerate unpleasant physical handicaps better than the untrained allows him to function more efficiently; and therefore, enables him to accomplish physically demanding tasks.

Various drugs have been tested in an attempt to reduce the severity of mountain sickness. *Acetazolamide* and *benzolamide* have been reported to reduce the severity of symptoms at 4,300 meters. Both drugs are classified as carbonic anhydrase inhibitors, and they act to increase renal excretion of bicarbonate. This means that at altitude the compensating increase in the rate of bicarbonate excretion generally taking place with respiratory alkalosis is accelerated by these drugs. It should be pointed out that although these agents are quite effective in reducing the severity of mountain sickness, the effects on work performance have not been adequately determined.

Severe cases of mountain sickness bring on symptoms similar to pneumonia; that is, fever, coughing, and congestion of the lungs (note that severe cases of mountain sickness can develop at elevations as low as 2,300 meters or 7,300 feet). In fact, several people have been known to die from severe cases of mountain sickness in recent years. This apparently occurred because the victims were believed to be suffering from pneumonia and, as a result, were given antibiotics while remaining at high altitude. Emergency treatment includes oxygen therapy and removal to lower altitude. The patient should see a physician at once.

V. SUMMARY

(1) As one ascends to high altitude, the decreased barometric pressure causes the partial pressure of oxygen to also be reduced. The decreased oxygen pressure decreases the arterial oxygen saturation of the blood which, in turn, decreases the amount of oxygen available to the working muscles.

(2) The decreased density of the air at altitude favors those performances (requiring a few seconds to 2 minutes) in which air resistance is a factor such as sprint-type activities, jumping, pole vaulting, weight throwing, and other high-velocity events which are powered mainly by anaerobic metabolism. Activities lasting more than 2 minutes in which aerobic (oxygen) energy is absolutely essential will be hampered at altitude.

(3) While the cooler air at altitude makes exercise more pleasant and comfortable, the dryer air at altitude can also increase the water loss from the respiratory tract which may contribute to dehydration.

(4) Physiological alterations induced by altitude acclimatization are as follows:

   (a) increased pulmonary ventilation,
   (b) increased number of red blood cells,
   (c) increased blood volume and hemoglobin,
   (d) increased diffusing capacity of the lungs,
   (e) increased vascularity of the tissues,
   (f) better distribution of blood to the active tissue cells,
   (g) greater ability of the cells to adjust to the low partial pressure of oxygen and make use of the available oxygen, and
   (h) increased myoglobin concentration.

(5) Although the time required to acclimatize to altitude is directly related to the individual as well as the preceding training state of the individual, it is generally agreed that a minimum period of approximately 2 to 3 weeks is needed for acclimatization to take place at altitudes of 2,300 meters (7,300) involving aerobic-type activities. At higher elevations, the period should be extended, while at lower elevation the time is slightly less. It is important to remember that no matter how well acclimatized an individual becomes, because lactic acid increases more steadily and at lower work loads, performance of aerobic activities will always suffer to a certain degree at high altitude. Acclimatization changes will be lost relatively quick following the return to sea level.

(6) While training programs similar to those used at sea level can be used for training at high altitude one should be aware that because muscular fatigue sets in earlier (lactic acid rises more readily and at lower work levels) at altitude, one is forced to accept a slower tempo as well as a reduced intensity and duration.

(7) Altitude training may improve performance at sea level for the unconditioned, nonathletic person, but because the training intensity and duration that is required for the highly trained athlete (in order to reach peak performance) cannot be achieved at altitude the same as it can at sea level, this improved performance is not found for highly conditioned athletes.

(8) Exposure to altitude may result in a functional disorder known as mountain or altitude sickness. Symptoms include nausea, vomiting, headache, insomnia, acceleration of heart rate, cyanosis, gastrointestinal disturbances, lack of appetites, apathy, euphoria, deterioration of neuro-muscular coordination, diminution of visual acuity, decrease in auditory perception, fatigue, and lowered stamina.

(9) Emergency treatment of severe mountain sickness involves oxygen therapy and removal to lower altitude. The patient should obtain the services of a physician at once.

VI. REVIEW REFERENCES

(1) Bhattacharjya, B. *Mountain Sickness,* John Wright and Sons, Ltd., Bristol, 1964.
(2) Dill, D. B., K. Braithwaite, W. C. Adams, and E. M. Bernauer. "Blood Volume of Middle-Distance Runners: Effect of 2,300-m Altitude and Comparison with Non-Athletes," *Medicine and Science in Sports,* 6:1-7, 1974.
(3) Evans, W. O., S. M. Robinson, D. H. Horstman, R. E. Jackson, and R. B. Weiskopf. "Amelioration of the Symptoms of Acute Mountain Sickness by Staging and Acetazolamide," *Aviation and Space Environmental Medicine,* 47:512-16, 1976.
(4) Goddard, R. F. (editor). *The International Symposium on the Effects of Altitude on Physical Performance,* The Athletic Institute, Chicago, 1967.
(5) Horstman, D. H., R. Weiskopf, and S. Robinson. "The Nature of the Perception of Effort at Sea Level and High Altitude," *Medicine and Science in Sports,* 11:150-54, 1979.
(6) Kollias, J., and E. R. Buskirk. "Exercise and Altitude," in *Science and Medicine of Exercise and Sport,"* 2nd edition, (W. R. Johnson and E. R. Buskirk, editors), Harper and Row, Publishers, New York, 1974.
(7) Krissoff, W. B., and B. Eiseman. "The Hazards of Exercising at Altitude," *The Physician and Sportsmedicine,* 3:26-31, 1975.
(8) Margaria, R. (editor). *Exercise at Altitude,* Excerpta Medica Foundation, New York, 1967.
(9) Ryan, A. J. "The Olympic Games at Altitude," in *American Academy of Orthopadic Surgeons Symposium on Sports Medicine,* The C. V. Mosby Co., Saint Louis, 1969.
(10) Sime, F., D. Penaloza, L. Ruiz, N. Gonzales, E. Covarrubias, and R. Postigo, "Hypoxemai, Pulmonary Hypertension, and Low Cardiac Output in Newcomers at Low Altitude," *Journal of Applied Physiology,* 36:561-65, 1974.
(11) Vogel, J. A., H. Hartley, J. C. Cruz, and R. P. Hogan, "Cardiac Output During Exercise in Sea-Level Residents at Sea Level and High Altitude," *Journal of Applied Physiology,* 36:169-72, 1974.
(12) Vogel, J. A., L. H. Hartley, and J. C. Cruz. "Cardiac Output During Exercise in Altitude Natives at Sea Level and High Altitude," *Journal of Applied Physiology,* 36:173-76, 1974.
(13) Weihe, W. H. (editor). *The Physiological Effects of High Altitude,* The Macmillan Co., New York, 1964.

9

NUTRITION, WEIGHT CONTROL AND PERFORMANCE

KEY CONCEPTS TO BE GAINED FROM THIS CHAPTER

(1) While carbohydrate and fat constitute the major fuels for muscular activity, the relative contribution of each to the total metabolism during work varies with the preceding diet, with the intensity and duration of work, and with the training of the subject.

(2) Although they are not considered as major energy nutrients, proteins, vitamins, minerals, and water are essential for the diet and maintenance of health.

(3) Composition of the pre-game meal does not effect muscular efficiency during short-term events, however, for long-term activity (such as an hour or longer), efficiency and performance is generally higher when the meal favors carbohydrates.

(4) Although the carbohydrate-loading technique may increase the glycogen content of a muscle and thus the endurance capacity of athletes, there are also disadvantages for which the person should be informed.

(5) The most effective method of losing weight is through a combined cardiorespiratory-endurance exercise and diet program over a relatively long period of time.

A basic understanding of nutrition and its effects upon health, weight control, and physical performance is essential for all people, including the coach, trainer, and athlete. An athlete's performance may be improved with good, sound nutrition, while at the same time, it may deteriorate with poor nutritional practices.

Overweight or obese is one of the major risk factors in cardiovascular disease, and inactivity is believed to be the primary cause of it. Underweight, while it does not appear to present the same type of health problems that overweight does, it still may cause nervous and respiratory disturbances. Individuals who experience a constant weight fluctuation may also be faced with a troubled endocrine system which plays a major role in controlling metabolism. At any rate, good nutrition plays an important part in maintaining proper weight control and in preventing possible diseases. The purpose of this chapter is to discuss nutrition and its effects upon weight control and athletic performance.

I. GENERAL NUTRIENTS OF THE DIET

As stated in Chapter 2, carbohydrates and fats constitute the major energy nutrients of the diet. However, proteins, vitamins, minerals, and water are also important and essential for the diet and maintenance of health.

A. CARBOHYDRATES

The main function of carbohydrates is to furnish energy to the millions of cells within the human body. Carbohydrates, which make up approximately 50 percent of the average American diet, are classified as either *monosaccharides, disaccharides,* or *polysaccharides.* All carbohydrates in the diet must be reduced to monosaccharides by way of digestion before they can be used by the body as a source of energy.

The most common or simplest monosaccharide (one that has a single 6-carbon sugar molecule) carbohydrate is *glucose* which can be oxidized and used directly by the body for energy, or it may be broken down by the digestive system and converted into *glycogen* (a polysaccharide) and stored in the muscle and liver for later use.

It is interesting to note that once the storage capacity for glycogen has been reached in the muscles and liver, the excess glucose is converted into fat and stored in the fatty (adipose) tissue of the body. This means, therefore, that even if a person is on a high carbohydrate and low fat diet, it is still possible, if excessive amounts of calories are consumed for that person to increase his or her body fat level.

In addition to glucose, there are two other monosaccharides that have the same chemical make-up and they are *fructose* and *galactose*. In the final products of carbohydrate digestion, glucose makes up about 80 percent, while fructose and galactose make up approximately 10 percent each. Glucose and fructose are found mainly in fruits (especially dried), pastries, candy, jams, and honey, whereas galactose is present primarily in the mammary glands of certain animals.

Disaccharide (unit that has two 6-carbon sugar molecules) carbohydrates include *maltose, sucrose,* and *lactose*. Maltose is produced during digestion of starches, while lactose is found in milk and it eventually breaks down to galactose and glucose during digestion. Sucrose (or table sugar) is normally found in cane sugar.

Polysaccharide (made up of three or more 6-carbon sugar molecules) carbohydrates in the diet include the *starches*. Starch is found mainly in potatoes, cereal and bread products such as rice, corn, wheat and barley along with beans and peas. Other polysaccharide products that are ingested to a slight extent in the diet are glycogen, dextrins, pectins, and cellulose, all of which are digested in basically the same manner as the starches. The digestion of carbohydrates is illustrated in Figure 9-1.

B. FATS

Fats have several major functions in the body. Briefly, they are: (1) energy storage which can be used as fuel as the body needs it; (2) carrier for fat soluble vitamins A, D, E, and K throughout the body; (3) as a soft cushion for protection against inside and outside shocks or blows to vital

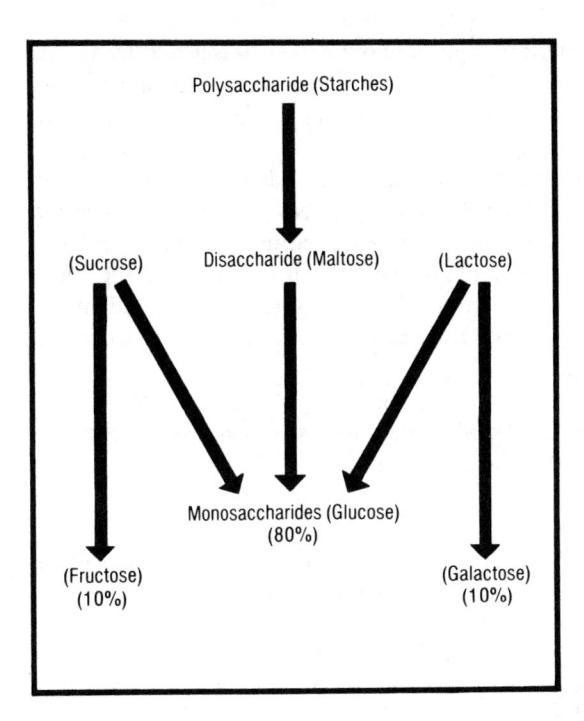

Figure 9-1 Schematic diagram of the digestion of carbohydrates.

organs such as the heart, lungs, kidneys, liver, spinal cord, etc.; (4) heat insulator to protect body against cold weather; and (5) after ingesting fats, its presence in the small intestines may have an effect of retarding or depressing hunger pangs.

Like the carbohydrate molecule, a fat molecule consists of carbon, oxygen, and hydrogen atoms only in different amounts. While fats contain less oxygen than carbohydrates, they also have more carbon and hydrogen. This obviously allows them to be greater fuel providers, but at the same time, a greater cost in terms of oxidation.

Chemically, a fat molecule is made up of two different groups of atoms; namely, *fatty acids* and *glycerol. Saturated* and *unsaturated* are terms used to describe the fatty acids. Fats are considered to be saturated fatty acids if the carbon atom chain contains as many hydrogen atoms as it will hold. In other words, the single bond link between the carbon atoms is completely saturated with hydrogen atoms and will not hold any more. On the other hand, fats are classified as unsaturated fatty acids if two or more hydrogen atoms, because of the presence of a double bond link between the carbon atoms, are missing from the carbon atom chain. Note that the carbon chain of unsaturated fats contain two less hydrogen atoms for each double bond. The fat molecule is referred to as *monounsaturated* if the carbon chain contains one double bond and *polyunsaturated* if two or more double bonds are present.

Fats are stored in the body in the form of *triglyceride* (three fatty acids joined with glycerol). Triglycerides, also known as neutral fats, are the most common fats of the diet. Other fats found in the body are *phospholipids* and *cholesterol,* both of which play important roles in maintaining the membrane structure of all cells. Phospholipids also plays an important role in blood clotting while cholesterol is needed for the production of both male and female hormones *androgen, estrogen,* and *progesterone.*

While fat plays an essential part in our diet, as was pointed out earlier, it is generally agreed that most Americans consume far more fat than they really need. Today, fat makes up about 42 percent of the total average American diet, while most experts in the area of nutrition agree that approximately 25 percent is adequate.

Although this is a highly controversial subject, there is suggestive evidence that a diet high in saturated fats may be directly or indirectly related to cardiovascular disease. It has been suggested that in order to perhaps avoid this potential risk, a portion of saturated fats should be replaced with unsaturated fats. This has been especially advisable for people who are overweight, those with a history of heart disease (especially middleage people), those people who have sedentary-type jobs, or people who hold highly-stressful type jobs. Obviously, more research is needed in this area before any final recommendations can be made.

Meats, cream, whole-milk, ice cream, butter, lard, margarine, egg yolks, cheese, lobster, and crabs are rich sources of saturated fats, whereas vegetable oils such as cottonseed oil, corn oil, peanut oil, and soybean oil are good sources of unsaturated fats.

C. PROTEINS

Proteins, unlike carbohydrates and fats, contain nitrogen in addition to carbon, hydrogen, and oxygen. Every cell in the body needs protein. In fact, proteins are found throughout the entire body with muscle tissue being their major location. Proteins are not used to any great extent for energy, but instead, they are considered to be the "building blocks" of tissue. That is, they provide not only the basic material for the structure of cells, enzymes, and hormones, but they also furnish the basic material that is essential for muscular contraction.

Proteins are made up of long chain-like nitrogenous compounds called *amino acids*. While there are over 20 different known amino acids in protein, 8 of these cannot be manufactured within the body, and therefore, must be obtained directly from the diet. These are referred to as *essential amino acids*. The remaining ones, called *nonessential*, can be synthesized within the body from the nutrients taken in from the diet. The 8 essential amino acids are: isoleucine, leucine, lysine, methionine, phenylalanine, threonine, tryptophan, and valine.

While there is some disagreement as to how much protein is needed daily, most nutritionists cheese, cereals, beans, nuts, and soybeans, it is interesting to note that the animal protein sources contains all of the essential amino acids, and therefore, are generally considered to be "high-quality" proteins. On the other hand, protein from vegetables and other sources tend to be "low-quality" protein because these foods may be missing one or more of these essential amino acids. A mixture of proteins from various vegetables and grain products may, however, furnish all the essential amino acids.

While there is some disagreement as to how much protein is needed daily, most nutritionist do agree that no more than one gram of protein per kilogram of body weight is needed each day. In fact, the United States Food and Nutrition Board has recommended a daily protein allowance of 0.9 grams per kilogram of body weight for adolescent and adult men and women. This means that a person who weighs 165 pounds (75 kilograms) would require, on a daily basis, approximately 67.5 grams of protein intake in order to meet the needs for tissue growth and maintenance. People who are heavier would naturally require a greater amount. It has also been suggested that women who are pregnant should raise their daily protein allowance by as much as 10 grams, whereas young mothers who are nursing young babies should increase their daily intake to 20 grams.

D. VITAMINS

Vitamins are organic substances that are essential for human life. Although vitamins are needed in only small amounts, they must be provided in either the diet or by way of supplements since the living cell cannot manufacture them.

Vitamins are generally classified as either water-soluble or fat-soluble. The fat-soluble vitamins are composed of carbon, hydrogen, and oxygen, whereas the water-soluble vitamins contain not only carbon, hydrogen, and oxygen, but also nitrogen as well as cobalt and sulfur. As might be expected, the water-soluble vitamins are not capable of being stored in the body to any significant degree as are the fat-soluble vitamins. As a result, they should be included in the daily diet, whereas daily ingestion of fat-soluble vitamins is not necessarily a "must" since they can be stored and retained within the body. Any excessive amounts of water-soluble vitamins is generally voided in the urine, while excessive amounts of fat-soluble vitamins may be kept and stored within the body tissues. In some cases, excessive dosages of fat-soluble vitamins may result in toxic side effects. Thus, most authorities agree that there is little or no value to ingesting large sums of vitamins over and above the daily recommended allowance. Vitamins taken over the recommended allowance should be done only under a physician's recommendation.

The water-soluble vitamins have been identified as the B-complex vitamins and vitamin C (ascorbic acid). The B-complex group includes thiamine (B_1), riboflavin (B_2), niacin (B_5), pyridoxine (B_6), biotin (B_7), folic acid (B_9), cyanocobalamine (B_{12}), pantothetic acide, and choline. The fat-soluble vitamins include vitamins A, D, E, and K. Table 9-1 describes some of the more important vitamin functions and their food sources, while Table 9-2 represents the recommended dietary daily allowances of both fat-soluble vitamins and water-soluble vitamins.

E. MINERALS

Minerals, like vitamins, provide no energy but they play an important part in an individual's diet. While the amount of each mineral in the body is relatively small, the diverse function of each mineral is vital for proper body functioning. Minerals are not only found in bones, teeth, muscles, cells, connective tissue, and body fluids, but they also are present in vitamins, hormones, and enzymes. Minerals make up approximately 4 percent of the body weight. Among those required for maintenance of health are: calcium (1.5%), phosphorus (1.0%), potassium (0.35%), sulfur (0.25%), sodium (0.15%), chlorine (0.15%), magnesium (0.05%), iron (0.004%), copper (0.00015%), iodine (0.00004%), and some small traces of cobalt, bromine, fluorine, manganese, molybdenum, and selenium. Table 9-2 illustrates the recommended dietary daily allowance for some of the above mentioned minerals.

While there is no solid evidence that mineral supplementation above the recommended daily allowance will improve physical performance, a substantial amount of evidence is available to show that mineral deficiencies can lower an athlete's efficiency. Also, since exercise and work (especially in hot climates) can alter the body's balance for certain minerals (such as sodium, chloride, potassium, calcium, magnesium, and phosphorus), it is absolutely essential that those depleted minerals be replaced by either the diet or through supplementation. Iron supplementation may also be required for the young adult woman during her menstrual period.

Table 9-3 illustrates the various functions of the different minerals along with their food source. Note that a discussion on sodium chloride, as an ergogenic aid, may be found in Chapter 10.

Table 9-1. Vitamins—Their Functions and Food Sources

Vitamin	Function	Food Sources
Water-Soluble		
C	Used in collagen formation for binding cells together and for tooth formation	Mainly in the fruit and vegetable group
Thiamine (B_1)	Coenzyme used for metabolism of carbohydrates	Mainly in the meat and bread group
Riboflavin (B_2)	Coenzyme whose reactions aid the release of energy in the cells	Mainly in the meat, milk and bread group
Niacin (B_5)	Coenzyme whose reactions aid the release of energy from the metabolism of of the various food nutrients of the diet (carbohydrates, fats & proteins)	Mainly in the meat and bread group
Pyridoxine (B_6)	Coenzyme used for metabolism of amino acids	Mainly in the bread group
Biotin (B_7)	Coenzyme used in the synthesis and breakdown of amino acids and fatty acids	Mainly in the meat group
Folic Acid (B_9)	Coenzyme used in normal growth and formation of red blood cells	Mainly in the meat and vegetable group
Cyanocobalamine (B_{12})	Coenzyme used in normal growth and formation of blood and nucleic acid	Mainly in the meat group
Pantothenic Acid	Coenzyme used for metabolism of carbohydrates, fats, and proteins	Mainly in the meat group
Choline	Coenzyme whose reactions aid in the formation acetylcholine	Mainly in the meat and bread group
Fat-Soluble		
A	Coenzyme used in normal growth and vision	Mainly in the fruit and vegetable group
D	Coenzyme used in bone calcification	Mainly in the milk, meat and fat group
E	Unclear in humans, but may be used in lipid metabolism	Mainly in the meat, cereal and vegetable group
K	Coenzyme used in blood clotting and coagulation	Mainly in the bread, fat and vegetable group

F. WATER

Although water makes up between 40 and 60 percent of the total body weight, it is like vitamins and minerals in that it is not classified as an energy nutrient. However, it has several important functions in the human body that relate to the area of nutrition. It not only provides the medium for all body chemical processes to take place in, but it also assist in forming blood plasma, digestion of foods, glandular secretion, and in waste elimination. Water is lost from the body through the skin, in urine, as water vapor in breathing, and in feces. The normal water

Table 9-2. Recommended Daily Allowances for Vitamins (Fat and Water-Soluble) and Minerals

	Ages	Fat-Soluble				Water-Soluble						Minerals					
		A (IU)	D (IU)	E (IU)	C (mg)	B_9 (ug)	B_5 (mg)	B_2 (mg)	B_1 (mg)	B_6 (mg)	B_{12} (ug)	Ca (mg)	PO_4 (mg)	I (ug)	Fe (mg)	Mn (mg)	Zn (mg)
Children	1-3	2000	400	7	40	100	9	0.8	0.7	0.6	1.0	800	800	60	15	150	10
	4-6	2500	400	9	40	200	12	1.1	0.9	0.9	1.5	800	800	80	10	200	10
	7-10	3300	400	10	40	300	16	1.2	1.2	1.2	2.0	800	800	110	10	250	10
Men	11-14	5000	400	12	45	400	18	1.5	1.4	1.6	3.0	1200	1200	130	18	350	15
	15-18	5000	400	15	45	400	20	1.8	1.5	2.0	3.0	1200	1200	150	18	400	15
	19-22	5000	400	15	45	400	20	1.8	1.5	2.0	3.0	800	800	140	10	350	15
	23-50	5000	—	15	45	400	18	1.6	1.4	2.0	3.0	800	800	130	10	350	15
	51+	5000	—	15	45	400	16	1.5	1.2	2.0	3.0	800	800	110	10	350	15
Women	11-15	4000	400	12	45	400	16	1.3	1.2	1.6	3.0	1200	1200	115	18	300	15
	15-18	4000	400	12	45	400	14	1.4	1.1	2.0	3.0	1200	1200	115	18	300	15
	19-22	4000	400	12	45	400	14	1.4	1.1	2.0	3.0	800	800	100	18	300	15
	23-50	4000	—	12	45	400	13	1.2	1.0	2.0	3.0	800	800	100	18	300	15
	51+	4000	—	12	45	400	12	1.1	1.0	2.0	3.0	800	800	80	10	300	15

Source: Food and Nutrition Board, *Recommended Dietary Allowances*, 8th edition, National Academy of Sciences, Washington, D.C., 1974.

Table 9-3. Minerals—Their Functions and Food Sources

Minerals	Function	Food Source
Calcium (Ca)	Combines with phosphorus to form bones and teeth; blood clotting; transport of fluids across cell membrane, maintaining normal function of muscle	Mainly in the milk group
Phosphorus (PO$_4$)	Combines with calcium to form bones and teeth; component of ATP and CP; helps regulate acid content of blood	Mainly in the meat group
Potassium (K)	An electrically charged ion that is part of three other minerals called an electrolyte which functions to control and maintain the correct rate of fluid within the several fluid areas of the body; maintain proper electrical gradient around the nerve membrane for transmission of nerve impulse	Mainly in the bread, fruits, and vegetable group
Sodium (Na)	Same as potassium	Same as potassium
Chlorine (Cl)	Same as potassium	Same as potassium
Magnesium (Mn)	Similar to calcium and phosphorus; also important in glucose metabolism, it aids the reaction of glucose to glycogen in liver and muscles	Mainly in the bread, fruits, and vegetable group
Iron (Fe)	Important in formation of hemoglobin, myoglobin, and other oxidative enzymes such as cytochromes, cytochrome oxidase, peroxidase, and catalase	Mainly in the bread, meat, and vegetable group
Copper (Co)	Important in the normal breakdown of nutrients (glucose, fatty acids, and amino acids) in the diet	Mainly in the bread group
Iodine (I)	Essential for formation of thyroxine which, in turn, is important for maintenance of normal metabolic rate in all cells	Mainly in the meat group (especially in seafood)
Sulfur (S)	Important in the normal breakdowns of nutrients (glucose, fatty acids, and amino acids) in the diet	Mainly in the bread group

consumption required to replace the lost water on a daily basis is around 2 to 3 quarts. For the interested reader, water is also discussed in Chapter 10 as an ergogenic aid.

II. DAILY FOOD REQUIREMENTS

As was pointed out in Chapter 2, the energy value of food as well as the work resulting from the energy can be described in terms of calories. One Calorie (spelled with a capital C) or kilocalorie represents the heat (energy) required to raise the temperature of one kilogram of water by one degree centigrade. Depending upon age, size, and sex, the average calorie intake needed for maintaining body weight for most people during a normal day varies between 1,500 to 3,000 kcal per day. As Table 9-4 illustrates, athletes during training and competition, in some cases, need and consume nearly twice the amount of calories that sedentary people do. Because some of these athletes (for example, the marathon runner) are extremely thin and low in percent body fat, it should be obvious to the reader that this high caloric intake is needed merely to satisfy the energy demands of their training and competition.

While it is rather difficult to give the exact breakdown on how much of the diet should be carbohydrate, fat, and protein, it is generally agreed that carbohydrates should contribute somewhere between 50 and 55 percent of the total food intake with fats contributing between 25 and 30 percent and protein between 12 and 20 percent. For example, a sedentary person working behind a desk all day that requires 2,400 kcal per day could have the following diet breakdown:

$$\begin{aligned} \text{Carbohydrate} &= 1{,}200 \text{ to } 1{,}320 \text{ kcal} \\ \text{Fat} &= 600 \text{ to } 720 \text{ kcal} \\ \text{Protein} &= 288 \text{ to } 480 \text{ kcal} \end{aligned}$$

On the other hand, an athlete who requires 6,000 kcal per day because of his or her training and competition could have the following daily food breakdown:

$$\begin{aligned} \text{Carbohydrate} &= 3{,}000 \text{ to } 3{,}300 \text{ kcal} \\ \text{Fat} &= 1{,}500 \text{ to } 1{,}800 \text{ kcal} \\ \text{Protein} &= 720 \text{ to } 1{,}200 \text{ kcal} \end{aligned}$$

Experts suggest that of the 25 to 30 percent total daily contribution of fats, saturated fats (meats, butter, cream, cheese, lard, etc.) should be held to about 10 percent or less.

Table 9-4. Estimated Daily Caloric Intake for Athletes in Different Sport Activities

Sport	Average Body Weight (kg)	Estimated Caloric Intake (kcal)
Cross-country skiing	67.5	6105
Bicycle racing	68.0	5995
Canoe racing	75.0	5995
Marathon racing	68.0	5940
Soccer	74.0	5885
Field hockey (men)	75.0	5720
Handball (European)	75.0	5610
Basketball	75.0	5610
Ice hockey	68.0	5390
Gymnastics (men)	67.0	5000
Sailing	74.0	5170
Fencing	73.0	5000
Sprinting (track)	69.0	4675
Boxing (middle and welter weight)	63.5	4675
Diving	61.0	4620
Pole vault	73.0	4620

Source: American College of Sports Medicine *Encyclopedia of Sport Sciences and Medicine*, Macmillan Publishing Co., Inc., New York, 1971.

III. THE ESSENTIAL FOOD GROUPS

The following food groups have been recommended by not only the American Association for Health, Physical Education and Recreation, but also the American Dietetic and Nutrition Foundation as being essential for ensuring the necessary daily requirements of carbohydrates, fats, proteins, vitamins, and minerals. Note that foods within each group may be exchanged or substituted for each other.

A. MILK GROUP

While whole milk is most commonly used, other forms such as powdered milk, buttermilk, skim milk, evaporated milk and cocoa are also valuable milk sources. The milk group is a major supplier of calcium, protein, fat, and vitamins (D and B_2).

B. MEAT GROUP

This group includes beef, lamb, pork, liver, chicken, fish, tuna, salmon, crab, lobster, oysters, shrimp, clams, sardines, cottage cheese, eggs, peanut butter, and cheese. All of these foods are major sources of protein, vitamins B_1, B_2, B_5, B_7, B_9, B_{12}, D, pantothenic acid, choline, and iron. The seafoods are especially good sources for iodine. Liver is also a good source for vitamin A.

C. DARK GREEN OR DEEP YELLOW VEGETABLES

Included in this group are broccoli, carrots, chicory, escarole, pepper, pumpkin, tomatoes, watercress, winter squash, lettuce, spinach, mustard greens, kale greens, turnip greens, beet greens, chard greens, dandilion greens, and collard greens. This group of vegetables is a major source of vitamins A, B_9, C, E, and K and minerals (iron, sodium, potassium, and magnesium). While lettuce and greens contain very little carbohydrates, the remaining vegetables do provide some carbohydrate energy.

D. CITRUS FRUITS

Sources in this group include oranges, orange juice, grapefruits, grapefruit juice, tangerine, tomato juice, and cantalopes. The citrus fruit group is an excellent source of vitamin C and minerals (sodium, potassium, and magnesium), while at the same time, it provides some carbohydrate energy.

E. OTHER FRUITS

Included in this group are apples, applesauce, apricots, bananas, blueberries, cherries, dates, figs, grapes and grapejuice, honeydew melon, mango, papaya, pears, pineapples and pineapple juice, peaches, plums, raisins, raspberries, prunes, strawberries, and watermelons. This group is a major supplier of vitamins (especially A) and minerals (sodium, potassium, and magnesium). The fruits in this group also provides some carbohydrate energy.

F. OTHER VEGETABLES

This group includes asparagus, beets, brussel sprouts, celery, cauliflower, cabbage, cucumbers, eggplants, mushrooms, onions, okra, green peas, rutabagas, radishes, string beans, summer squash, sauerkraut, and turnips. These foods are good sources for vitamins A and B_9 and sodium, potassium, and magnesium. The beats, onions, green peas, and turnips are good sources for carbohydrate energy. Brussel sprouts are also a good source for vitamin C.

G. BREAD GROUP

Included in this group are enriched or whole grain breads, pizza, muffins, cornbread, cooked or dry cereals, spaghetti, noodles, macaroni, saltine crackers, graham crackers, dried or cooked beans and peas, baked beans, corn, rice or grits, parsnips, potato, potato chips, pretzels, french fries, sweet potatoes or yams, spong or angel cake, and ice cream. These foods are excellent sources of carbohydrates in both sugar and starch forms. These sources are also suppliers of protein as well as vitamins B_1, B_2, B_5, B_6, K, choline, and minerals (sodium, potassium, magnesium, and iron).

H. FAT GROUP

Although much controversy still exist concerning this food group, it is still an important part of the daily diet in that it helps to metabolize certain vitamins in the diet such as A, D, E, and K. This group includes bacon, butter or margarine, cream, cream cheese, french dressing, mayonnaise, olive oils, and vegetable oils (safflower, sunflower, sesame, soybean, corn). One tablespoon per day is generally considered to be sufficient for this group and it is recommended that it be prepared and consumed either as cooking oil or in the form of either butter or margarine or perhaps even vegetable or olive oil spread on breads and salads.

I. SUGARS

Included in this group are sugars, jellies, honey, syrup, carbonated beverage, and hard candy. This group is a supplier of carbohydrates.

IV. SPACING AND NUMBER OF MEALS

The influence of spacing and number of meals have been investigated experimentally in relation to work performance. Because research has shown that blood sugar levels tend to decrease along with efficiency after approximately 2 to 3 hours of eating, experts have recommended that the minimum number of meals that a person should have each day is three. In fact, the results from research indicate that frequent feeding may be more desirable. Five smaller than normal meals a day appear to be superior to three regular size meals and three regular size meals appear to be superior to two large size meals a day with respect to physical performance. With the more frequent feedings, an individual is better able to maintain their normal blood sugar level and blood lipid level (with smaller amounts of fat being stored) throughout the day. It should be emphasized, however, that if frequent feedings are going to be undertaken by the athlete or by the general population, caution should be taken that "junk" foods are not substituted in place of the more nutritive foods for the in-between-snacks. Also, depending upon your age, size, sex, and physical activity, the total overall daily number of calories should remain the same regardless of whether you are having three meals per day or five meals per day. In other words, do not increase your total number of calories per day just because you may be eating more often. The problem of overweight and obesity is always present if eating between your three regular meals gets out of control.

V. PRE-GAME MEAL

From the standpoint of digestion, there is excellent rationale for the last meal prior to an athletic event (regardless of the meals content) to be consumed three hours or more before the start of the contest. This has generally been the practice. Most physiologists believe that by doing this, the food will have had time to clear the stomach and thus eliminate an added drain on the circulatory sytem that might be brought about by the working muscles competing with the digestive system for the available blood.

Another reason for consuming the food several hours before the event is that emotions or nervousness witnessed by some performers prior to the contest is less likely to interfere with the digestive processes if this meal is consumed well in advance. Gastric emptying and gastrointestinal motility are known to be slowed down considerably among nervous athletes prior to an athletic performance. Therefore, the pre-game meal should be light and easy to digest. Steak is not recommended since it is heavy, has very little fuel value, and is very slow to digest.

Athletes who are taking part in events that last 30 minutes or longer should consume a pre-game meal that is made up of mainly carbohydrates (at least approximately 80 to 90 percent). The reason for this is simple: (1) carbohydrates are able to be digested quicker than either fats or proteins; (2) carbohydrates can be converted as an energy source with the least amount of effort; (3) the normal blood plasma glucose level can be maintained easier on a diet that is high in carbohydrates; and (4) a diet high in carbohydrates will increase the stored carbohydrates in the muscles and liver, and therefore, allow the athlete to exercise longer.

Because there is probably very little physiological benefits from the pre-game meal in events lasting less than 30 minutes, individual food preference should probably be allowed provided that the athlete knows from experience what food and how much of it he or she can eat without it causing discomfort and nausea. A factor that cannot be ignored is the psychological effect of the pre-game meal. In most cases, the psychological effect of the pre-game meal probably plays a bigger part than the actual physiological. If the athlete really feels that what he is eating is going to help his performance, then there is a good chance that it might. At the same time, if he is not happy and does not like the pre-game meal (regardless of whether it is high in nutritive values or not), then chances are he will perform poorly. Many coaches and athletes have recently found that the use of liquid formula meals to be very satisfactory since they are easy to digest and are less likely to bring about nausea and abdominal cramps. Presently, this appears to be a very favorable pre-game meal.

VI. DIET AND PERFORMANCE

A. CARBOHYDRATE AND FAT

While it has been well established over the years that carbohydrate and fat constitute the major fuels for muscular activity, it has also been generally well established that their relative contribution during work apparently varies not only with the actual intensity and duration of the work load, but also with the training of the subject. For example, light sustained work loads utilizing 70 percent or less of maximum oxygen uptake calls upon a greater proportion of fat for its energy needs than it does carbohydrates while prolonged heavy work loads utilizing over 75 percent of maximum oxygen uptake relies more on carbohydrates (glycogen) than it does on fat for its energy needs. As was just mentioned, training (especially endurance) also apparently plays an important role in determining carbohydrates and fats relative contribution during work. For instance, the literature is well documented that during endurance training, an individual develops a greater muscle cell capacity and rate for using free fatty acids as a source of energy. At the same time, training apparently raises the intramuscular resting pool of glycogen for which the person, during work, may call upon early for its energy source until fatty acid sources can become available and take over.

In addition, while over the years it has also been pretty well established that carbohydrate yields less than half as many kilocalories per gram as does fat (4.1 to 9.3, respectively), it has also been well documented that the burning of carbohydrate yields more kilocalories of energy produced per liter of oxygen than does the burning of fat (5.05 to 4.74, respectively). Keeping the above information in mind, one might theoretically expect that in any sport or activity in which the duration and intensity level (over 75 percent of maximum oxygen uptake) is so high that the oxygen supply to the tissues is a limiting factor, a diet high in carbohydrates would be advantageous.

Indeed, as early as the 1930's, laboratory scientists noted that endurance type work could perhaps be increased if the diet was high in carbohydrates and, at the same time, they noticed that endurance was decreased if the diet was high in fat. Because of this reported finding between diet and performance, a number of interested nutritionists and exercise physiologists started conducting extensive research in this area. In the 1960's, researchers noted that when subjects were exercised to exhaustion, their blood sugar level was always down. Later, muscle biopsy studies confirmed these findings by noting that when subjects worked to exhaustion, their muscle glycogen stores were completely depleted. Typically, other studies have illustrated that as work continues to fatigue, muscle glycogen stores becomes low and eventually completely depleted. From these findings have resulted two major types of research to examine the possible advantage of a specific type of diet on physical performance: (1) those in which exercise following the ingestion of single meals of the desired composition, and (2) those in which the subjects were fed for several days a certain diet high in a given component (carbohydrate, fat, protein) and low in the others to "saturate" the body with one particular type of food prior to performance in the postabsorptive state.

Although the majority of available evidence indicates that the composition of the pre-exercise meal does not affect performance during short-term exercise (such as 100-yd sprint swimming and running), there is better evidence in favor of a high carbohydrate diet for prolonged heavy exercise. For example, researchers working in the first area have generally found that in events lasting 30 minutes or longer, work efficiencies are increased (as much as 10 percent or more) as well as endurance capacities when the pre-exercise meal is high in carbohydrates.

In muscle biopsy* studies where investigators kept subjects for several days prior to exercise on either high fat diets, high carbohydrate diets, or mixed diets, results indicated that endurance, when performed on a bicycle ergometer, was by far the greatest when the subjects were on the high carbohydrate diet as compared to when the same subjects were on the other two diets. This is illustrated in Figure 9-2 where work performance is directly related to the amount of glycogen found in the muscle. From these findings as well as the fact that glycogen stored in small amounts (note that the normal amount of glycogen stored in the muscle is around 13 to 15 grams per kilogram of muscle as compared to a storage capacity of 40 or more grams per kilogram of muscle) and that only a small amount can actually be taken in from the intestine during exercise or competition, it is quite evident that the consumption of a diet high in carbohydrates several days before competition (for the purpose of enhancing the glycogen stores of the muscles) can be to the athlete's advantage in endurance-type events.

---

*The muscle-biopsy technique involves the use of a special-type of needle which is placed in an individual's muscle while under local anesthesia. A small section of the muscle is actually removed for the measurement for muscle glycogen.

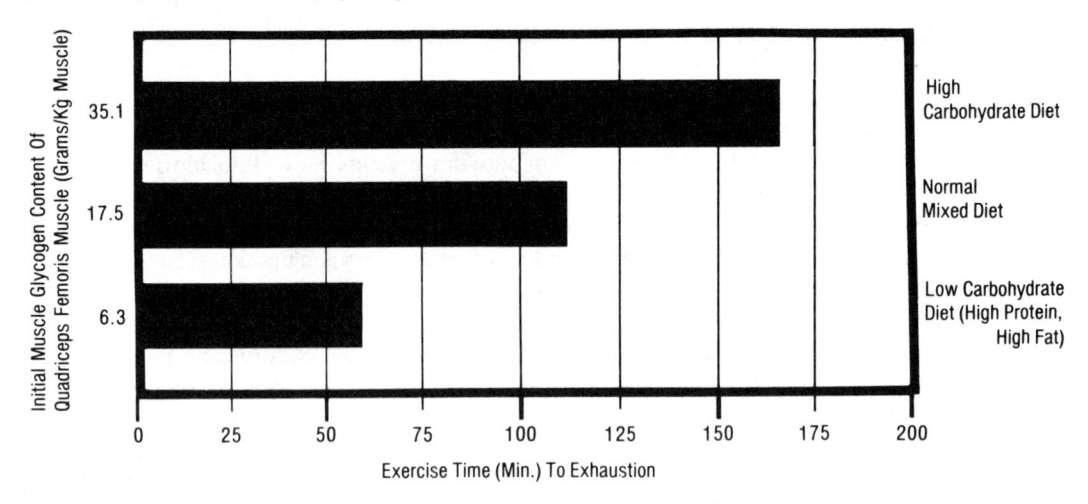

Figure 9-2 The effects of three different diets (high fat, high carbohydrate, or mixed) on endurance, when performed on a bicycle ergometer.

A recommended procedure has been prescribed in the literature for allowing maximal glycogen storage. This technique is commonly referred to as *carbohydrate loading* and the following steps are recommended:

(1) Deplete the glycogen stores. That is, approximately 7 days prior to competition, the athlete should exercise vigorously over a prolonged period of at least 60 to 90 minutes. The glycogen stores should be kept as low as possible during this 7-day period by consuming a low carbohydrate diet (diet should contain mostly protein and fat) and with continued exercise and training. Remember, the greater the depletion of glycogen, the greater the ability for storing glycogen.

(2) Three to four days prior to competition when the athlete's work has tapered off, the diet should become predominantly carbohydrate. Also, additional fluids should be taken in along with the high carbohydrate diet since each gram of stored glycogen is associated with an increased storage of about 3 to 4 grams of water. While this procedure has been proven to more than double the glycogen content of the muscle and thus increase the endurance capacity of participants, it should be pointed out, however, that this type of dietary program carries some risk with it. For example, some investigators have found marathon runners to actually suffer angina-like pain and electrocardiographic abnormalities after using this technique. It is now well established that an increased glycogen storage is generally associated with an increased water storage (in fact, about 3 times as much water as glycogen), and that this increased storage of water and glycogen in the muscle may cause a feeling of heaviness and stiffness in the athlete.

It has also been suggested that the technique of carbohydrate loading may alter somewhat the supply and utilization of fat as sources of energy during work. For example, carbohydrate loading has been found to decrease glycerol and plasma free fatty acid concentrations, while increasing ketone body concentration as well as insulin and growth hormone levels. It is also known that glycogen can destroy muscle fiber, although this usually only occurs during disease states such as an acid maltase deficiency. One important question that remains unanswered is what happens to the muscles and heart of the athlete who does not use all of the stored glycogen as a result of loading. Longitudinally, we also do not know what the effects of this technique may or may not have over a competitive lifetime. Thus, in summary, while the carbohydrate-loading technique may improve athletic performance, there are also disadvantages for which the athlete should be informed.

B. PROTEIN

It was once believed that a high protein diet was essential because some people had the notion that during muscular contraction, the muscle was actually consuming itself as a source of energy and that the protein was needed to restore and rebuild the consumed muscle tissue. As was pointed out earlier in this chapter, it is now well documented that protein is not used as a fuel to any great extent when the caloric supply is adequate. In fact, protein supplies only about 5 to 15 percent of the body's total energy. Exercise, even to exhaustion, has very little effect on protein metabolism. Therefore, consuming a large amount of protein prior to an event or contest from the viewpoint of energy metabolism is not supported.

While the performance of heavy work does not increase protein requirements, the increase in muscle mass associated with training does, like other growth processes, require an adequate supply of protein. However, contrary to popular opinion, consuming large amounts of protein over and above the normal daily requirements has very little effect on bringing about increased lean muscle mass and strength. Apparently, the normal daily protein intake (0.9 grams/kg of body weight) along with training is sufficient to bring about increased muscle mass and strength changes.

It should be pointed out that during the early part of training (especially involving heavy muscular work when muscle mass is increasing) when the athlete is expending and consuming several thousand kilocalories over his or her normal daily expenditures, it is important to continue consuming the proper proportion (or perhaps a little more than normal) of protein from the total overall caloric intake in order to prevent possible anemia and iron deficiencies from occurring. Otherwise, if the vigorous training is continued without adequate protein consumption, a decrease in hemoglobin concentration will eventually be experienced by the athletes.

It should be pointed out that while most animal and human studies have not demonstrated any benefits from eating excessive amounts of protein, one of the most impressive developments in clinical nutrition in recent years, as reported by Nelson, has been the treatment of chronic renal disease by cutting down on protein intake. This program has apparently kept people working and feeling good (even though they may have kidney malfunctions), while at the same time, keeping them from being bedridden in the hospitals. If these benefits are possible by lowering protein intake, is excessive protein intake healthy for normal people? Is there perhaps even some degree of danger in consuming too many proteins? While human evidence is lacking, animal research does support such a thought. In fact, evidence is available to indicate that some animals nearly double their life span when protein intake is halved. Because most of the research has not demonstrated any benefits from eating excessive amounts of protein, and because animal research shows that there may be a health hazard in overconsumption of protein, it is highly recommended that there is no place in the training program of athletes for high protein diets or protein or amino acid supplements.

C. VITAMINS

While the need for vitamins in the human diet is well known, it is by far, one of the most common offenders in use today as an ergogenic aid. In fact, the sale of unnecessary and perhaps even harmful vitamin supplements have been reportedly the biggest fraud by unethical promoters in the United States today. This is not to imply that some people do not need vitamin supplements, only that most people do not. Because of their role in energy metabolism, it is easy to understand why some people including coaches, athletes, and trainers feel that additional vitamins will improve performance. Vitamins are materials that serve as coenzymes in the body and most of them are required for ATP production. In other words, they are needed in order that other enzymes in the body can do their function. Without vitamins, ATP production would be impossible.

Are vitamins ergogenic aids? Will massive does of any one vitamin above the recommended daily allowance bring about better performance in an athlete or laborer? To date, there is no clear scientific evidence that indicates that extra vitamins will enhance physical performance. However, research with vitamins B_1, C, and E have resulted in contradictory evidence, and some of the results seem to indicate that they may have some ergogenic properties. As a result, these are the ones that will be discussed here.

Vitamin B_1 (Thiamine)

Because thiamine is involved in the chemical removal of carbon dioxide from pyruvic acid prior to pyruvic acid entering the citric acid cycle (also known as the Krebs cycle), it plays an important part in fat and carbohydrate metabolism. The literature in this area has shown that deficiencies in thiamine have resulted in poor athletic performance while thiamine supplementation has shown to improve performance as well as have no influence on performance. It would appear that if a healthy person is on a well-balanced diet, thiamine supplementation would not be beneficial since thiamine is quickly excreted in the urine once its concentration passes a threshold level in the body. More solid scientific research is needed in this area before any final conclusion can be made concerning whether vitamin B_1 is an ergogenic acid.

Vitamin C (Ascorbic Acid)

Vitamin C not only plays an important role in maintenance of cartilage and bone tissue as well as dentin of teeth, but it also has an important influence on muscle metabolism. Available evidence indicates that deficiencies in vitamin C results in a decrease in physical performance due to muscle glycogen reduction and in weak muscle contractions. It is also believed that vitamin C may play an important part in production of certain hormones from the adrenal glands that serve as protection against certain stress agents. The literature is well documented that exercise brings about a reduction in vitamin C in the adrenal glands. While it may be to the individual's advantage to take vitamin C during stress conditions such as exercise, it should be kept in mind that there is no conclusive evidence available to suggest that supplementation of a nutritionally adequate diet with vitamin C will improve muscle metabolism or physical performance. Although most of the studies show no beneficial effects of massive dose of vitamins C on performance, a few have shown vitamin C supplementation to bring about an improved endurance capacity. It would seem that if a healthy person is on a well-balanced diet, vitamin C supplementation would not be beneficial since it is not stored, and instead, it is quickly excreted in the urine if an excess is ingested. Further well-controlled research would appear to be needed in order to clarify its role as perhaps an ergogenic aid for endurance performance.

Vitamin E (Alpha-Tocopherol)

Over the past several years, vitamin E (an antioxidant) has received considerable attention as a possible ergogenic aid. Vitamin E is a fat-soluble vitamin found in meats, cereal, and vegetables.

Vitamin E is believed to play an important role in lipid metabolism. It has also been reported that vitamin E may play a role in preventing atherosclerosis by not allowing a cholesterol buildup in the blood vessels of the body. The evidence shows that deficiencies in vitamin E results in a reduction of creatine phosphate in the muscles as well as weak muscular contraction. It would appear, therefore, that vitamin E supplementation would increase the level of creatine and thus make muscle contraction stronger and improve performance. However, like the two previous vitamins, the hard scientific research is conflicting in regards to the influence of vitamin E on physical performance. Some have found improvements in strength and endurance performance, while others have illustrated little or no effect. Therefore, we must reserve judgment at this time until additional studies are more conclusive on whether or not vitamin E can be considered as an ergogenic aid for improving physical performance.

VII. WEIGHT CONTROL AND EXERCISE

There are two components to the weight control equation; namely, the number of calories that you consume and the number of calories that you burn. Under normal conditions, the objective in weight control is to achieve a balance between the two. If an imbalance does occur it will generally result in either a loss or possibly a gain in weight. For example, if more calories than needed for energy expenditure are taken in, a weight gain usually results. The reverse is also true.

An individual can lose or gain weight in one of three ways: (1) by manipulating the number of calories taken in; (2) by manipulating the number of calories burned up; and (3) by manipulating both the intake and the expenditure. Most people, when attempting to lose a few pounds, generally think of cutting down on their caloric intake (by dieting) while giving very little attention to the number of calories that they burn. Although the result is usually some weight loss and a reduction in lean body weight, its generally just for a short period of time and is usually not retained. Under this system where weight loss is accomplished only by dieting, a feeling of deprivation and resentment is usually developed over a period of time. What normally happens is that people often revert back to their old previous eating habits and gain weight in terms of body fat. Most nutritionists and exercise physiologists agree that a combination of reduced intake and increased expenditure is generally considered the best. In fact, the majority of research in recent years has concluded that the best method of losing weight is through a combined exercise (progressive cardiorespiratory-endurance type) and diet program over a relatively long period of time. This type of weight-reduction program is designed to allow for a slow and gradual weight loss of between 1 and 2 pounds per week without a large reduction in the daily food intake. Note that medical experts suggest that individuals should not lost more than 2 pounds per week. A weight loss of 2 pounds per week is a considerable amount when one considers that this would total around 104 pounds if carried on for 12 months or one year. It should also be mentioned that this combined exercise and diet long-range program is also designed to not only reduce body weight to optimum levels without necessarily lowering lean body weight, but also to perhaps create new and long lasting eating and exercising habits.

At this point, it should be mentioned that in some circles a general misconception concerning exercise and weight control is that exercise is not really effective in weight reduction because appetite is automatically increased in direct proportion to the increased exercise. There is no doubt that laborers such as lumberjacks and farmers who perform daily 8 hours of hard physical work consume twice as many daily calories as sedentary people. Also, athletes such as marathon runners and cross-country skiers who devote a considerable amount of time (in some cases, 8 hours or more) to strenuous training consume a large amount of calories per day (around 6,000 kcal) as compared to sedentary (between 2,000 and 3,000 kcal) people. Apparently, this high caloric intake for these athletes, however, are needed to meet their energy demands for training since some of the athletes have very low percent body fats.

On the other hand, there is a considerable amount of evidence available to indicate that if exercise is performed for short to moderate periods of time (such as one hour per day) daily, appetite and food intake is not increased regardless of whether the work is mild or vigorous. But instead, most people's appetite will generally decrease (especially if they are used to sedentary style living). Figure 9-3 reflects this relationship between caloric intake and exercise from sedentary to light to heavy work. Animal studies show quite clearly that when rats are exercised for one hour each day, they eat less than sedentary rats who are not exercised. At the same time, studies show that rats who are exercised more than one hour each day, actually eat more than sedentary rats.

Another misconception concerning exercise and weight control is the amount of time required by exercising to reduce body weight. In other words, some people claim that a person

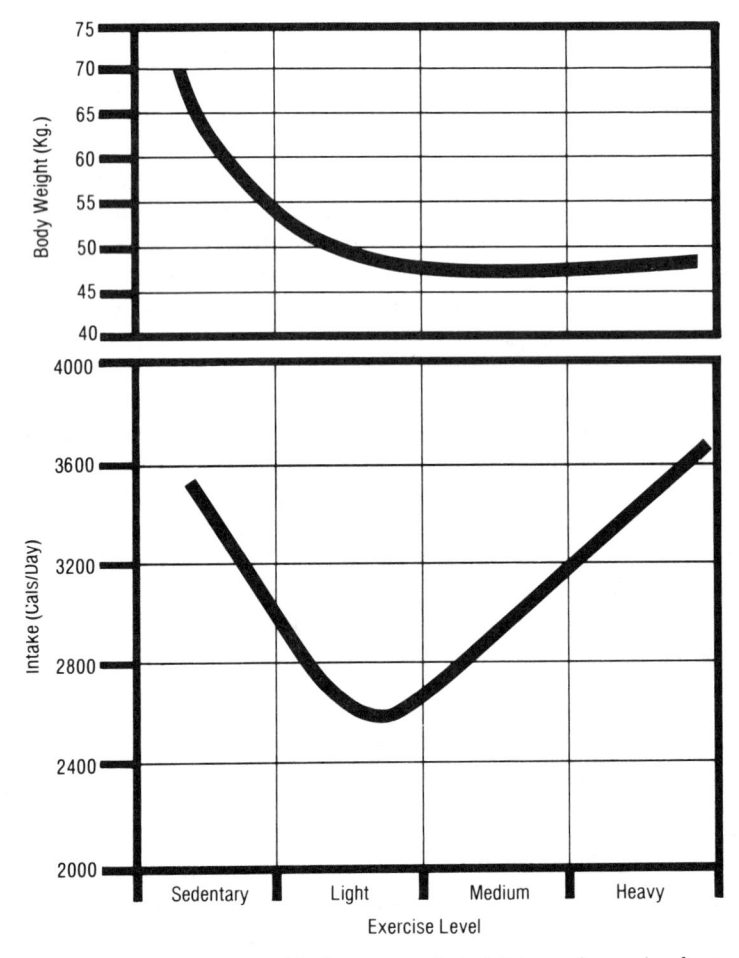

Figure 9-3 The relationship between caloric intake and exercise from sedentary to light to heavy work.

must spend an unbelieveable amount of time and effort to lose just one pound of fat. On a short-time weight-reduction exercise program, this is probably true since in order to lose a pound of stored fat, a deficit of 3,500 kcal is equal to 3,087 ft-lb of work. What this actually means in terms of physical activity is playing golf (walking and not riding in a cart) for something like 20 hours, leisure walking for something like 20 to 25 hours, or performing some other ridiculous feat of work. From these figures, it is understandable why a person who is overweight and wants to lose 10 to 20 pounds would become very discouraged and upset if he thought that he had to spend that much time in one or two days or even in a week in order to lose one pound. In fact, he probably would choose dieting over exercising if he felt that it was going to require that much time. On the other hand, what most people tend to forget is that the number of calories expended during physical activity is cumulative and may take place over a prolonged period of time. In other words, a caloric deficit of 3,500 kcal is equal to one pound of weight loss no matter if it occurs in one day, over a one-month period, or in one year.

From a realistic point of view, it makes much more sense to think in terms of exercise, for the purpose of reducing weight, to be spread out over several days or weeks. In other words, in order to take one pound of fat off, it makes much more sense to walk and play 9 holes of golf (approximately 2 hours) two times per week for 5 weeks than to think of spending 20 straight hours on the golf course. Or, if an individual could just average walking and playing one 18-hole round of golf (approximately 4 hours) each week for one year, he would be able to see a weight reduction of a little over 10 pounds. This, of course, would only hold true if daily caloric intake was held constant. Clearly, the long-range approach (combining exercise with diet), as was pointed out earlier, is by far the most practical and successful in losing weight.

It is important to remember that the speed by which an effective weight loss can be brought about will naturally depend upon the individual's personal goals, their motivation, how much they reduce the intake of food, and how much exercise they actually get involved in.

Figure 9-4 illustrates some typical caloric values of several physical activities. Remember, however, that they are only average energy values for normal people and should not be interpreted as absolute values since the number of kilocalories expended for any physical activity will fluctuate from person to person. These values can be used as a helpful guide in calculating how much extra daily activity one needs in a weight reducing program. Procedures for determining desired body weight may be found in a later section in this chapter.

VIII. BODY COMPOSITION

It is well known that a high percentage of fat in relation to the total body weight is detrimental and may lead to obesity. While the standards vary from one source to another, it is generally believed that the normal percent body fat for young men and women should not exceed 15 and 25 percent, respectively. Values over these are considered to be above normal and may lean toward obesity. Note that an individual may be overweight without necessarily being obese.

It is well known that obesity is generally brought about by overeating and lack of exercise. It is interesting to note that research has shown that along with obesity comes an increase in the number of adipose cells as well as an increase in their size. The difference in number of adipose cells appear to be more variable during the early years before reaching adulthood, whereas the size of the cells appear to be more variable during the adult stage. This is illustrated quite clearly in Figure 9-5, whereby a comparison between obese, normal, and lean subjects in terms of cell size and cell number was made. Although it is disturbing, it is also interesting and important to note

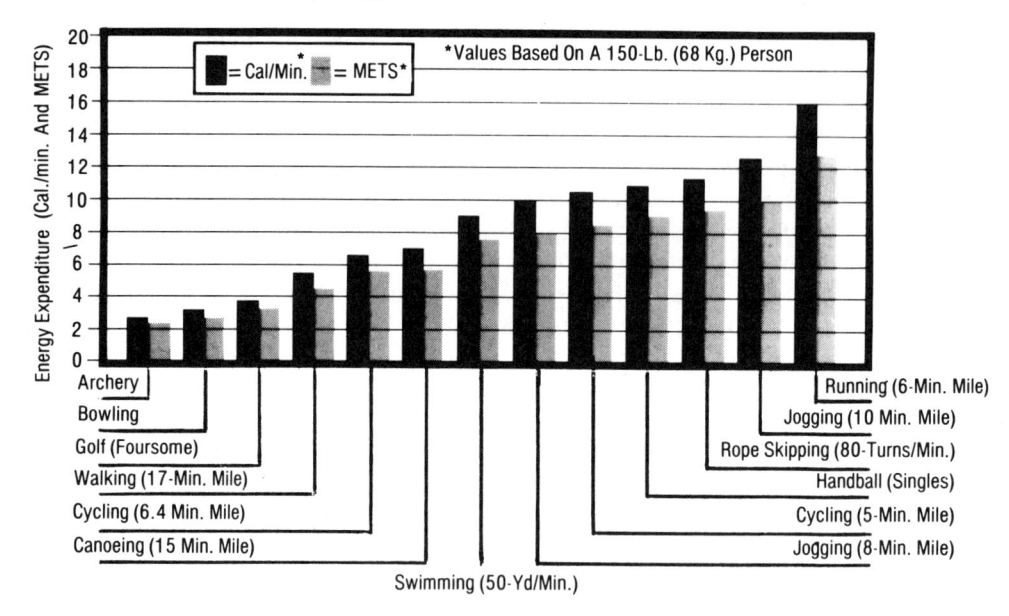

Figure 9-4 Schematic illustration of some typical caloric values of various selected physical activities.

that it has been found that young babies (during their first year) who add weight by increasing the number of adipose cells more rapidly than normal are more likely to become overweight and obese in their adult years. Published reports indicate that 50 percent of obese adults were obese babies and 80 percent obese juveniles will end up being obese adults. Also, research shows that there is a strong possibility that children who have obese parents (either one or both) will more than likely be obese themselves.

The smaller the fat content of the body, the larger the so-called "fat-free" or lean body weight. A substantial amount of evidence is available to indicate that the relative degree of fat-free body weight is not only valuable from a health point of view (overweight and obesity are clearly associated with hypertension and heart disease), but it is also an important factor contributing to higher levels of physical performance in activities where the total body weight must be moved. In addition, studies have shown that high percentages of body fat not only serves as dead weight, but it also lessens the relative ability to supply oxygen to the working muscles thus cutting down on one's cardiovascular endurance.

As was pointed out earlier in this chapter, exercise and diet in a long-range weight control program can bring about a reduction in both total body weight and percent fat. However, it should be pointed out that it is not unusual for an indvidual who is overweight and is just starting out in their exercise program to experience a weight gain and not a weight loss. This is often experienced by individuals who are low in strength and muscular development. What happens is that body or adipose tissue is replaced by lean muscle tissue. This is illustrated quite clearly in Figure 9-6 where adolescent girls and boys trained daily for 5 months and noticed a significant increase in lean body tissue and a decrease in excess body fat. It is also clear that those who did not take part in the training program did not notice any such changes. Figure 9-7 illustrates the percent body fat for a number of male and female trained athletes, all of which are below the normal untrained values. The evidence is also substantial showing that trained athletes also have higher levels of lean body tissue than non-trained subjects of similar age.

It should be pointed out that if weight loss is the primary motivating factor, then the overweight person may be somewhat disappointed at the end of the program. However, he or she should keep in mind that it is the body composition (the amount of fat-free weight) that is important and not so much total body weight. Although no weight loss may be seen, inches are usually lost around the waist, hips, and other parts of the body thus resulting in perhaps a more trimmer and nicer appearance. Whether or not total body weight is reduced depends largely upon the combined efforts of restricting caloric intake and caloric expenditure, as was pointed out earlier. It is certainly possible that a balance could be obtained between a gain in lean body tissue and a loss in body fat, thus resulting in no change in total body weight.

Ordinarily, normal weight is predicted from standard height-weight tables that have been developed by insurance companies and the military services. By the use of such tables, gross errors are not uncommon in assessing normal weight. For example, when 51 male USAF personnel were tested by two different standards, it was noticed that 15 of the subjects who were not found to be 15 percent overweight according to the standard weight tables were nevertheless found to be obese (more than 20 percent body fat). In addition, it was noticed that 6 of the subjects who would have been considered overweight by the standard tables were found to have less than 20 percent body fat, and consequently were not really obese. This means that 21 of the 51 subjects would have been incorrectly classified by the conventional tables alone. Similar findings have been reported

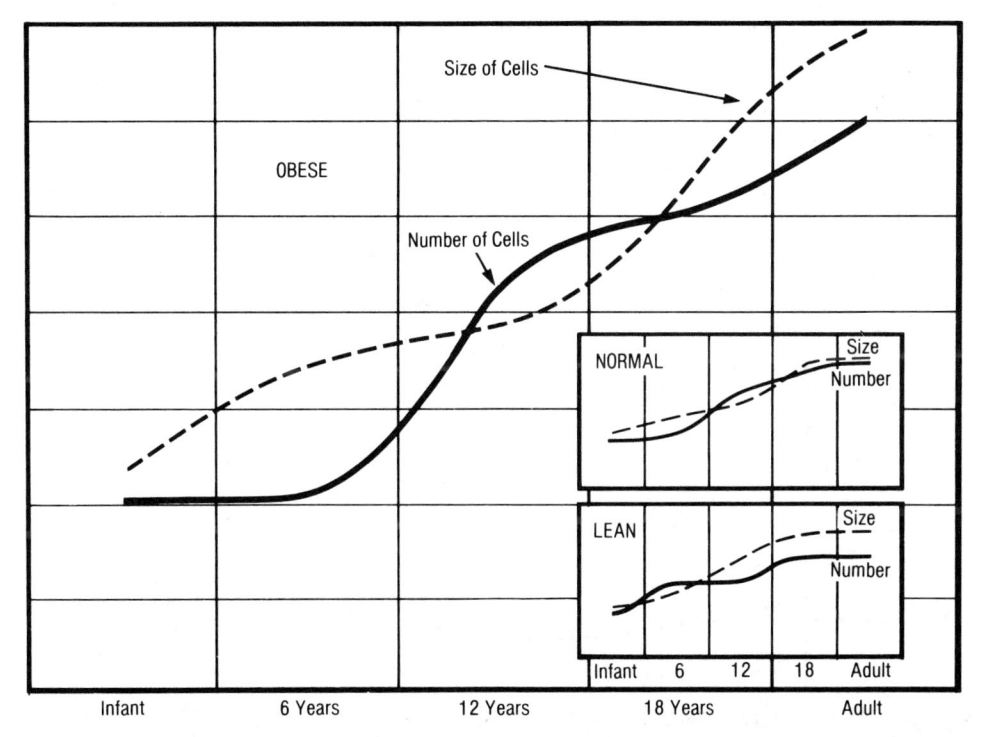

Figure 9-5 Schematic illustration of cell size and cell number from early childhood to adulthood for obese, normal, and lean subjects.

throughout the literature. This clearly indicates the need for determination of body composition, rather than a complete reliance upon tables made up of age, height, weight, etc. Fortunately, methods have been developed for determining body composition and a select few are reported here.

IX. METHODS FOR ASSESSING BODY COMPOSITION

A. UNDERWATER WEIGHING

Since fat tissue is less dense than other tissue (outside of lung tissue), it should be obvious that fat people float better than thin people. Consequently, as the quantity of fat deposit increases, density (defined as the mass of a substance per unit of volume) decreases. It has been well demonstrated that underwater weighing not only provides measures of body density (or specific gravity), but it also provides accurate estimates of the proportions of lean body weight and body fat tissue.

In this procedure, the subject is first weighed on land and then again in water when the subject is submerged completely (either in a water tank or a swimming pool), with the help of 15 or 20 pounds of lead weight (note that this is to ensure submersion of those who would normally float at the surface). Figure 9-8 illustrates the underwater weighing procedures. This method for determining body volume is based on Archimedes' principle that says an object submerged in water is buoyed up by a force equal to the weight of the water it displaces. By use of the following equation, the individual's body density is calculated.

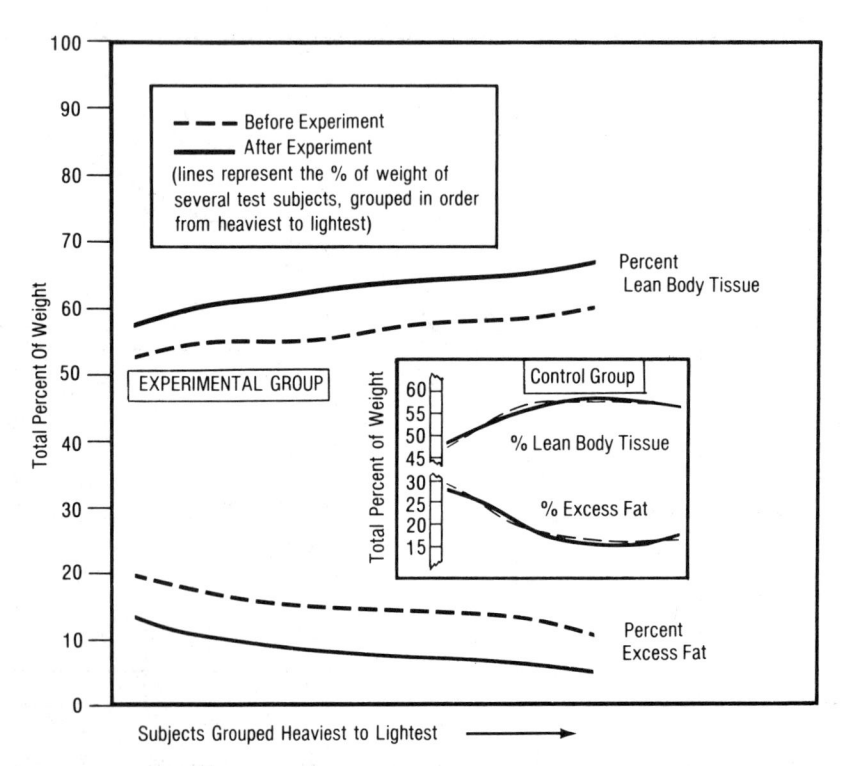

Figure 9-6 The effects of 5 months of training on adipose tissue and lean muscle tissue.

Nutrition, Weight Control and Performance

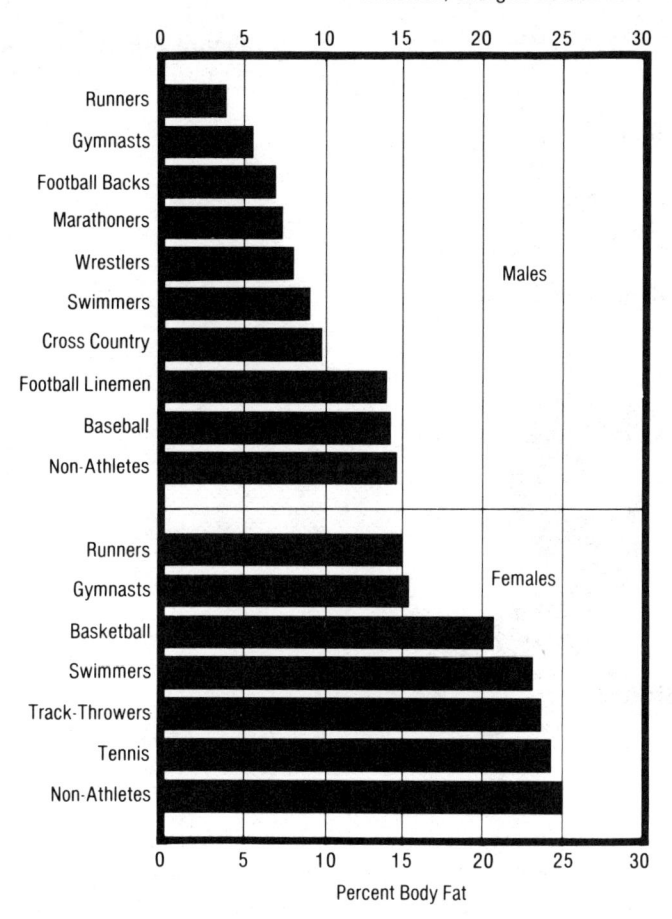

Figure 9-7 Percent body fat for a number of male and female trained athletes.

$$\text{Body density (gm/cc)} = \frac{\text{weight of subject in air}}{\frac{\text{weight of subject in air} - \text{weight of subject in water}}{\text{density of water}} - RV}$$

where: Weight of subject in air in grams,
Weight of subject in water in grams,
Density of water at the temperature recorded during underwater weighing (conversion factor is found in Table 9-5),
RV = residual volume in cc.

Since the lungs act as a built-in flotation device that reduces the weight of the body in water, it is extremely important that residual lung volume be measured or estimated at the time of land weighing. The measuring of residual volume requires the use of expensive respiratory apparatus. If the special equipment is available, the calculated residual volume values should be used. If not, however, then residual volume (air left in the lungs following a maximal expiration) may be closely estimated from their vital capacity (BTPS) which is the maximum amount of air that can

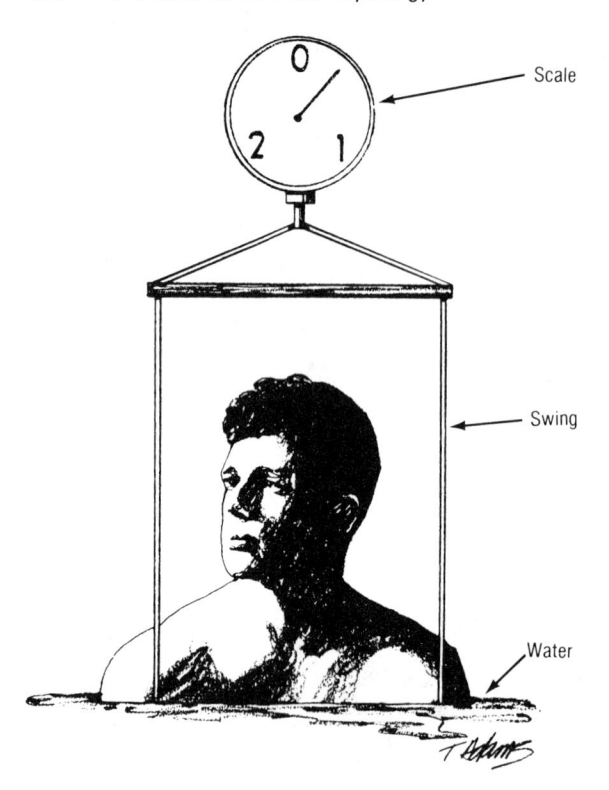

Figure 9-8 Schematic illustration of the underwater weighing procedures.

be exhaled following a maximum inhalation. For males, multiply vital capacity by the constant 0.24 and females by the constant 0.28. The estimated values should be around 1,300 ml for males and 1,000 ml for females. Very little accuracy is lost by assuming these values. Once body density has been determined, one may then compute percent of body fat by using the standardized equation below or some similar one.

$$\text{Percent body fat} = \left(\frac{4.570}{\text{body density}} - 4.142\right) \times 100$$

Once percent body fat has been determined, the following equation can be used to calculate the total weight of fat in either pounds or kilograms.

$$\text{Total weight of fat (kg)} = \frac{\text{weight (kg)} \times \text{percent fat}}{100}$$

Lean body weight (LBW), the quantitative expression of the lean body mass (LBM) includes all of the body tissue such as bone, muscle, nerve fiber coverings, etc. With the exception of stored "depot" fat, as was pointed out earlier, the LBW generally remains relatively constant while most body weight changes are brought about by changes in fat content. LBW can be determined by use of the following equation:

$$\text{LBW (kg)} = \text{total body weight (kg)} - \text{total weight of fat (kg)}$$

Below is an illustrative example of the underwater weighing procedures when determining (a) body density, (b) percent body fat, (c) total weight of fat, and (d) lean body weight (LBW).

Example:

Bill, a 160-lb male, was weighed in the laboratory and then was given a vital capacity test. Following this test, he was completely submerged in the water tank and his weight was then recorded. The following data were obtained for determining his body density, percent body fat, absolute fat, and lean body weight:

Body weight in air = 160 lb (73 kg) or 73,000 gm
Underwater weight = 8.85 lb (4 kg) or 4,000 gm
Vital capacity (BTPS) = 5,000 cc
Residual volume = 0.24 × 5,000 cc (vital capacity) = 1,200 cc
Density of water 30°C = 0.9957 gm/ml

$$\text{Body density (gm/cc)} = \frac{73{,}000 \text{ gm}}{\left(\dfrac{73{,}000 \text{ gm} - 4{,}000 \text{ gm}}{0.9957}\right) - 1{,}200 \text{ cc}}$$

$$= \frac{73{,}000 \text{ gm}}{\left(\dfrac{69{,}000}{.9957}\right) - 1{,}200 \text{ cc}}$$

$$= \frac{73{,}000 \text{ gm}}{69297.98 - 1{,}200 \text{ cc}}$$

$$= \frac{73{,}000 \text{ gm}}{68097.98} = 1.0720 \text{ gm/cc}$$

Table 9-5. Density of Water at Various Temperatures

Temperature (°C)	Density of Water* (grams/ml)
21	0.9980
22	0.9978
23	0.9975
24	0.9973
25	0.9971
26	0.9968
27	0.9965
28	0.9963
29	0.9960
30	0.9957
31	0.9954
32	0.9951
33	0.9947
34	0.9944
35	0.9941
36	0.9937
37	0.9934
38	0.9930
39	0.9926
40	0.9922

Source: Weast, R. C. (editor). *Handbook of Chemistry and Physics,* 54th edition, The Chemical Rubber Co., Cleveland, 1967, p. F-11.
*Rounded to 0.0001.

Percent body fat (%) = $\left(\dfrac{4.570}{1.0720} - 4.142\right) \times 100$

$ = (4.263 - 4.142) \times 100$
$ = 0.121 \times 100$
$ = 12.1\%$

Total weight of fat (kg) = $\dfrac{73 \text{ kg} \times 12.1}{100}$

$ = \dfrac{883.3}{100}$

$ = 8.83 \text{ kg}$

Lean body weight (kg) = 73 kg – 8.83 kg
$ = 64.17 \text{ kg}$

B. SKINFOLD MEASUREMENTS

This method is probably the most widely used of all and it is based on the fact that about one-half of the total adipose tissue is kept in specialized cells within the subcutaneous areas beneath the skin. A fold involving two layers of skin and subcutaneous structures can be held between the thumb and index finger while the skinfold calipers are being applied. The quantity of stored fat will determine the thickness of the fold. While this method is widely used, it should be pointed out that taking skinfold measurements requires a considerable amount of practice and expertise (especially if the data is being collected for research purposes) in order to obtain consistent and accurate measurements. If the person taking the measurements has the knowledge and knowhow, then the skinfold technique can provide some useful information on body composition.

Although several skinfold sites have been used for determining body density, only a few have been found to be of value and these are illustrated in Figure 9-9. Specific instructions for taking skinfold caliper measurements, as illustrated in Figure 9-9, are as follows:

Men Measurements

(1) Abdominal skinfold — at the midaxillary line at waist level.
(2) Chest skinfold — at the level of the xiphoid in the midaxillary line.
(3) Arm skinfold — at the midposterior, midpoint between the tip of the acromion and the tip of the olecranon with the arm hanging at the side.

Women Measurements

(1) Arm skinfold — same as described above for the men.
(2) Iliac skinfold — at the iliac crest in the midaxillary line.

Note that in taking skinfold measurements, all determinations should be made on the right side of the body. The calipers should be applied about 1 cm from the fingers holding the skinfold and at a depth that is about equal to the thickness of the fold. All measurements should be taken with the skinfold in a vertical position, except where the natural folding of the skin is in opposition, in which case the measurement is made with the skinfold along the lines of the natural folding. All readings should be recorded in millimeters.

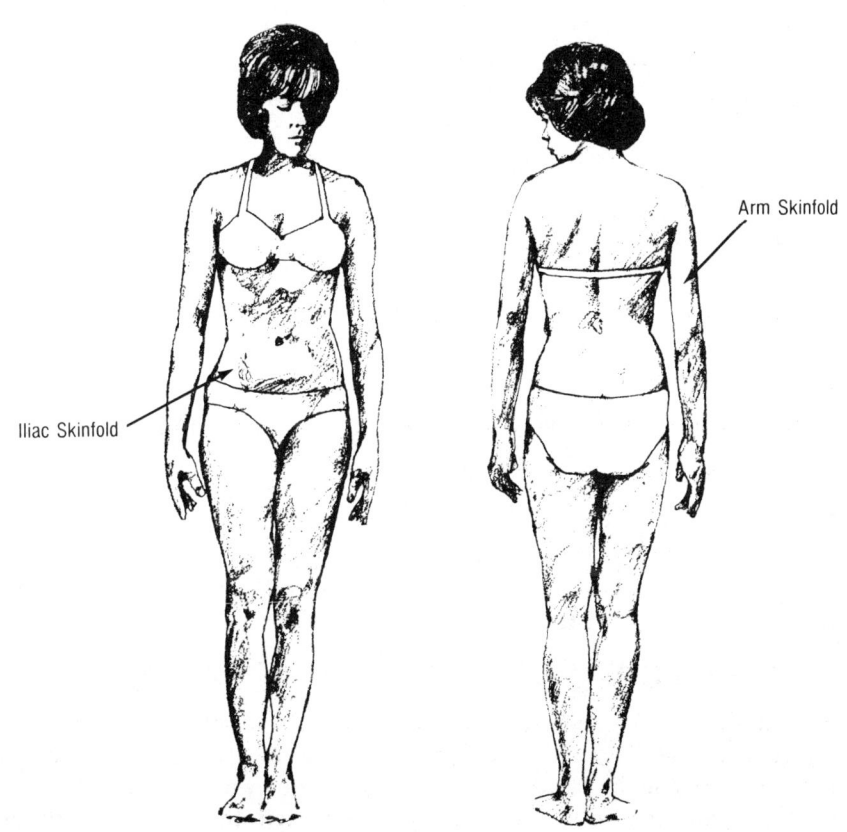

MEN MEASUREMENTS

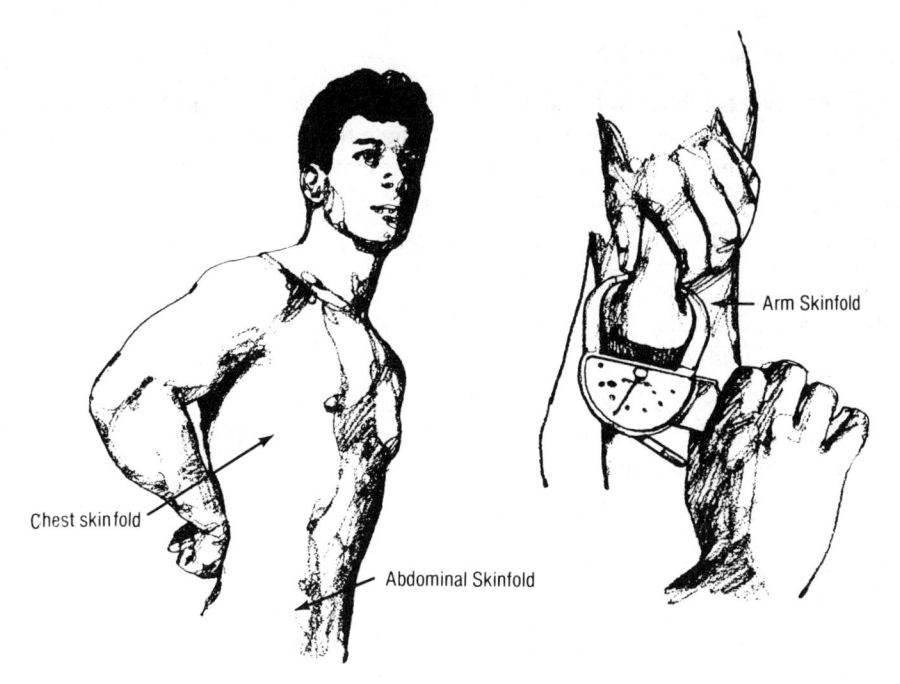

WOMEN MEASUREMENTS

Figure 9-9 Schematic illustration of several skinfold measurement sites.

Since both percent body fat and its distribution are sex-linked characteristics, several equations have been developed for both men and women for the assessment of body density from skinfold measures. Although only two formulas are presented here, both have been found to give good estimates. The following is applicable for men:

$$\text{Density} = 1.1017 - (0.000282) \times (A) - (0.000736) \times (B) - (0.000883) \times (C)$$

where (A) = abdominal skinfold
(B) = chest skinfold
(C) = arm skinfold

Once body density has been determined, the percent of body fat, total weight of fat, and lean body weight (LBW) can then be computed from the equations given previously for the underwater weighing technique. The following formula has been devised and is applicable for women:

$$\text{Density} = 1.0764 - (0.00081) \times (A) - (0.00088) \times (B)$$

where (A) = iliac skinfold
(B) = arm skinfold

Below is an illustrative example of the skinfold procedures when determining (a) body density and (b) percent body fat.

Example:

Men

$$\begin{aligned}
\text{Body density} &= 1.1017 - (0.000282) \times (15 \text{ mm}) - (0.000736) \times (9 \text{ mm}) - (0.000883) \times (12 \text{ mm}) \\
&= 1.083 \text{ gm/cc}
\end{aligned}$$

$$\begin{aligned}
\text{Percent body fat} &= \left(\frac{4.570}{1.0803} - 4.142\right) \times 100 \\
&= 8.8\%
\end{aligned}$$

Women

$$\begin{aligned}
\text{Body density} &= 1.0764 - (0.00081) \times (21 \text{ mm}) - (0.00088) \times (17 \text{ mm}) \\
&= 1.0444 \text{ gm/cc}
\end{aligned}$$

$$\begin{aligned}
\text{Percent body fat} &= \left(\frac{4.570}{1.0444} - 4.142\right) \times 100 \\
&= 23.4\%
\end{aligned}$$

C. ANTHROPOMETRIC MEASUREMENTS

Several anthropometric measurements and techniques have been used over the years to assess body composition. The anthropometric technique involves taking breath or diameter measurements of different body segments at various sites with sliding calipers. While this technique is simple and easy to use, it is extremely important that the measurements be taken carefully and with some degree of accuracy since small errors (in anthropometric readings) will result in large body composition inaccuracies. The following formula has been found to be very satisfactory for determining lean body weight from selected anthropometric measurements:

$$LBW = D^2 \times h$$

where LBW = lean body weight in kilograms
     h = height in decimeters
     D = sum of d values divided by 8 (where $d = c/k$)
     c = measured values in centimeters
     k = conversion constant

Eight measures of skeletal diameter are required and these are illustrated in Figure 9-10. Note that these measures are converted into d values by dividing by a constant k. Table 9-6, along with the k values for both men and women, illustrates the computational procedure for determining lean body weight and percent body fat by the anthropometric technique.

Table 9-6. Determination of Lean Body Weight from Anthropometric Measurements

Measurements	Constants (k) Male	Constants (k) Female	Measured Values (c)	Calculated Values (c/k)
Biacromial diameter	21.6	20.4	38.4	1.78
Bitochanteric diameter	17.4	18.6	31.5	1.81
Chest width	15.9	14.8	29.9	1.88
Bi-iliac diameter	15.6	16.7	26.5	1.70
Knee widths (R + L)	9.8	10.3	17.3	1.77
Ankle diameter (R + L)	7.4	7.4	14.5	1.96
Elbow widths (R + L)	7.4	6.9	12.8	1.73
Wrist diameter (R + L)	5.9	5.6	11.9	2.02

Subject = Male
Height = 160 cm (16.0 decimeters)
Weight = 63 kg

Sum of $d(c/k)$ = 14.65

$$D = \frac{\text{Sum of } d}{8} = \frac{14.65}{8} = 1.83$$

$$LBW = D^2 \times h$$
$$= (1.83)^2 \times 16.0$$
$$= 3.35 \times 6.0$$
$$= 53.6 \text{ kg}$$

$$\text{Percent fat} = \frac{\text{body weight} - LBW}{\text{body weight}} \times 100$$

$$= \frac{63 \text{ kg} - 53.6 \text{ kg}}{63 \text{ kg}}$$

$$= \frac{9.4 \text{ kg}}{63 \text{ kg}} \times 100$$

$$= 14.9\%$$

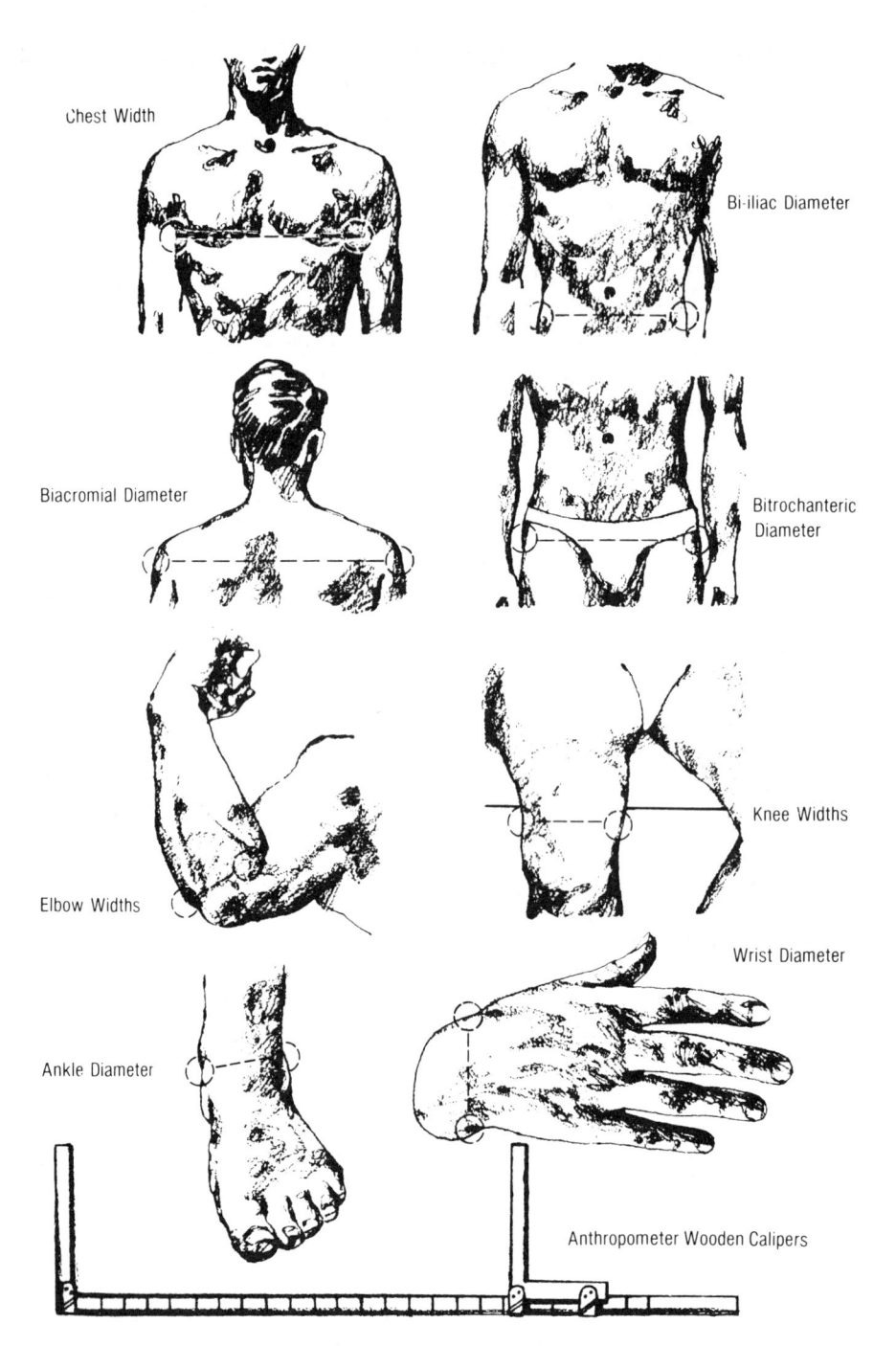

Figure 9-10 Schematic illustration of various anthropometric measurement sites.

While both the skinfold and the anthropometric procedures have been shown to be fairly accurate, it should be remembered that the formulas for these procedures have been found to be population-specific. That is, they have been found to be more accurate for specific groups or populations that are similar in sex, age, nationality, and even in general levels of physical fitness. Therefore, if maximum accuracy is wanted, it is highly recommended that the samples to which the formula is being applied is very similar to the one from which it was devised. In other words, do not use an equation that was developed from a group of middle-aged women for the determination of body composition of a group of young teen-age girls. If you do, maximum accuracy should not be expected.

X. DETERMINING YOUR DESIRED WEIGHT

As was mentioned earlier, predicting normal weight from the standard height-weight tables have resulted in gross errors in the past and more and more people are now using body composition as the determining factor for estimating normal weight. Once the percentage of body fat has been determined by one of the previously mentioned methods (underwater, skinfold, or anthropometric), and by comparing this figure to the standardized recommended body fat figures of either 15 percent for men or 25 percent for women, a very close estimate of desired weight can then be determined. For example, if a young woman weighs 115 pounds (52 kg) and her percentage of body fat is calculated as 30 percent, by multiplying the body weight (52 kg) times the percent body fat (0.30) results in 15.6 kg of body fat and 36.4 kg of "fat-free" weight or lean body weight (52 kg − 15.6). To determine the young woman's body weight at the standardized 25 percent body fat figure, divide the computed lean body weight (36.4 kg) by 0.75 (100% − 25% or 1.00 − 0.25). This results in a value of 48.5 kg or 107 pounds as the young woman's ideal body weight. Remember, this is only an estimate. However, it should be helpful for setting personal goals for losing weight.

XI. SUMMARY

(1) Carbohydrates and fats constitute the major fuels for energy production while proteins (which consist of amino acids are utilized primarily in muscle hypertrophy).

(2) Vitamins, minerals, and water are essential for proper nutrition. Deficiencies in any of them may result in poor health and below par in physical performance.

(3) For short-term anaerobic type activities, the make-up of the pre-game meal does not affect physical performance, while on the other hand, efficiency and physical performance during long-term events such as running a marathon is higher when the meal is high in carbohydrates.

(4) The technique called carbohydrate loading is where an individual is consuming a low amount of carbohydrates in their diet during 7 days prior to the event while training vigorously. Then, approximately 3 days prior to their contest or event when the persons work has tapered off, their diet becomes heavy in carbohydrates. Such a practice is not needed nor recommended for athletes competing in short events such as sprinters or field-event athletes.

(5) While carbohydrate loading may actually increase the glycogen content of the muscle and thus the endurance of athletes, there are also disadvantages for which the athlete should be aware. For example, some athletes undergoing this technique have experienced angina-like pain, electrocardiographic abnormalities, muscles feeling heavy and stiff with the increased storage of water and glycogen.

(6) Contrary to popular opinion, consuming large amounts of protein over and above the normal daily requirements has very little effect on bringing about increased lean muscle mass and strength. The normal daily protein intake (0.9 gm/kg of body weight) along with training is sufficient to bring about increased muscle mass and strength changes.

(7) While the evidence is contradictory concerning the influence of spacing and number of meals on work performance, the results generally favor frequent, small feedings over a few, large meals. From the standpoint of digestion, it is generally agreed that the last meal before an athletic event should be consumed three or more hours before the start of the contest.

(8) The most effective way of taking off weight and keeping it off is through a program that combine exercise (progressive cardiorespiratory endurance type) and diet over a relatively long period of time which will result in a gradual weight loss of between 1 and 2 pounds per week.

(9) Contrary to what some people think, evidence is available to show that appetite does not automatically increase as one exercises. In fact, if exercise is performed for short to moderate periods of time (such as one hour per day), appetite and food intake generally decreases. Laborers or highly competitive athletes who work or train heavy for several hours a day may show an increase in appetite and food intake. For these individuals, however, the high caloric intake is apparently needed to meet their energy demands for working and training. Some of these athletes (like the marathon runner) have the lowest percent body fat of any athletes.

(10) Evidence indicates that obesity brings about an increase in not only the number of adipose cells, but also in their size. Nutrition in early childhood has been illustrated to be critical in the development of new adipose cells.

(11) Physical training increases the amount of active tissue (lean body mass) while decreasing the amount of adipose tissue.

(12) Several methods are available for assessing body composition. They are (a) underwater weighing, (b) skinfold determinations, and (c) anthropometric measurements.

XII. REVIEW REFERENCES

(1) Ahlborg, G., and P. Felig. "Substrate Utilization During Prolonged Exercise Preceded by Ingestion of Glucose," *American Journal of Physiology,* 230:E188-E194, 1977.
(2) Astrand, P. O., and K. Rodahl. *Textbook of Work Physiology.* 2nd edition, McGraw-Hill Book Co., New York, 1977.
(3) Behnke, A. R. "Quantitative Assessment of Body Build," *Journal of Applied Physiology,* 16:960-68, 1961.
(4) Brook, C. G. D., J. K. Lloyd, and O. H. Wolf, "Relation Between Age of Onset of Obesity and Size and Number of Adipose Cells," *British Medical Journal,* 2:25-27, 1972.
(5) Brozek, J., and A. Henschel (editors). *Techniques for Measuring Body Composition,* Washington, D.C.: National Academy of Sciences, Research Council, 1961.
(6) Edington, D. W., and V. R. Edgerton. *The Biology of Physical Activity,* Houghton Mifflin Co., Boston, 1976.
(7) Food and Nutrition board. *Recommended Dietary Allowances,* 8th edition, Washington, D.C.: National Academy of Sciences, 1974.
(8) Foster, D., D. L. Costill, and W. J. Fink. "Effects of Preexercise Feedings on Endurance Performance," *Medicine and Science in Sports,* 11:1-5, 1979.

(9) Getchell, B. *Physical Fitness: A Way of Life,* 2nd edition, John Wiley & Sons, Inc., New York, 1979.
(10) Hickson, R. C., M. J. Rennie, R. K. Conlee, W. W. Winder, and H. O. Holloszy. "Effects of Increased Plasma Free Fatty Acids on Glycogen Utilization and Endurance," *Journal of Applied Physiology: Respiratory, Environmental, and Exercise Physiology,* 43:829-33, 1977.
(11) Ivy, J. L., D. L. Costill, W. J. Fink, and R. W. Lower. "Influence of Caffeine and Carbohydrate Feedings on Endurance Performance," *Medicine and Science in Sports,* 11:6-11, 1979.
(12) Katch, F. I., and W. D. McArdle. *Nutrition, Weight Control, and Exercise,* Houghton Mifflin Co., Boston, 1977.
(13) Lamb, D. R. *Physiology of Exercise: Responses and Adaptations,* Macmillan Publishing Co., New York, 1978.
(14) Mayer, J. *Overweight: Causes, Cost, and Control,* Prentice-Hall, Englewood Cliffs, New Jersey, 1968.
(15) Mayer, J., and Bullen, B. A. "Nutrition, Weight Control, and Exercise," in *Science and Medicine of Exercise and Sport,* 2nd edition, (W. R. Johnson and E. R. Buskirk, editors), Harper and Row Publishers, New York, 1974.
(16) Mirkin, G. "Carbohydrate Loading: A Dangerous Practice," *Journal of American Medical Association,* 223:1511-12, 1973.
(17) Nelson, R. A. "What Should Athletes Eat? Unmixing Folly and Facts," *Physician and Sportsmedicine,* 3:66-72, 1975.
(18) Sloan, A. W., J. J. Burt, and C. S. Blyth. "Estimation of Body Fat in Young Women," *Journal of Applied Physiology,* 17:967-70, 1962.

10
ERGOGENIC AIDS IN EXERCISE AND SPORTS

KEY CONCEPTS TO BE GAINED FROM THIS CHAPTER

(1) A number of diet and food supplements as well as various drugs and hormone stimulants are used quite frequently in athletics as ergogenic aids to enhance performance without knowledge of the long-term (and in some cases, short-term) side effects.

(2) The effects of ergogenic aids are highly specific to not only the individual, but to the activity as well.

(3) The American Medical Association and the International Olympic Committee as well as most other medical and sporting control bodies have established strict regulations outlawing the use of drugs in sports. Participants who are known to use them will be disqualified.

(4) There are psychological as well as physiological effects of some ergogenic aids, and the coach, athletic trainer, or physical educator must be able to differentiate between the two.

For years the facilitation of physical work performance by use of various ergogenic aids has been of interest to not only coaches and athletes, but also to scientific investigators concerned with exercise and sports. This is certainly understandable since improvements of only several tenths of a second or perhaps a few inches can make the difference between winning and losing in athletics.

An ergogenic aid is generally defined as something that improves physical work performance. A review of the literature reveals that various diets, drugs, hormones, certain foods, vitamins, water, oxygen, and many other substances have been tried as ergogenic aids. Some have been studied more than others either because they have shown to have some benefit, or perhaps because their ergogenic properties suggest that they should improve work performance. As might be anticipated, ergogenic aids appear to affect people differently. That is, some studies have found either beneficial effects, no effects, or dangerous side effects. Thus, it is apparent that no ergogenic aid is absolutely certain to improve physical work performance in every individual.

The purpose of this chapter is to present in alphabetical order some of the more commonly used aids, and to discuss why each aid has been believed to be beneficial to work performance. A brief summary of what the available literature has generally found for each aid will also be presented.

I. ALCOHOL

Although alcohol, in some circles, is believed to be a central nervous system stimulant, it is really a depressant and if consumed in large quantities, it may bring about partial or complete loss of sensibility.

Numerous studies have been conducted to observe the effects of alcohol on strength, local muscular endurance, psychomotor skills, aerobic and anaerobic work capacities. While there appears to be agreement that large amounts of alcohol (such as 6 ounces or more) may be detrimental to physical performance, there is no general agreement as to the effects of small and moderate amounts on work performance. Some studies, in using small and moderate amounts of alcohol, found performance to be either enhanced, retarded, or unchanged. This should be apparent, however, since the tolerance varies from person to person, and probably from time to time in the same person. In conclusion, since alcohol is considered to be a habit-forming drug, it cannot be recommended as an ergogenic aid.

II. ALKALIES

It is well known that during strenuous work, an individual's level of performance depends a great deal upon his or her ability to tolerate a large oxygen debt. A large oxygen debt, on the other hand, relies somewhat upon an individual's ability to tolerate a large lactic acid level, which when increased, will result in a decrease in blood pH (acidosis state). Of course, the ability of an individual to tolerate a large lactic acid level and a below normal pH during exercise depends upon the alkaline reserve in the body for buffering the lactic acid. It is easy to understand why some experimenters feel that increasing the size of alkalies in the body for buffering purposes would lead to an improved work performance.

The available evidence indicates that artificial alkalinization in the human being does result in improved work performance. While there appears to be strong agreement for the benefits of alkaline salts in untrained to moderately trained subjects, the evidence is not near as conclusive for the highly trained athlete. For the highly trained athlete, some of the studies have shown improved performance and some found no difference in performance. One explanation for the different findings between the trained and untrained subject is that the highly trained athlete may have already increased his alkaline reserve as a result of training, and as a result, he has less room for further improvement through alkali ingestion than the untrained person.

Also, it would appear from the available evidence that proper administration of alkali may play a vital part in noticing any improvement in performance. For example, the greatest improvement has been shown to result from 2 to 4 doses per day after meal-time beginning 2 days prior to the test and ending 5 hours before the actual test. More research is needed (especially comparing trained with untrained subjects) before any final conclusions can be made on whether or not alkaline ingestion can improve performance of athletes who are already in a highly trained state.

III. AMPHETAMINES

It appears that amphetamine is the most widely used drug by athletes today. Legally, it can be purchased only by prescription and is sold in drugstores under a variety of trade names in ampules, tablets, and sustained-release capsules. The three most popular forms of amphetamines are: (1) *amphetamine (Benzedrine)*, (2) *d-amphetamine sulfate (Dexedrine)*, and (3) *methamphetamine hydrochloride (Methedrine)*. The combination of amphetamines with barbiturates (often referred to as a "greenie") are often used by athletes. The terms "bennies," "uppers," "dexies," "speed," and "pep pills" are also often used to identify amphetamines. The presence of barbiturates apparently alleviates some of the nervousness and shakiness felt as side effects of the amphetamines alone.

The chemical make-up and physiological action of this drug are similar to those of epinephrine. That is, it is capable of causing increased blood pressure and heart rate, vasoconstriction, increased muscle tension, respiratory stimulation, pupillary dilation, elevated blood sugar, and smooth muscle relaxation in the bronchi, according to researchers working in this area. The normal therapeutic dosage given for cortical stimulation is between 5 and 10 mg.

This drug has the ability to depress appetite, to reduce or abolish the sense of fatigue (especially when this has been brought about by lack of rest and sleep), and to increase the fatigued person's performance of tests calling for skill, dexterity, and concentration, according to Golding. However, since most people (especially competitive athletes) are seldom sleepy or tired prior to competition, there should be no need to abolish this kind of fatigue. In fact, medical authorities warn against the use of this powerful and dangerous drug as a solution for sleepiness or fatigue, or to increase work performance, because of the following possible side effects: psychological dependence, paranoia, high blood pressure, rapid pulse, ulcers, insomnia hallucinations, strokes, heart attack, liver damage, mental confusion, possible blood cell abnormalities, compulsive and aggressive behavior, constipation, irritability, and nutritional problems.

Although the literature contains scattered reports that amphetamine inhibits fatigue during isometric and isotonic contraction, increases work output on a bicycle ergometer, improves sprinting performance, and increases the strength of forearm flexion, the weight of good solid scientific evidence in athletic performance studies indicates quite clearly that amphetamines do not enhance physical performance in terms of oxygen uptake capacity, oxygen debt capacity, and reaction time and movement time.

Since the majority of the experimental studies do not demonstrate increased physical performance, and since the side effects of large doses of drugs can be harmful, why is amphetamine still widely used by athletes? It appears, according to survey interviews and observations, that the primary purpose for athletes taking amphetamines is because it seems to get them "up" for their event or contest. That is, to "key" them up and make them mentally alert and ready for the event which is desirable for optimal performance. According to Golding, increased psychological preparedness is apparently the only rational justification for the continued use of amphetamine. However, if this is true, then scientific evidence should be available to support this notion.

Double-blind type studies investigating the psychological effects of both amphetamine sulfate and a tranquilizer meprobamate have shown that subjects could not distinguish which substrate they had actually taken. When given a questionnaire concerning whether they were on amphetamines or placebos, the subjects were apparently unable to identify the drug from the placebo. Results from these studies seem to suggest that perhaps the psychological effect of amphetamines is probaby self-induced by the fact that the subject is expecting to feel "keyed up" and ready to act. It appears, in light of this information, that more work needs to be done in order to demonstrate not only the psychological benefits of expecting to feel good, but also its subsequent effect on physical performance.

In summary, evidence not only indicates that amphetamines do not improve physical performance, but coaches, athletic trainers, team-physicians, and other athletic controlling bodies feel that the use of this drug is harmful, undesirable, and has no place in athletics. In fact, rules have been made by various governing bodies and International Olympic Committees to disqualify any athletes caught using amphetamines.

IV. ANABOLIC STEROIDS

Anabolic steroids is another group of drugs that is commonly used by many athletes (primarily wrestlers, weight-lifters, shot-putters, discus throwers, and javelin throwers) today in the belief that it will increase weight, size, and strength. While it is difficult to know for sure, it is generally believed that 70 percent or more of the aforementioned athletes are using these substances. Interviews with athletic champions in the United States and Canada and with athletes at the World Pentathlon Games and at the 1972 and 1976 Olympic Games showed that the majority of championship-level athletes taking part in weight and strength oriented events used steroids at some time during training.

Legally, this group of drugs can only be purchased with a written prescription of a physician, and is generally sold in drugstores under a variety of trade names (such as *Dianabol, Androyd, Nilevor, Maxibolen,* and *Winstrol*) in tablet form. Warnings that the drug should not be taken by healthy individuals for the sole purpose of gaining an advantage in sports is usually found on most of the anabolic steroids.

The chemical and functional characteristics of androgenic-anabolic steroids are quite similar to those of the male sex hormone, testosterone. Testosterone is a steroid that has both anabolic (nitrogen retention-protein building) and androgenic (refers to masculinity) properties that promote both muscular development and the male secondary sex characteristics, respectively. It is well known that the synthetic androgenic steroids have the same identical physiological effects as testosterone. That is, they stimulate growth and possible weight gain, bone maturation, and virilization. It is because of this that has led people to believe that ingestion of anabolic steroids will increase size, strength, and improved physical performance.

Investigations on the androgenic-anabolic steroids as they relate to physical performance are conflicting and not clear. Some published experiments have not only been poorly designed and controlled, but have used only one or two subjects. At the same time, however, some of the more well-designed and controlled clinical studies have even differed in their final conclusions. One reason for lack of agreement may be due to the different amounts of dosages that the subjects have been given from one study to another. Unfortunately, the majority of the clinical studies reported to date have not administered the same amount of anabolic steroids that most athletes ingest. The clinical studies are well below the massive doses that most athletes take. While it may be that massive doses of anabolic steroids do in fact increase size, strength, and physical performance, the potential dangers far outweigh any possible benefits that an individual may gain from their use.

In addition to the psychological side effects of breaking the rules and regulations, there have been many toxic side effects reported in the literature, such as premature epiphyseal closure, impotency, masculinization of the female, possible atrophy of the male testes, possible tumors, liver disorders, and possible cancer and leukemia. High blood pressure is also associated with ingestion of anabolic steroids. The one fact that coaches, trainers, sports-physicians, athletes, and researchers should not forget is that no one knows exactly what the long-term physiological or psychological chronic side effects of these steroids can be. The medical profession feels that there are so many unknown factors and possible serious consequences that to use these powerful and dangerous drugs in normal healthy individuals is totally ridiculous.

The American College of Sports Medicine made a comprehensive survey of the world literature concerning the use and abuse of anabolic-androgenic steroids in sports and as a result of that survey, it is their position that:

(1) "The administration of anabolic-androgenic steroids to healthy humans below age 50 in medically approved therapeutic doses often does not of itself bring about any significant improvements in strength, aerobic endurance, lean body mass, or body weight.
(2) There is no conclusive scientific evidence that extremely large doses of anabolic-androgenic steroids either aid or hinder athletic performance.
(3) The prolonged use of oral anabolic-androgenic steroids (C_{17}-alkylated derivatives of testosterone) has resulted in liver disorders in some persons. Some of these disorders are apparently reversible with the cessation of drug usage, but others are not.
(4) The administration of anabolic-androgenic steroids to male humans may result in a decrease in testicular size and function and a decrease in sperm production. Although these effects appear to be reversible when small doses of steroids are used for short periods of time, the reversibility of the effects of large doses over extended periods of time is unclear.
(5) Serious and continuing effort should be made to educate male and female athletes, coaches, physical educators, physicians, trainers, and the general public regarding the inconsistent effects of anabolic-androgenic steroids on improvement of human physical performance and the potential dangers of taking certain forms of these substances, especially in large doses, for prolonged periods."

In summary, we must conclude that the ergogenic effects are—at best—debatable and that the potential dangers involved are tremendous. Because anabolic steroids are generally taken out of season (which means that any weight and strength increase occurs well before the event), the problems of their control still remains unsolved. However, strict regulations have been established by various International Olympic Committees and other governing and medical bodies to disqualify participants who are caught or known to use these dangerous aids.

V. ASPARTIC ACID SALTS

Aspartic acid salts have been used experimentally by the medical profession in the treatment of fatigue. The major reason for their use involves the ability of the urea cycle to remove ammonia from the blood. Blood ammonia in the body may result from either foods that have ammonia compounds, metabolism, or skeletal muscular contraction. It is generally known that blood ammonia levels are raised following physical exertion, and that increased blood ammonia is one of the causes for fatigue. The urea cycle is responsible for returning the elevated blood ammonia concentrations to its normal values (note that this is accomplished because the urea cycle converts the excess ammonia to urea, which is then eliminated from the body). As Golding has already pointed out, however, the urea cycle may not be able to remove all the ammonia. It has been suggested that perhaps the weakest part in the urea cycle for the conversion of ammonia to urea is aspartic acid, and as a result, it is generally believed that a faster and more functional conversion process in the urea cycle would be possible if the aspartic acid concentration was increased (via exogenous sources of aspartic acid salts). If this is true, then following exercise, the increased blood ammonia concentration could then be converted much more rapidly to urea, thus preventing a large build-up of blood ammonia. It would appear that this decrease in blood ammonia would, in part, prevent the onset of fatigue and perhaps improve physical performance.

Several studies (human and animal) have been carried out in the laboratory to examine the effects of aspartic acid salts (namely, potassium, magnesium, or ammonium carbonate) on physical performance. The results from these investigations conflict, however, since some found blood ammonia levels to be reduced while others did not. In summary, although aspartic acid salts may have some application for the relief of subjective fatigue, there is not enough good conclusive evidence available to state any generalizations about their ergogenic effects on physical performance. Because aspartic acid salts, in normal doses, are not harmful and present no serious contraindications, additional research should be conducted.

VI. BLOOD DOPING

Blood doping (or blood boasting) is the injection of either whole blood or packed red blood cells (RBC's) into the participant the day prior to competition in the hope of increasing the blood volume and its oxygen carrying capacity, and thus improving endurance performance. Blood doping may be the injection of an individual's own blood which was withdrawn several weeks prior to reinjection. Training continues and this apparently allows time for the body to regenerate new RBC's in which to restore the normal hemoglobin level.

In reviewing the literature, differences of opinion do exist as to the influence of blood doping on physical performance. Some studies have illustrated some improvement in maximal oxygen uptake and endurance while others have found no significant improvements. While some results suggest a somewhat ergogenic effect from blood doping, it is considered to be unethical by most sports governing bodies and its potential dangers, when attempted by untrained people, far outweigh any potential benefits that might be found and should be condoned by physicians. The potential dangers include infections, intravascular blood clotting, and even mismatched transfusions.

VII. CAFFEINE

Caffeine, along with cola and tea are considered as xanthines often consisting of *theophyline* and *theobromine* and a few other alkaloids of little or no practical concern. Caffeine is used in the medical profession not only as a central nervous system (CNS) stimulant, but also as a diuretic. In small doses, it has shown to have a beneficial effect upon psychic processes. That is, it generally eliminates the feeling of fatigue and drowsiness, while at the same time, promoting alertness and clearer feelings. Caffeine also effects the blood vessels and the heart. For example, it causes general vasoconstriction, with simultaneous dilatation of the coronary artery, and increases the contractile strength of the heart muscle. As a group, long-term side effects of coffee drinkers have been closely associated to those with a somewhat higher incidence of coronary heart disease, intravascular blood clotting, and ulcers.

Medical dosage varies from 100 to 500 milligrams (mg) while a cup of coffee usually contains about 150 mg. Although the caffeine of tea (about 120 mg) leaves surpasses that of the coffee bean, more dilution is generally found in a cup of tea. A cola drink contains about 55 mg of caffeine and some theobromine.

In regards to physical performance, results indicate that ingestion of caffeine, when administered to healthy subjects, not only will increase endurance performance, but it also results in faster recovery times from fatigue. Anaerobic work, on the other hand, is apparently not affected by caffeine. Research has also shown recently that ingestion of caffeine also increases the rate of metabolism by about 25 percent. This is apparently brought about because of theophyline's inhibited effect on the enzyme *phosphodiesterase,* which has a function of breaking down *cyclic adenosine monophosphate* (cAMP). Note that because cAMP normally increases the metabolic activity of both lipids and glycogen, inhibition of phosphodiesterase by theophyline naturally facilitates the metabolic action of cAMP.

The findings are controversial concerning the effects of caffeine on psychomotor performance. For example, while several cups of coffee may be detrimental to fine motor coordinations such as in target shooting, writing, simple visual reaction time, and simple reaction time to a sound stimulus, other studies show improvement in these skills following ingestion of caffeine. In summary, caffeine is far from being an ergogenic aid and because of the potential long-term health risks involved, it should probably be eliminated from an individual's diet.

VIII. DIET

The use of carbohydrates, fats, proteins, and vitamins for the purpose of improving physical performance has already been discussed earlier in Chapter 9.

IX. OXYGEN

It is well known that some coaches, in an effort to improve performance, administer oxygen to their athletes either (a) immediately prior to the contest or event, (b) during time outs or breaks in the contest, or (c) immediately following the event or contest. Before reporting the evidence on oxygen as a potential aid, it is first necessary to consider the physiological factors by which greater than normal concentrations of oxygen could have an influence on physical performance.

It is well known that one of the major limitations in obtaining maximal work capacity for an individual is the oxygen transport system. Several factors play vital roles in controlling the oxygen supply to the working muscles. They are: (a) breathing oxygen from the atmosphere to the alveoli (pulmonary ventilation); (b) the diffusion of oxygen from the alveoli into the pulmonary capillary blood; (c) the amount of blood pumped from the heart per minute (cardiac output); (d) peripheral blood flow to the working muscles; and (e) the diffusion of oxygen from the systemic capillaries to the working muscles. While all of these factors are important, as Wilmore has suggested in an earlier publication, only a, b, and e is apparently effected by supplementing the oxygen supply during exercise.

Because of the combined effects of the above factors, each person is limited to a certain degree as to the greatest amount of oxygen that he or she can transport to the working tissues during maximal exertion. This limit is referred to as the maximal oxygen uptake or aerobic capacity. Thus, it would appear that by increasing this maximal oxygen uptake via supplemental oxygen breathing while reducing pulmonary ventilation and anaerobic metabolism would increase one's capacity for physical work and perhaps enhance the recovery process following work.

Studies in which oxygen was administered within one minute prior to exercise of short duration (anaerobic-type work) have shown to have some benefits as illustrated by an increase in the total amount of work done and the rate of work performed. Submaximal work was completed with lower heart rates following the ingestion of oxygen. At the same time, exercise in excess of 2 minutes or if the time interval between oxygen inhalation and performance is longer than 2 minutes, then the benefits of breathing oxygen is not noticed. The lack of sufficient oxygen storage in the body is apparently reflected in these findings.

Because the normal stores of oxygen, glycogen, and creatine phosphate should be adequate to supply the necessary energy for short work periods of one minute or less, it seems highly possible that the benefits of breathing oxygen prior to this type of exercise is psychological since researchers have been able to demonstrate an improved performance by having subjects breath from an empty tank that was marked "oxygen." Or, it may be due to the individual's desire merely not to breathe. For example, if the later is true, then the increased oxygen supply along with the lower level of carbon dioxide in the extracellular fluids would bring about a decrease in stimulation of the respiratory centers of the brain.

The fact that oxygen breathing must take place within one minute prior to actual competition means that oxygen inhalation before the event or contest has little or no practical value since just about all competitive events take longer than one minute for preliminary instructions.

Researchers administering oxygen during exercise generally agree that performance is improved if the work periods are 2 minutes or more. In work periods below 2 minutes, improvements are not noticed. This is apparently due to the lag in the circulatory system. Thus, this lag has been suggested as a major limiting factor for oxygen supply to the tissues during the early stages of work. Results of these studies indicate an increase in the amount of exhaustive work performed as well as the rate of work. During submaximal work, heart rates are significantly lower, thus indicating less stress on the individual. Because it is impractical and against the rules to wear an oxygen outfit during most athletic competition, breathing oxygen during this period has little or no real value to the competitive athlete. However, in certain professional job situations such as fire-fighters fighting fires, certainly has some value. For those people who have respiratory problems and are restricted in their work and activities, the value of breathing oxygen for them is obvious.

Studies concerning the effects of oxygen breathing during recovery following exercise are contradictory. Unfortunately, not enough well-controlled research has been conducted to merit any generalizations abut the ergogenic effect of oxygen during the recovery period. However, it appears that there is a beneficial effect from breathing oxygen during the postexercise periods, it's very small and probably has no physiological value in regard to subsequent performance.

X. SALT (SODIUM CHLORIDE)

It is a well-known fact that excessive sweating (such as football, wrestling, distance running, and military recruits) can cause, in addition to a water deficit, a substantial loss in salt (sodium chloride) which may lead to heat cramps and even perhaps serious heat illnesses. For years, salt tablets have been administered by coaches, military personnel, and others to counteract the excessive loss of water and salt through sweating. While salt replacement in sweat is certainly desirable, extreme care must be taken to make sure that excessive amounts are not ingested.

It is unfortunate that some military personnel, coaches, and trainers still believe today that overloading the body with salt tablets can be responsible for extra energy and improved performance in recruits and athletes in general. This is absolutely not supported by evidence and could be extremely dangerous. Salt loading via indiscriminate administration of salt tablets to athletes prior to physical activity may lead to serious potassium depletion and increased water retention, which in turn, may lead to poor performance and even heat injuries.

In summary, most experts agree that the problems attributed to salt excess and lack are probably over emphasized because normally, the dietary intake of salts will more than adequately offset the salt loss in a single bout of exercise. At the same time, however, it is generally felt that when athletes take part in hard training over several days in hot weather, they may experience a salt deficit that can best be corrected by ingesting, in moderation, commercial salt and electrolyte beverages such as Gatorade, Sportade, ERG, or other equivalent salt and electrolyte fluids. The athlete may also add extra salt to their food during this time. The athlete and coach should be cautioned, however, not to expect any better benefits from the commercial beverages containing salt and electrolytes than from regular water. As Karpovich and Sinning point out, salt added to the diet is only a precautionary measure to insure a normal output of energy which may be decreased if there is an excessive amount of sodium chloride lost.

XI. TOBACCO SMOKING

During the past, numerous studies have been conducted to determine the effect of cigarette smoking on physical performance. Many of the studies have reported detrimental effects of smoking on various individual physiological adjustments to exercise. In general, they have found: (a) a decrease in airway conductance; (b) a decrease in lung diffusing capacity; (c) an increase in airway constriction in lung bronchioles; (d) a decrease in the efficiency of the heart as determined by a higher heart rate and lower stroke volume; (e) an increase in the oxygen cost of breathing; (f) a larger oxygen debt for a standardized work load; and (g) an increase in blood pressure.

At the same time, in reference to competitive athletics or sports performance, the evidence is somewhat unclear and inconclusive. Some studies have found decreased performance while others have found improved performance. However, most of the research reported in the literature show no difference in performance. In summary, while the evidence concerning selected physiological parameters is rather conclusive in terms of smoking having a detrimental effect, not enough solid evidence is available to draw any final conclusion involving the ergogenic effect of smoking upon actual competitive athletics or sport performance. However, because of smokings tremendous potential for causing lung cancer and heart disease, it should obviously be discouraged and banned from active use.

XII. WATER

Although it is well documented that water ingestion facilitates the physical performance of man working in hot, humid environments, it has only recently been alluded to as a possible ergogenic aid. Much of the research has been confined to observing the influence of fluid ingested prior to and during the performance of exercise. One of the major criticisms that is often heard concerning fluid consumption prior to as well as during performance is that it tends to stretch the stomach, thus obstructing the respiratory processes and muscular exertion. There is no scientific evidence that ingesting as much as a quart or more of water several minutes before physical performance has any adverse effects associated with a full stomach. On the contrary, substantial amount of evidence is available to indicate water ingestion prior to and during prolonged exercise (30 minutes or longer) in the heat not only reduces the increase in body temperature, but it also allows the subject to exercise longer and perform better with lower heart rates. For short anaerobic-type exercise, it does not make sense to have to ingest large amounts of water prior to or during the exercise since the body's thermoregulatory system is generally able to regulate its temperature within safe ranges.

During strenuous work in heat such as in long-distance running when severe dehydration is inevitable and often dangerous, and since research shows that people's voluntary thirst does not necessarily drive them to replace the water that is lost, athletes should be instructed to ingest more water than they think they need. Water ingestion prior to exercise and during performance should be encouraged by coaches and trainers. It has been suggested that athletes, during prolonged work in heat, should drink about 200 milliliters of cool liquid every 15 minutes. The interested reader is referred to Chapter 7 for a more complete discussion on exercise in heat.

To summarize, while the consumption of fluids prior to and during exercise is beneficial in lowering the body temperature and cardiac stress associated with prolonged work in the heat, it apparently provides little if any ergogenic value to people during short-term work. There is no evidence available to justify the restriction of fluids prior to and during physical work. In fact, participants performing in hot weather should be encouraged to ingest cold fluids in excess of thirst demands to minimize the potential of heat injuries and to insure top performance.

XIII. SUMMARY

(1) The evidence is clear that large amounts of alcohol may be detrimental to physical performance, but there is no general agreement as to the effects of small and moderate amounts on work performance. Alcohol is considered to be a habit-forming drug and is not recommended as an ergogenic acid.

(2) Evidence indicates that amphetamines do not improve physical performance. Furthermore, coaches, athletic trainers, team-physicians, and other athletic controlling bodies feel that the use of this drug is harmful, undesirable, and has no place in athletics. Rules have been made and passed by various governing bodies, the International Olympic Committees, and the American Medical Association to disqualify any athletes caught using amphetamines.

(3) The ergogenic effects of anabolic steroids are—at best—debatable and the potential dangers involved are tremendous. Strict regulations have been established by the International Olympic Committee and various other governing bodies to disqualify participants who are caught or known to use these dangerous aids.

(4) While aspartic acid salts may have some benefits for the relief of subjective fatigue, there is not enough good solid evidence to state any generalizations about their ergogenic effects on physical performance. More research is recommended since they are not harmful and present no serious contraindications, when given in normal doses.

(5) While some results suggest an ergogenic effect from blood doping, it is considered to be unethical by most sports governing bodies and its potential dangers (including infections, intravascular blood clotting, and mismatched transfusions), when attempted by untrained people, far outweighs any potential benefits that might be found and should be condoned by physicians.

(6) Caffeine is far from being an ergogenic aid. It is more commonly used by office workers than by athletes. Long-term side effects of coffee drinkers have been closely associated to those with a somewhat higher incidence of coronary heart disease, intravascular blood clotting, and ulcers.

(7) Oxygen, when administered immediately prior to a short exercise bout (less than 2 minutes in length) or during the actual performance, appears to be beneficial. Not enough solid research is available to make any generalizations about the ergogenic effect of oxygen during the recovery period. If there is a beneficial effect, it is very small and probably has no physiological value.

(8) Salt loading via indiscriminate administration of salt tablets to athletes prior to activity may lead to serious potassium depletion and increased water retention, which in turn, may lead to poor performance and possible heat injuries. While salt replacement in sweat is desirable, extreme care must be taken to make sure that excessive amounts are not ingested.

(9) Salt deficit can usually be best corrected by ingesting commercial salt and electrolyte beverages such as Gatorade, Sportade, ERG, etc., or by extra salt added to the table food or both.

(10) While the evidence on smoking as an ergogenic aid is conflicting, because of smoking's tremendous potential for causing lung cancer and heart disease, it should be discouraged and banned from active use.

(11) Water ingested prior to and during physical work is beneficial in lowering body temperature and in lowering heart rate during prolonged exercise. There is no evidence to justify the restriction of water prior to and during physical work.

(12) Participants performing in hot weather should be encouraged to ingest cold fluids in excess of thirst demands to minimize the potential of heat injuries and to insure top performance.

XIV. REVIEW REFERENCES

(1) American College of Sports Medicine. "Position Statement on The Use and Abuse of Anabolic-Androgenic Steroids in Sports," *Medicine and Science in Sports,* 9:xi-xiii, 1977.
(2) Chandler, J. V. "The Effects of Amphetamines of Selected Physiological Components Related to Athletic Success," *Medicine and Science in Sports,* 10:38, 1978.
(3) Costill, D. L., G. P. Dalsky, and W. J. Fink. "Effects of Caffeine Ingestion on Metabolism and Exercise Performance," *Medicine and Science in Sports,* 10:155-58, 1978.
(4) Edington, D. W., and V. R. Edgerton. *The Biology of Physical Activity,* Houghton Mifflin Co., Boston, 1976.
(5) Engs, R. C. *Responsible Drug and Alcohol Use,* Macmillan Publishing Co., Inc., New York, 1979.
(6) Golding, L. A. "Drugs and Hormones," in *Ergogenic Aids and Muscular Performance,* (W. P. Morgan, editor), Academic Press, New York, 1972.
(7) Golding, L. A., and J. E. Freydinger. "Weight, Size, and Strength-Unchanged With Steroids," *Physician and Sportsmedicine,* 2:39-43, 1974.
(8) Ivy, J. L., D. L. Costill, W. J. Fink, and R. W. Lower. "Influence of Caffeine and Carbohydrate Feedings on Endurance Performance," *Medicine and Science in Sports,* 11:6-11, 1979.
(9) Karpovich, P. V., and W. E. Sinning. *Physiology of Muscular Activity,* 7th edition, W. B. Saunders, Co., Philadelphia, 1971.
(10) Lamb, D. R. *Physiology of Exercise: Responses and Adaptations,* Macmillan Publishing Co., New York, 1978.
(11) Percy, E. C. "Ergogenic Aids in Athletics," *Medicine and Science in Sports,* 10:298-303, 1978.
(12) Rogozkin, V. "Metabolic Effects of Anabolic Steroid on Skeletal Muscle," *Medicine and Science in Sports,* 11:160-63, 1979.
(13) Williams, M. H. "Blood Doping—Does It Really Help Athletes?" *Physician and Sportsmedicine,* 3:52-56, 1975.
(14) Williams, M. H. *Drugs and Athletic Performance,* Charles C. Thomas, Springfield, Illinois, 1974.
(15) Wilmore, J. H. "Oxygen," in *Ergogenic Aids and Muscular Performance,* (W. P. Morgan, editor), Academic Press, New York, 1972.

11
SEX DIFFERENCES IN EXERCISE

KEY CONCEPTS TO BE GAINED FROM THIS CHAPTER

(1) There are certain anatomical and physiological sex differences which favor both the male and female for specific activities.

(2) Training data indicates that similar training effects leading to a greater work capacity can be obtained in both sexes following similar-type training programs.

(3) Gynecological evidence indicates that exercise is beneficial in relieving pain and in improving and preventing dysmenorrhea.

(4) Important consideration should be given to vigorous training and competition during pregnancy.

One of the most interesting developments in sport and physical education during the decades of the sixties and seventies has been the tremendous growth in the number of girls and women taking part in competitive athletics. Prior to this time, the female's physiological responses to athletic performance has not been as extensively studied as those of men. However, with the increased interest being shown in the past several years in providing competitive sports programs for girls and women on a equal basis to that of men, a number of research studies have been conducted and published on the female athlete. In addition, several conferences have been held throughout the United States and other countries to discuss this topic.

Because participation by girls and women in competitive athletics is increasing at such a rapid pace, every physical educator and coach as well as administrator should be aware of the available knowledge concerning the female in competitive sports. It is hoped that the information found in this chapter will provide the reader with a greater insight and understanding regarding the female in sports.

I. STRUCTURAL CHARACTERISTICS

A. SKELETAL

The most accurate method of determining maturity is to measure by way of X-rays the degree of ossification (process by which bone salts are deposited in the intercellular center of bone, producing a hardening of the bone itself and a closure or bony union between the primary and secondary growth centers) of the carpal and metacarpal bones as well as the phalanges. It is well known that the carpal and metacarpal bones ossify sooner in the female than in the male. X-ray assessment of the pisiform indicates that this bone is usually completely ossified in the female at the ages of 9 and 10 years, whereas complete ossification in the male does not take place until around the age of 13 years. In addition, complete ossification of the metacarpals and phalanges in the female and male is around the age of 16 and 19 years, respectively. It appears that the growth patterns of the long bones (especially the length of them) for both sexes are very similar with the female's being completed 1 to 3 years sooner than the males. According to authorities working in this area, this earlier ossification of the bones in the female suggests a more rapid calcium metabolic rate than in their male counterpart. Generally speaking, a growing girl at any age has reached greater maturity than a boy of the same age. It should be pointed out, however, that the rate of ossification can be changed by health, nutrition, endocrine secretions, and other factors.

Also, an examination of the male and female skeleton at full maturity reveals that the skeleton of the male is more rugged, the bones are more massive and of greater density, and the long bones are somewhat longer. In addition, the joints of the male are slightly larger and thus present a greater articular surface. From the above information, it would appear that the male may have a slight advantage over the female in terms of leverage and angular of movement.

B. TRUNK, SHOULDER WIDTH, AND PELVIS

In regards to the trunk, the male has wider shoulders in relation to the width of his hips (which results in a wedge-shaped appearance) while the female generally has a wider pelvis as compared to the width of her shoulders (note that the female pelvis is also more shallow than that of the male). Between the ages of 11 and 15 years the female has relatively wider shoulders than the male. However, after the age of 15, the shoulder width of the male continues to increase until at the age of 19 years it is somewhat larger than that of the female.

The pelvis is comprised of two parts with each consisting of three bones, the ischium, which is below and to the rear; the pubis, which is below and forward; and the ilium, which is above and on the side of the hip. The entire pelvis is held together by several strong ligaments. Although the two pubis bones in the front are separated by a cartilaginous disc, they are securely held together by other strong ligaments. During the period of pregnancy, the female experiences some degree of movement at the symphysis pubis (joint between the two pubis bones) and therefore expansion of the pelvis. This is made possible because during this time the action of certain hormones permit the ligaments to become soft and relaxed. Although this phenomenon generally occurs during menstruation, it is not quite as noticeable as during recovery.

C. CHEST

The male exhibits a greater chest circumference except perhaps at the ages of 12 and 13 years, at which time the female, due to the adolescent spurt, will usually equal or surpass him. In addition, the maximum thoracic index (calculated by dividing chest depth into chest width and multiplying by 100) for girls and boys is generally obtained around the age of 11 and 14 years, respectively. Beyond these ages, the girl only experiences slight increases in the index, whereas the index for the boy continues to increase rather rapidly so that at the age of 16 years he shows a broader chest than the female.

D. ABDOMEN

The female has a larger abdominal cavity than the male. This is due to the fact that this area contains relatively larger visceral organs as well as the additional organs of reproduction.

E. UPPER AND LOWER EXTREMITIES

In terms of upper and lower limbs, when males and females of the same height are compared, the male generally shows not only a longer upper arm, but also a longer forearm. The male also exhibits a longer length in the lower extremity. Research evidence is available to indicate that men's leg length is approximately 52 percent of their height as compared to about 51.2 percent for women. Between the ages of 7 and 12 years, the girl's leg is longer than the boy's. However, after 12 years of age, the boy takes over for the remainder of his life. The lower leg of the female is also much shorter than that of the male. Finally, measurements of the foot indicate that the male has a greater length and breadth than that of the female.

F. HEIGHT AND WEIGHT

Between the ages of 1 and 9 years, there is very little, if any, difference between males and females in terms of height. However, after the age of about 9 or 10 years, the female takes the lead and with the onset of puberty (which results in a rapid growth), the girl may outgrow her male counterpart as much as 2 inches. On the other hand, around the age of 15 years, the boy experiences his growth spurt and thus takes over the lead and never relinquishes it. In fact, males generally continue to grow until the age of about 20 to 23 years, whereas females stop growing in height around the ages of 18 and 20 years. From all indications, the average male is somewhere around 5 to 6 inches taller than that of the average female.

A similar pattern is seen in terms of body weight. During pubertal growth, a girl may weigh as much as 4 to 5 pounds more than that of the male. Again, the boy catches up and surpasses the girl around the age of 15 years. Upon reaching full maturity, the boy may have a total weight advantage of somewhere between 30 and 40 pounds and between 40 and 50 pounds in terms of lean body weight.

G. CENTER OF GRAVITY

Center of gravity (point within the body at which the total weight of the body is concentrated) is an important concept in physical education and sport because it determines ones balance. Man's mean center of gravity is found at a point around 56.7 percent of his height above ground, whereas woman's is located at 56.1 percent of her height. Apparently, man's greater height, shorter trunk, wider shoulders, and narrower pelvis account for the 0.6 percent difference. The lower center of gravity found in the female (due to shorter legs and broader hips), however, gives her an advantage over the male in terms of better balance for activities such as gymnastics or tumbling. Thus, in order to obtain a comparable degree of balance, the male, in most situations, would have to widen his stance to a certain degree.

H. ADIPOSITY

At the time of full maturity, the average female has considerable more absolute subcutaneous fat than the average male (25% as opposed to 15% relative body fat). The female generally accumulates more fat in the hips, in the thighs, and in the breasts than the male. The male, on the other hand, carries a greater amount of fat in the upper areas of the body and in the abdominal region.

Between the ages of 18 and 22 years, the average female's relative body fat will be somewhere between 22 and 26 percent as compared to 12 and 16 percent for her male counterpart of similar age. The higher figures for the female are obviously due to her higher absolute levels of subcutaneous fat as well as her lower absolute levels of lean body weight. It is now well documented that the larger amounts of the estrogen hormones found in the female are reponsible, in part, for her larger amounts of body fat. At the same time, its well-known that the larger amounts of the androgen hormones found in the male are responsible for his larger lean body weight. Exactly what part environmental and cultural factors play in these differences is not clear and conclusive at this time.

This high percentage of body fat poses some disadvantages as well as advantages for the girl athlete. For example, the female shows some 10 percent greater buoyancy (which favors swimming) than her male counterpart, and she loses much less body heat in cold water. At the same time, the female is less able to deal with hot environments than the male. Note that this is covered in more detail later in the chapter.

Figure 9-7 illustrates some typical relative body fat figures for both male and female athletes of various sports. It is interesting to note that mean relative body fat values as low as 6 to 10 percent has been found for trained women distance runners. These values are better than half of the value found in sedentary females. In addition, these values are as good, if not better, than most of those found for trained male athletes. It is also interesting to note in Figure 9-7 that values as low as 4 percent have been found for trained male distance runners. Thus, it is obvious that training (endurance type) can not only lower the percent body fat in both men and women, but it also appears from the evidence that the female athlete, with the opportunity and proper training and diet can lower her relative body fat levels nearly to the same level as that of her male athlete counterpart.

In terms of body build (on the basis of somatotyping), the average untrained female generally favor endomorphy (fatness), whereas the average untrained male generally favors either ectomorphy (thin) or mesomorphy (muscular).

I. HEART SIZE

Measurements of the transverse diameter of the heart indicate that with the exception of the 12th and 13th year, the male heart is larger than that of the female. Mean measurements for men are around 12.13 cm while recordings for women are around 10.67 cm. The fact that the male is physically larger and has a higher percentage of lean muscle mass as opposed to the female's high percentage of adipose tissue may well account for this difference.

Calculations on the ratio of heart weight to body weight also indicate that between the ages of 10 and 60 years, the average value for the female is only about 85 to 90 percent of the value for the male, whereas after the age of 60, the values are similar for both sexes.

J. STRENGTH

Since the male possesses a larger muscle mass, and since strength potential is directly related to the physiological cross section of the muscle itself, it is obvious that the male has greater absolute strength (males are approximately 30 to 40 percent stronger than females). In other words, the male's strength-to-weight ratio is greater. The reason for the female's lower strength-to-weight ratio is, of course, the greater adiposity in relation to lean muscle mass. Figure 11-1 illustrates that when average strength of several different muscle groups are plotted as percentages of maximum strength, the female's closest approximation of the male's strength takes place between the ages of 8 and 12 years, after which time the male notices a much greater improvement in strength as compared to the female. This difference is believed to be due to the influence of the males sex hormone, testosterone, which brings about muscle growth.

The illustration in Figure 11-1 shows that both sexes, after the age of 12, continue to get somewhat stronger until they reach their twenties. The female reaches her peak in the early-to-middle twenties, whereas the male obtains his peak somewhere in the middle-to-late twenties. Following these periods, strength gradually decreases with increased age. It is interesting to note that girls below the age of 12 years often surpasses the boys of similar age in terms of strength performance (such as sprints, jumps, etc.). However, from the ages of 12 to 18 years, the boys, because of their tremendous muscle growth, are considerably more stronger in terms of absolute strength than the girls. This is especially true of upper body strength, where the male is approximately 50 to 70 percent stronger as compared to leg strength where the strength levels of the two sexes are nearly identical. At the same time, however, when leg strength is expressed relative to body size, the two sexes are the same. Also, when leg strength is calculated in terms of relative to lean body weight (to more closely approximate muscle mass), the male is slightly weaker (approximately 5.8%) than the female. From the above information, it appears, therefore, that the quality of muscle in terms of its ability to contract and exert force is identical in both sexes. Leg strength similarities between the sexes are probably the result of similarities in use (such as in walking, riding bicycles, climbing stairs, etc.), whereas on the other hand, the female traditionally has not used her upper body to the same degree as the male in masculine activities

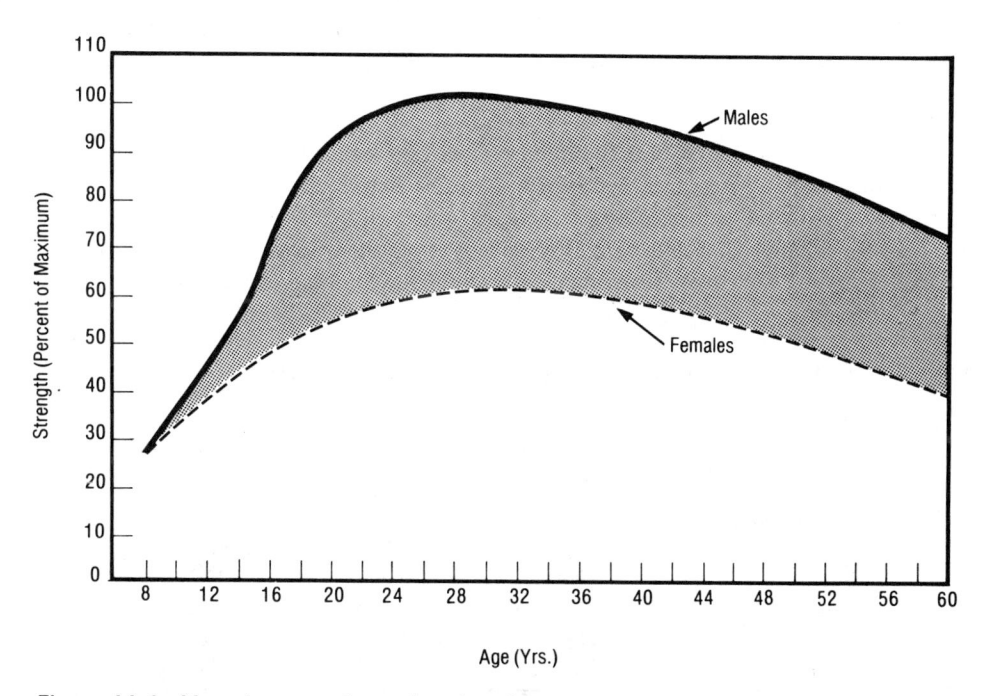

Figure 11-1 Muscular strength as a function of age and sex.

such as throwing, lifting, rope climbing, etc., and as a result, she is much weaker in upper body strength.

It is apparent that the male enjoys an advantage over the female in activities where strength (especially upper body strength) is a factor. This advantage, along with the advantages he has in respect to leverage and angles of motion, makes it nearly impossible and unfair for the female to compete with the male in activities where strength in the upper body plays an important role. At the same time, an important question in this area is can the female attain the same (or nearly the same) levels of strength as the male from strength training exercises? This topic is covered in a later section on the "trainability of the female."

II. PHYSIOLOGICAL CHARACTERISTICS

A. CARDIOVASCULAR SYSTEM

Blood Volume and Hemoglobin

Table 11-1 illustrates quite clearly that the male (trained and untrained) has a greater blood volume as well as a greater total hemoglobin count than the female (trained and untrained). In fact, the male, on an average, has about 15 percent more hemoglobin per 100 milliliters of blood than the female. In addition, the male has an average resting red blood cell count of about 5,000,000 per cubic millimeter as compared with 4,500,000 in the female. These factors indicate that the male has a greater oxygen-carrying capacity than the female.

Blood Pressure

Prior to menopause, the systolic and diastolic blood pressures in women are generally about 5 to 10 mmHg lower than men of the same age. However, after menopause the female blood pressure tends to increase slightly over that of the male.

Heart Rate

It has already been stated that the male possesses a larger heart than the female, perhaps because he has more muscular tissue which requires better circulation than the contrasting proportion of adipose tissue in the female. Note in Table 11-1 that the male also has a greater heart volume than the female. This heart size difference is apparently the cause for the 5 to 10 beats per minute faster resting heart rate in women. Although the maximal heart rate in both men and

Table 11-1. Cardiovascular Measurements of Trained and Untrained Men and Women

Subjects*	Heart volume (ml)	Blood Volume (liters)	Total Hemoglobin (grams)
Untrained			
Males	769	5.3	805
Females	560	4.1	555
Trained			
Males	986	7.5	1130
Females	691	4.8	632

*Subjects were between the ages of 24 and 38 years.

women at a given age is very similar, the heart rate of women during submaximal work has been found to be considerably higher. This indicates that for any given exercise, the female works at a higher percentage of her maximal heart rate per oxygen uptake rate than the male. In other words, the female's heart has to work harder by pumping more blood in order to achieve a given oxygen uptake rate than the male. This relationship of heart rate to oxygen uptake is illustrated in Figure 11-2.

Stroke Volume and Cardiac Output

Recall from Chapter 4 that cardiac output is defined as the volume of blood pumped by the heart in one minute, and is generally expressed in liters per minute or milliliters per minute. It is the product of heart rate times stroke volume (the amount of blood pumped with each beat of the heart).

At rest, in the supine position, the normal cardiac output in adults is around 5 liters per minute. In the upright position, cardiac output is about 1 to 2 liters per minute smaller (due to the fact that blood generally pools in the lower portion of the body under the influence of gravity when assuming a sitting or standing position, and thus results in a drop in venous return to the heart).

Stroke volume of an adult untrained man at rest and in the supine position is around 70 to 100 ml per beat depending upon the body size. Because of the smaller size heart in women, their stroke volume is usually around 25 percent lower. In a standing position, stroke volume is about 30 percent smaller in both men and women. Several investigators have found that at submaximal work loads, cardiac output per liter of oxygen uptake is higher in women than in men (around 1.5 liters higher) of adult ages. Stroke volume for women is also lower during submaximal work than

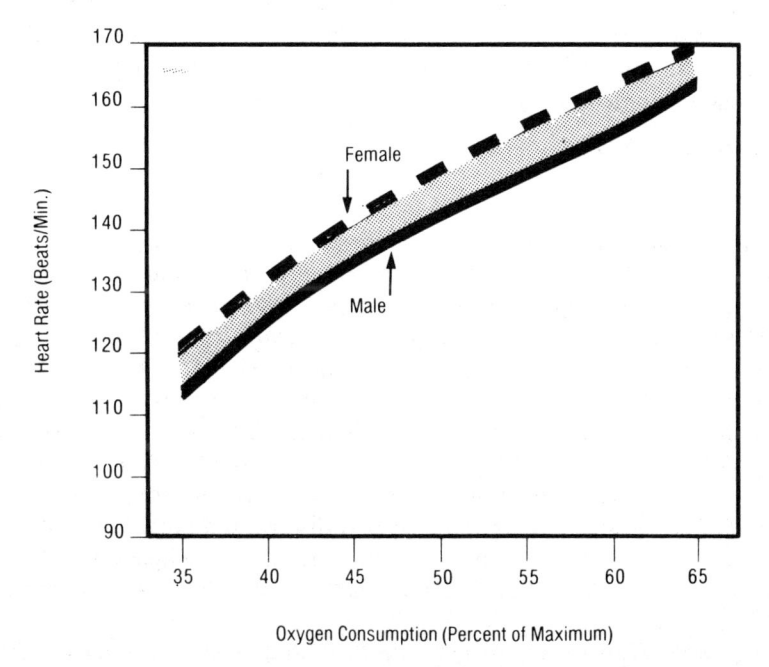

Figure 11-2 Schematic diagram of the relationship of heart rate to oxygen uptake during exercise for male and female subjects.

for men. In addition, it is well documented that both maximal cardiac output and maximal stroke volume is lower in the female during exercise than they are for the male. Maximal arteriovenous oxygen difference (a-$\bar{v}_{O_2}$ diff—represents how much oxygen is extracted by the tissues from each 100 ml of blood perfusing them) is also lower for the female during exercise.

Why do women have a higher cardiac output than men at submaximal work loads? As stated earlier, the hemoglobin concentration in women is lower than that of men and so is their arterial oxygen content. Therefore, to compensate for this, the female's cardiac output has to be larger than the males at each submaximal load in order that she might receive adequate oxygen (the product of cardiac output and arterial oxygen content).

Because submaximal stroke volume is the same as maximal stroke volume (in terms of its size) during exercise, the difference between men and women on this variable as well as the man's higher maximal cardiac output can be explained by the greater heart and blood volume of the male.

Oxygen Pulse

Oxygen pulse is generally defined as the amount of oxygen taken out of blood per heart beat, and it is calculated by dividing the amount of oxygen consumed during a given period of time by the number of heart beats during the same period. This calculation is another measurement that is used quite often in determining the efficiency of the heart. During work, the oxygen pulse generally reaches its maximal value of 11 to 17 cc at heart rates of about 130 to 140 beats per minute. With additional increases in heart rate, the oxygen pulse may, however, decrease, thus indicating that efficiency is dropping. At the same time, it should be pointed out that values of 27.2 cc has been found for well-trained athletes during heavy exercise.

While oxygen pulse values are about the same for both sexes (for similar work loads) between the ages of 12 to 15 years, from the age of 15 to 25 hears, the male's values continue to improve until they are almost double the size of the female's. The female's values remain relatively the same with very little increase after the age of 15 years.

B. RESPIRATORY SYSTEM

Vital Capacity

Vital capacity is defined as the maximal volume of air which a person can expel from his lungs by a forcible expiration after the deepest possible inspiration. Vital capacity is related to age, body weight, height, and skin surface area. Lung capacity for the normal, healthy female is approximately 10 percent smaller than that of her male counterpart of similar age and size. This difference may be due, in part, to the female's lower metabolic rate, which demands less oxygen. On the other hand, some authorities in the area feel that since women generally have a higher per minute respiratory rate than most men, difference in lung capacity is not due to the female's lower metabolic rate. Other authorities have suggested that the difference may be explained by the male's more developed respiratory musculature. It is well known that men, on the average, have a tendency to breathe somewhat slower and deeper with their abdominal and diaphragm muscles than women. At the same time, women tend to breathe faster and hgher up in their chest region using the intercostal muscles. Studies show that diaphragmatic breathing can be increased in the female as a result of training.

The average vital capacity in normal untrained adult men is around 4 liters, and for the untrained woman, around 3.5 liters. Some researchers have found average vital capacities of between 4.5 and 6.0 liters for well-trained college women and men, respectively. It should be pointed out that although vital capacity can be increased with training, it is not related very high to one's ability to perform work. For example, there have been superior athletes with low vital capacities and poor ones with large capacities. These findings suggest that an athlete should probably only have at least a normal vital capacity in relation to their overall body size.

Maximal Voluntary Ventilation

Maximal voluntary ventilation (MVV), or maximal breathing capacity (MBC) is defined as the maximum volume of air that can be moved in and out of the lungs per unit time. It is usually measured over a period of 15 or 30 seconds and converted to liters per minute. The mean value for healthy, untrained men (25 years of age) is about 140 liters per minute, with a range from 100 to 180 liters per minute. For women, the normal values range somewhere between 70 and 120 liters. It is well documented that MVV can be increased by training. In fact, it is not unusual to find values as high as between 200 and 250 liters per minute in well-trained athletes which indicates their ability to move air quickly.

Maximum Oxygen Uptake

Maximum oxygen uptake (or maximum aerobic power) is defined as the greatest oxygen uptake attained by an individual while breathing air at sea level during the performance of physical work, and it is considered by most exercise physiologists as the best single measure of an individual's cardiorespiratory capacity. Figure 11-3 illustrates quite clearly that up to the ages of between 10 and 15 years, there is very little difference in maxium oxygen uptake between girls and boys. However, in adult life, the capacity of women is considerably below that of men. These differences are probably due, in part, to the female's lower hemoglobin count and lower maximal

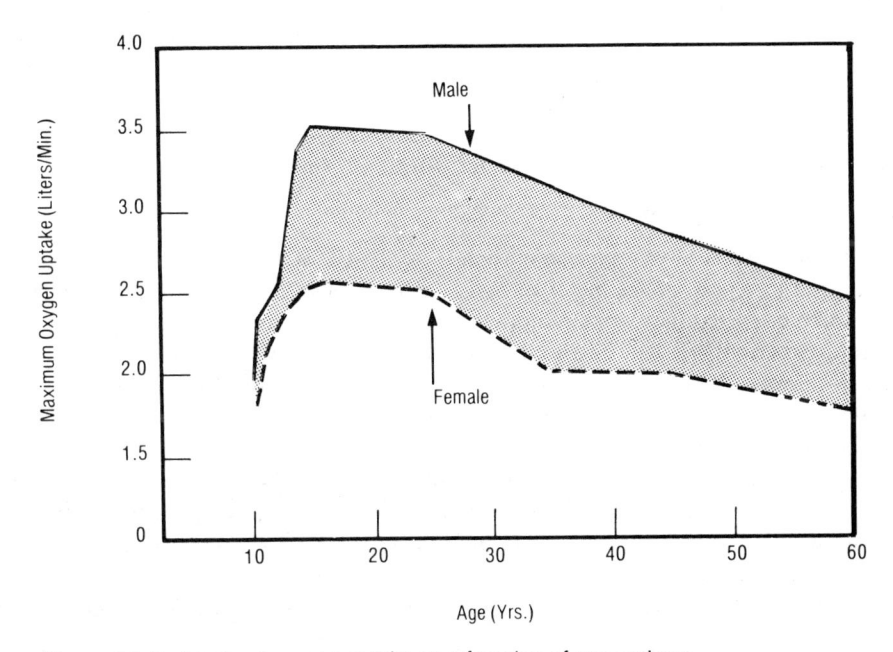

Figure 11-3 Maximal oxygen uptake as a function of age and sex.

cardiac output (which results in a lower oxygen-carrying and delivery capacity than the male), as was pointed out earlier. At the same time, however, part of the difference may also be due to the female's sedentary life style that society imposes on her once she reaches menarche. Because there is very little difference in maximal oxygen uptake up to the ages of between 10 and 15 years can perhaps be explained by the fact that both sexes are very similar in hemoglobin and maximal cardiac output up to puberty, at which time the differences began to show up. Figure 11-3 also shows that both sexes peak at around the ages of 18 to 20 years, followed by a progressive decline throughout the remaining years.

Maximal oxygen uptake is sometimes expressed in liters per minute, as Figure 11-3 illustrates, however, because it is influenced greatly by body size, it is better for comparative purposes to express it in terms of milliliters of oxygen per kilogram of body weight per unit of time (ml/kg/min). For untrained college women, typical maximal oxygen uptake is between 30 and 44 ml/kg/min, whereas for untrained college-age men, average values range between 45 and 53 ml/kg/min.

Figure 11-4 illustrates maximal oxygen uptake values for both men and women athletes in various sports. The highest recorded individual value for a female has been reported to be 74 ml/kg/min for a cross-country skier from Russia, while the highest individual value (94/ml/kg/min) for a male has also been found to be a cross-country skier from Norway. While Figure 11-4 shows that the female athlete's maximal oxygen uptake values are somewhat below those of the male athlete, the illustration also shows that most of the endurance trained female values are considerably greater than those found for the average untrained female and male as well as some of the "non-endurance" trained male athletes.

It is interesting to note that when maximal oxygen uptake is expressed relative to lean body weight instead of to total body weight, the female values are much closer to the male values. This is because women have a higher relative body fat than men. For example, instead of the usual 20 to 25 percent difference (favoring the male) in maximum oxygen uptake when expressed relative to body weight alone, the difference between the sexes has been found to be only around 8 to 10 percent when expressed relative to lean body weight. This probably has very little significance, as Drinkwater has pointed out, since the female must still carry her entire body weight, including her adipose as well as her lean tissue, as part of her workload (such as in jogging).

C. BASAL METABOLIC RATE

Recall from Chapter 3 that basal metabolic rate (BMR) is defined as the minimum amount of energy required for each square meter of body surface area during a state of complete rest. It is generally well recognized that women oxidize their food approximtely 5 to 10 percent slower than men; therefore, their BMR will be about 5 to 10 percent lower than their male counterpart at all ages. The differential begins to increase slightly at puberty and continues until around the age of 20 years at which time a gradual decline commences. This is illustrated in Figure 2-17 in Chapter 2. Between the ages of 20 and 40, women usually average about 35 kcal/m^2 of body surface area per hour in caloric expenditure, which over a period of 24 hours, will result in basal rates ranging from 1,200 to 1,400 kcal. Men, on the other hand, between the same ages and comparable body structure show values around 38 kcal/m^2 of body surface area and basal rates for a 24-hour period of somewhere around 1,668 kcal. The greater proportion of adipose tissue in the female to her lean body mass is probably responsible, in part, for this difference as well as the smaller overall size of the female.

It should be pointed out, however, that when BMR is expressed in terms of lean body mass instead of body surface area, the sex difference is no longer noticed. In general, this suggests that the BMR sex difference only has significance in terms of heat dissipation during resting conditions while contributing little or no value to exercise efficiency.

D. HEAT ADAPTATION

A substantial amount of evidence has been published indicating that the temperature regulating mechanism of both men and women are somewhat different. For example, it is well

MALES

Sport	Range
Cross-Country Skiing	70-94
Long-Distance Running	65-85
Rowing	58-75
Bicycling	55-70
Long-Distance Swimming	48-68
Gymnastics	48-64
Speed Skating	50-75
Ice Hockey	50-60
Football	45-64
Baseball	45-55
Tennis	42-56
Sedentary College Students	45-53
Sedentary Middle-Aged	35-38

FEMALES

Sport	Range
Cross Country Skiing	56-74
Long-Distance Running	55-72
Rowing	41-58
Distance Swimming	45-60
Speed Skating	40-52
Sprinting	38-52
Basketball	35-45
Sedentary College Students	30-44
Sedentary Middle-Aged	30-35

Maximum Oxygen Uptake (Ml/Kg/Min.)

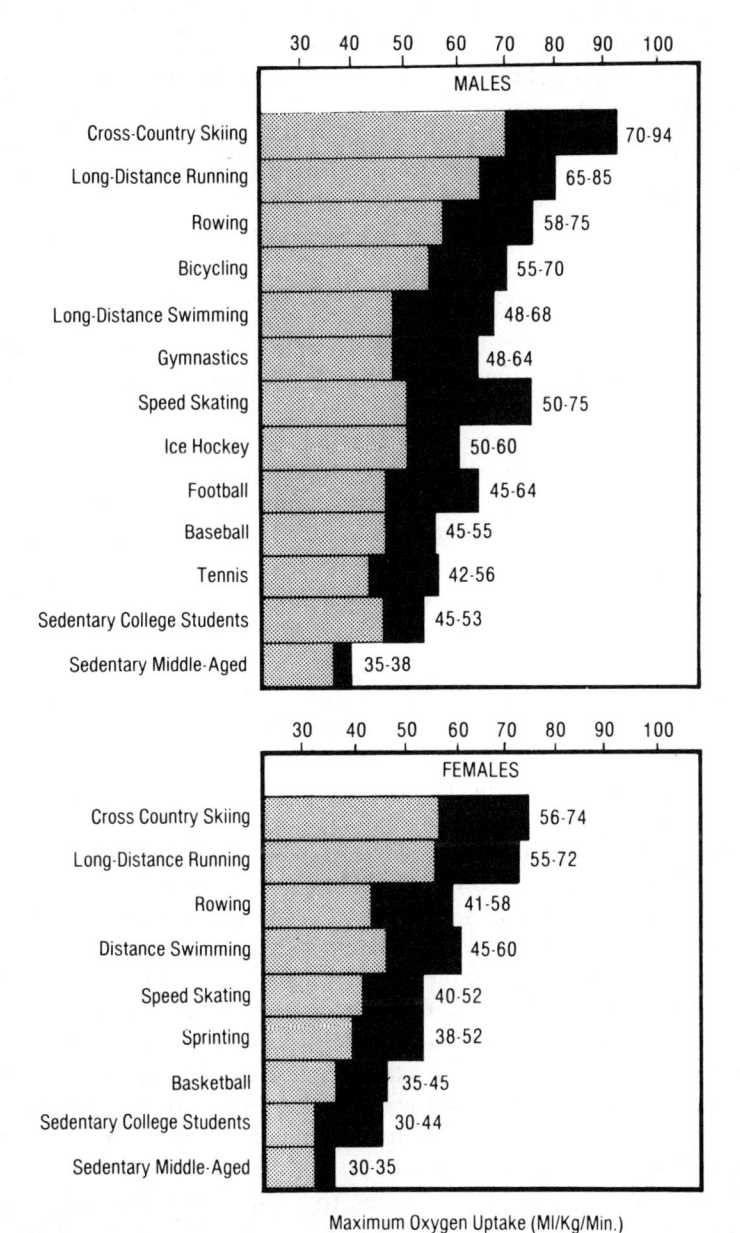

Figure 11-4 Maximal oxygen uptake values for male and female athletes of various sports.

documented that estrogen, the female sex hormone, inhibits (instead of promoting) sweating to some degree. As a result, the female possesses about a 2° to 3°F higher sweating threshold than the male. This means that the female does not commence sweating until the environmental temperature is 2° to 3°F above the male's sweating threshold. As a result, her sum of sweating at higher temperatures will be less than that of the males. Another difference between sexes in terms of heat adaptation is that the temperature gradient from core to skin appears to be smaller for the female. Recall also that the female has about 10 percent more adipose tissue than the male which serves as good heat insulation. These combined findings indicate that in a hot climate, the physiological cost of maintaining heat balance is not only greater for the female, but it apparently hinders her physical performance more significantly than it does for the male. On the other hand, it should be pointed out that because the female has approximately 10 percent more adipose tissue than the male, she is somewhat better able to cope with cold conditions than the male. In other words, the larger amount of adipose tissue may be to the female's advantage in activities such as channel swimming or snow skiing where the temperatures may be very cold.

III. GYNECOLOGICAL FACTORS

In the past, it has been generally believed (without scientific evidence) that participation in strenuous exercise and sports during menstruation could be physiologically harmful. Only recently has it been established somewhat clearer that vigorous athletic training and competition do not adversely affect either the menarch, menstruation, or subsequent obstetric and gynecologic history. When a large population of Hungarian women athletes were surveyed, it was found that there were no disturbances of the onset of menarche or during the menstrual period as a result of vigorous athletic activity. In another report when a large group of active and former Swedish champion girl swimmers were tested and interviewed, it was noted that not only was none of the active athletes injured by their vigorous conditioning, but that the obstetric and gynecologic history of the former swimmers was also normal. Other surveys taken at the Tokyo Olympics supports these findings.

In addition, there has been no evidence of dysmenorrhea (painful or difficult menstruation) of any consequence as the result of exercise or athletic competition. In fact, there have been recent reports to indicate complete absence of menstruation in women who are undergoing training for long-duration running. While complete absence of menstruation is the exception and not the rule for all women in all sports, there is a substantial amount of evidence available to indicate that exercise is beneficial in relieving pain and also in improving and preventing dysmenorrhea. Light to strenuous exercises are quite often recommended as part of a postpartum exercise program for mothers who are undergoing back pain following delivery. Thus, excusing a young menstruating girl from physical education classes requiring mild physical activities is apparently not justified. It is worth noting that research shows that the number of girls experiencing dysmenorrhea is much lower among the active athletes than among the more sedentary women.

It has been well established that the hormonal cycle, which brings about menstruation, may have either a positive or negative effect on athletic performance. However, the time when the actual effect is greatest is not completely known since the individual variability is so tremendous. For example, some investigators have found no decrement in terms of motor performance as a result of the menstrual cycle, whereas others report that physical performance is superior in the post-menstrual period, slightly poorer during menstruation, and at its lowest in the two or three days preceding menstruation. In fact, International and Olympic records have apparently been set by the female during all phases of the menstrual cycle.

As a general rule, most medical experts recommend regular participation in sports activities during the menstrual period provided the level of performance by the athlete does not drop below that which they are accustomed to performing. At the same time, however, the majority of physicians also agree that women should avoid vigorous athletic training and competition (especially activities that cause excessive jarring, torque, or strain to the pelvic area) during the first 2 days of the menstrual period since the womb is generally not only filled with blood during this time, but it is also somewhat heavier. It is usually during this period that the female's body is not only undergoing hormone adjustments, but she is also experiencing such psychological symptoms as fatigue, irritability, depression, nervousness, and water retention.

There is some evidence available to indicate that swimming during the menstrual period may be undesirable. The presence of pathogenic bacteria in the vagina has been found in a number of female swimmers along with a relatively high number of complaints dealing with the lower abdominal area. A higher percentage of menstrual and inflammatory diseases are generally experienced amng skiers, gymnasts, tennis players, divers, and swimmers than among the other athletic groups. Evidence indicates that physical performance efficiency among this group of athletes during menstruation also appears to decline somewhat.

Research also indicates that women's strength decreases a few days prior to the start of menstruation, and continues to remain at a somewhat inferior level throughout the menstrual period. Medical authorities have suggested that any deviation frm the normal rhythmic pattern may be one of the first indications of overconditioning. As deVries mentions, it would appear to be a good policy from the standpoint of good health and better performance for women coaches and physical educators to advise the members of their teams and classes to keep accurate and up-to-date records of their menstrual cycles. Consultation on the part of the girls should be encouraged whenever deviations occur.

Of all the elements that influence individual performance, none seems more variable in its effect than menstruation. However, it would appear from the available evidence that physical performance during this period is fairly well tolerated and appears to have a beneficial effect. More precise measures of studying blood flow before, during, and after menstruation would be welcome.

IV. EFFECTS OF TRAINING AND ATHLETIC COMPETITION ON PREGNANCY, CHILDBIRTH, AND THE POSTPARTUM PERIOD

A major argument against female participation in vigorous exercise and athletic competition has been that the physical stress and strain from such activity should be avoided because they could perhaps lead to permanent damage of the reproductive organs. However, scientific studies have shown that this point of view is not valid. In fact, it is well known that the reproductive organs are quite well protected against external forces. The female's breasts, on the other hand, are in a more likely position to be injured. However, even here, injuries are very rare.

Considerable evidence has shown that the practice of training and athletic competition has no harmful effect on pregnancy, childbirth, and the postpartum period. At the same time, however, most sport physicians agree that vigorous training and competition should be curtailed during pregnancy because of the tremendous risk involved for both mother and child. To start with, it should be pointed out that during pregnancy, the liver and kidneys of the expectant mother operates with little or no reserve capacity. In addition, it has been well established by research that exercise causes the cardiovascular and respiratory systems of the healthy, non-pregnant female to increase their work output more than twice what they normally do during rest (note that this is referring to light to moderate exercise). Such a demand for increased circulation and nourishment during exercise, along with the additional cardiorespiratory, muscular, and metabolic requirements of the fetus during pregnancy can obviously bring about a tremendous health risk for both the mother and the child. The risk is even higher for the expectant mother who has perhaps an unknown heart defect.

It was also once believed that female athletes developed tense abdominal walls that interfered with normal delivery. However, research shows that women athletes have no particular problems in regard to childbearing and childbirth. In a gynecological study conducted a few years ago with female athletes, it was found that the duration of labor was considerably shorter than the average in 87 percent of the women athletes when compared with controls, and complications per se were not above normal. When a group of female Olympic athletes were studied recently, it was noted that the majority had quick and relatively easy deliveries with very little pain. In addition, the athletes had both shorter delivery and convalescent periods. Following childbirth, many of the women showed considerable improvement in their physical performances. Similar results were reported recently by Zaharieva, who studied 150 female athletes between the years 1952 and 1972. In another investigation in which 15 female athletes were studied, 5 dropped out of sports activities following pregnancy because of their new responsibilities, 2 maintained equal performance, and 8 demonstrated record improvements in performance. Following pregnancy, all of the women agreed that they had more strength and endurance and felt stronger. The fact that most of the females cited in the above studies had a relatively easy time in giving birth and the fact that they showed considerable improvement in their performance following childbirth might be due, in part, to the female hormones that were activated during exercise and pregnancy. Also, since pregnancy places an increased demand on the cardiovascular, respiratory, muscular, and metabolic systems, it should be viewed as a source of physical conditioning and training.

In summary, it would appear from the available research that there is no need for concern regarding the effects of vigorous exercise before or after childbirth. On the other hand, because of the added requirements of fetal circulation during pregnancy, very limited training and competition is recommended (especially during the later part of pregnancy) during this period of time. At the same time, however, physical conditioning for the sake of general health and fitness is recommended and should be continued during a normal pregnancy.

V. FEMININITY

It is well known that inherent endocrinological and morphological factors are responsible for femininity and masculinity and not strenuous exercise as some people would like to believe. There is no evidence to indicate that participation in vigorous exercise and sports will masculinize women. On the contrary, it is a generally accepted fact that such activity tends to make a woman more graceful and feminine because it brings about better muscle tonus, replaces fatty tissue with firm musculature, and improves overall fitness, just to mention a few. Most authorities in this area agree that femininity is the general rule among today's female athletes rather than the exception.

In addition, available evidence indicates quite clearly that young girls and women should not be afraid that vigorous exercise and training during early youth will result in unsightly bulging muscles and in masculinity of build. Substantial evidence has been reported showing that girls and women, as a result of physical training, can gain muscular strength with no significant increase in muscle hypertrophy. The fact that physical training such as weight-lifting does bring about large increases in the female's body strength without a concomitant gain in muscle bulk is probably due to her low overall level of testosterone as compared to her male counterpart. Females who do notice an increase in muscle hypertrophy along with increased strength undoubtedly have naturally high levels of testosterone in their body. These young ladies are generally overall stronger and they generally possess certain mechanical advantages in athletic ability over young girls who may rate low in masculinity as well as young boys who may rate high in femininity.

VI. FEMALE INJURIES IN SPORTS

As was reported earlier in this chapter, it is well documented that there is a considerable difference (in favor of the male) in the locomotor structures of the female compared with the male. For example, not only is the female bones, muscles, tendons, and ligaments more delicately constructed than that of the male, but she also possesses a smaller proportion of muscle to adipose tissue. Lack of training on the female's part after puberty as a result of cultural demands may also play an important part in the higher incidence of athletic injuries found in women. Females, in general, after puberty have stayed away from vigorous exercise that would have a strength training effect because they have been taught that they were unfeminine. The literature is well documented that trained athletes can undergo vigorous competitive training and competition without injury. whereas the poorly trained person is more likely to incur injuries.

The scope of this text does not permit detailed presentation of the many sport injuries, however, it has generally been found that the greatest percentage of all female injuries is found in track and field events that require explosive efforts such as the sprints and the long jump. In one study involving comparable groups of men and women, it was noted that athletic injuries in women was found to be nearly double that of men. The study reported that the overstrain-type injuries (such as inflammations of tendons, contractures, tendon sheaths, bursae, foot deficiencies, and periosteal injuries) was nearly 4 times more common in females than in males. The available evidence seems to indicate that perhaps the female's musculoskeletal system is not as well suited for activities that require quick, explosive power as the male is. If the female is to compete in activities that call for quick, explosive efforts, then it is highly recommended that she undergo a vigorous training program for developing strength, speed, and quickness in the specific muscles that are used for the specific skill. This will help eliminate many of the injuries that are normally experienced by the female.

VII. FEMALE RESPONSE TO STRESS

Although in the past, it has been generally believed that women are emotionally unstable in stressful situations and that highly competitive events might cause unfavorable responses, there is no scientific evidence to support this assertion. In fact, there is no information to indicate that females are more psychologically or emotionally unstable than their counterparts. In fact, as Klafs and Lyon point out, stress reactions are usually quite similar in both sexes.

In a study of college-age women in competitive sports and scholastic competition, it was found that the female's emotional control in stressful situations was generally well stabilized in all cases. The report suggested that stress was more of a psychological than a physiological manifestation. Also, in a year-long study of young girl competitive swimmers between the ages of 12 and 16 years (a period that is normally considered to be somewhat emotionally unstable for young teen-agers), no nervous symptoms or emotional instability that could be attributed to intensive training or competition was found in the young swimmers. Other studies have found similar results. Thus, the notion that females are emotionally unstable in stressful situations is not supported by evidence.

VIII. TRAINABILITY OF THE FEMALE

Although it was once believed that girls and women are less responsive to strength training than men, the results of several investigations in more recent years indicate that girls and boys of similar age who take part in identical testing and training programs show the same relative amount of improvement in strength. In fact, in some cases, the female shows greater relative increases in strength than the male. Research conducted in Germany indicate that there is no difference in the rate of relative increase of strength per week for men and women as well as boys and girls taking part in the same type of training program. For example, when over 50 paralyzed muscles of both boys and girls were trained over a 10-week period, no sex difference was found in the rate of increase of strength relative to the state of training. These results indicate that age, muscle group, and sex have no influence on the rate of relative increase in strength.

Studies conducted in the United States on comparing nonathletic males with nonathletic females on the same identical training program indicate that the females, in most cases, exhibit greater gains in strength in selected muscle groups than the males. Although the female's initial strength levels were generally lower than that of the males (and therefore, had theoretically more room for improvement), it appears that the female has perhaps the same potential for relative strength development as the male of comparable size. At the same time, however, does the female have the same potential for development in terms of absolute strength? Recall from earlier discussion that strength potential is directly related to the physiological cross section of the muscle itself, and that an increase in body size and muscle bulk is primarily determined by the hormone called testosterone which is found predominantly in the male. Since the rate of testosterone production is considerably higher in normal healthy males than in normal healthy women, it is doubtful that the female will ever obtain the same absolute strength levels as that of their male counterpart.

In relation to cardiorespiratory endurance, the available evidence suggests that there are no sexual differences in trainability. It has been suggested by several authorities working in this area that if the body's fat content is disregarded, both sexes have about the same maximal aerobic power per kilogram of body weight following a cardiorespiratory endurance training program. At the same time, if maximal aerobic power is expressed in percent of capacity per kilogram of total body weight, improvement is slightly lower in women. Research shows that female champion distance runners who run somewhere between 50 and 100 miles per week in training not only have a greater ventilatory capacity than average, but also a maximum aerobic capacity approaching that found in male champion long-distance runners.

IX. PERFORMANCE COMPARISONS IN WORLD RECORDS (MALE VS FEMALE)

Table 11-2 illustrates a comparison of women's and men's world records (based on performances through August of 1979) set in the various running events. In reviewing the table, it can be seen that the records for the men in the 100- and 200-meter events averages around 9 percent faster than for their female counterparts, while the times for the 400-meter to the mile run vary from 8 to 17 percent in favor of the men. The difference in the two fastest times for the marathon event (distance of 26 miles, 385 yards) is approximately 10 percent in favor of the men.

The men's and women's world records for swimming are shown in Table 11-3. When compared to the running world records, it can be seen that the swimming times are closer and extend from a low of 6 percent difference (for the 400 and 800 meter free-style in favor of men) to a high of 11 percent (for the 100 meter free-style and breast stroke in favor of the men). The

Sex Differences in Exercise 227

Table 11-2. Comparing Men's and Women's World Records in Track Events*

Event	Men	Women
100 M	9.95	10.88
200 M	19.83	21.71
400 M	43.86	48.94
800 M	1:42.40	1:54.90
1,500 M	3:21.10	3:56.00
Mile	3:49.00	4:22.10
3,000 M	7:32.10	8:27.20
5,000 M	13:08.40	15:08.80
10,000 M	27:22.50	31:45.10
Marathon+	2:08:33.60	2:32:30.00

*As of August, 1979.
+Note that because of the varying severity of courses throughout the world, there is no official marathon record.

Table 11-3. Comparing Men's and Women's World Records in Swimming*

Event	Men	Women
(Free-Style)		
100 M	49.44	55.41
200 M	1:49.83	1:58.43
400 M	3:51.41	4:06.28
800 M	7:56.49	8:24.62
1,500 M	15:02.40	16:06.63
(Breast Stroke)		
100 M	1:02.86	1:10.31
200 M	2:15.11	2:28.36
(Butterfly Stroke)		
100 M	54.18	59.46
200 M	1:59.23	2:09.77
(Back Stroke)		
100 M	55.49	1:01.51
200 M	1:59.19	2:11.93
(Individual Medley)		
200 M	2:03.29	2:14.07
400 M	4:20.05	4:40.83

*As of August, 1979.

world record for the English Channel, on the other hand, is held by a 15-year-old girl. The difference for this event is about 1.4 percent or 8 minutes. It is interesting to note that the world records established by the female swimmers surpass those set by the men just a few years ago, and yet faster times are still predicted for the female swimmers. There is no doubt that the combination of improved training and coaching techniques, more young girls now competing at all levels, improved and more attractive swimming facilities for recruiting young swimmers into the various swimming programs, and finally, the females high level of buoyancy has all helped and played an important part in allowing the female to experience such tremendous advances in swimming.

Table 11-4 illustrates the men's and women's world records for various field events. It is clear that these activities yield the widest performance range in favor of the men. For example, the high jump has a 14 percent difference, the long jump 20 percent and the javelin 27 percent. Even though the female uses a shotput that is about 55 percent lighter than the male, she only compares about equal to the male in this activity and in the discus throw.

In summary, it should be obvious to the reader that the field events that require great explosive power (such as the discus throw, high jump, long jump, javelin, and shotput) are more of a limiting factor for the female than for the male. Here the male's greater size and strength as well as perhaps speed undoubtedly give him an advantage. With additional training, better equipment and facilities, improved coaching, and a much larger number of females participating in sports, it is apparent that the female athlete should continue to improve and set new records in probably all sports that they take part in. Undoubtedly, the tremendous gap that was once seen between the male and female performance will gradually change and will probably favor the female as she continues to gain equal recognition in the world of sports that was once dominated by the male.

X. SUMMARY

(1) While the female at any age, reaches greater skeletal maturity than the male of similar age, the longer and slower growing process experienced by the male results in a greater density, longer, larger, more rugged and more massive structure. Therefore, the male possesses mechanical and structural advantages over the female, especially in activities where the upper body is involved. In addition, the joints of the male are slightly larger, and therefore present a greater articular surface. In events calling for speed and force (such as throwing, striking, and explosive types of activities), the male, due to his longer leverage, heavier bones, and greater arc of movement, has a decided advantage over the female.

(2) Because of the female's body proportions (shorter and lighter with a lower center of gravity along with less muscle mass and more fatty tissue than males), she has an advantage over the male in buoyancy (which favors swimming), flexibility, balance, and stability (excellent for gymnastics).

(3) With the exception of strength and power, the female compares favorably to the male on most all other physiological parameters.

(4) Physical training and conditioning evidence indicates that similar training effects leading to a greater work capacity can be obtained in both sexes following similar-type training programs.

Table 11-4. Comparing Men's and Women's World Records in Field Events*

Event	Men	Women
High jump	7 ft, 8 in	6 ft, 7 in
Long jump	29 ft, 2½ in	23 ft, 3¼ in
Shot put	72 ft, 8 in	73 ft, 2¾ in
Javelin	310 ft, 4 in	228 ft, 1 in
Discus throw	233 ft, 5 in	232 ft, 0 in

*As of August, 1979.

(5) Evidence indicates that athletic training and competition do not adversely affect either the menarche, menstruation, or subsequent obstetric history.

(6) Gynecological data indicates that exercise is beneficial in relieving pain and also in improving and preventing dysmenorrhea.

(7) Research shows that the practice of training and athletic competition has no harmful effect on pregnancy, childbirth, and the postpartum period: At the same time, however, most sport physicians agree that vigorous training and competition should be curtailed during pregnancy because of the tremendous risk involved for both mother and child.

(8) The female is capable of great endurance. She apparently has not achieved her potential in terms of physical performance (when compared to the male) and is obviously capable of reaching much greater heights. With increased training, better equipment and facilities, improved coaching, and a greater emphasis on females in sport, it is quite possible that the gap (in terms of performance) between the sexes will continue to close.

(9) Evidence indicates that the female is no more psychologically or emotionally unstable in stressful situations than the male.

(10) The anatomical and physiological differences between the sexes should be carefully considered when selecting physical activities and sports for the female. The activities should be designed in such a way to take advantage of the female's body structure and physiological functions.

XI. REVIEW REFERENCES

(1) Burke, E. J., and F. C. Brush. "Physiological and Anthropometric Assessment of Successful Teenage Female Distance Runners," *Research Quarterly,* 50:180-87, 1979.
(2) Daniels, J., G. Krahenbuhl, C. Foster, J. Gilbert, and S. Daniels. "Aerobic Responses of Female Distance Runners to Submaximal and Maximal Exercise," *Annuals New York Academy Science,* 301:726-33, 1977.
(3) deVries, H. A. *Physiology of Exercise for Physical Education and Athletics,* 2nd edition, Wm. C. Brown Co., Dubuque, Iowa, 1974.
(4) Drinkwater, B. L. "Physiological Responses of Women to Exercise," in *Exercise and Sport Science Reviews,* (J. H. Wilmore, editor), Academic Press Inc., New York, 1973.
(5) Edington, D. W., and Edgerton, V. R. *The Biology of Physical Activity,* Houghton Mifflin Co., Boston, 1976.
(6) Freedson, P., V. L. Katch, S. Sady, and A. Weltman. "Cardiac Output Differences in Males and Females During Mild Cycle Ergometer Exercise," *Medicine and Science in Sports,* 11:16-19, 1979.
(7) Klafs, C. E., and M. J. Lyon. *The Female Athlete: Conditioning, Competition, and Culture,* The C. V. Mosby Co., Saint Louis, 1973.
(8) Krahenbuhl, G. S., C. L. Wells, C. H. Brown, and P. E. Ward. "Characteristics of National and World Class Female Pentathletes," *Medicine and Science in Sports,* 11:20-23, 1979.
(9) Pedersen, P. K., and K. Jorgensen. "Maximal Oxygen Uptake in Young Women with Training, Inactivity, and Retraining." *Medicine and Science in Sports,* 10:233-37, 1978.
(10) Plowman, S. "Physiological Characteristics of Female Athletes," *Research Quarterly,* 45:349-62, 1974.
(11) Ryan, A. J. "The Female Athlete: Gynecological Considerations," *Journal of Health, Physical Education and Recreation,* 46:40-44, 1975.
(12) Wilmore, J. H. *Athletic Training and Physical Fitness: Physiological Principles and Practices of the Conditioning Process,* Allyn and Bacon, Inc., Boston, 1977.
(13) Wilmore, J. H. "Exploding the Myth of Female Inferiority," *Physician and Sportsmedicine,* 2:54-58, 1974.
(14) Zaharieva, E. "Olympic Participation by Women—Effects on Pregnancy and Childbirth," *Journal of American Medical Association,* 222:992-95, 1972.

12

THE PREADOLESCENT AND COMPETITIVE SPORTS

KEY CONCEPTS TO BE GAINED FROM THIS CHAPTER

(1) There is no solid longitudinal evidence to show that highly competitive sports or prolonged periods of strenuous training adversely affects the normal physical growth of children.

(2) Evidence indicates that there is little reason to believe that the physiological stress and strain placed on young participants who are taking part in a competitive sports program that is highly-organized and well supervised is likely to be physiologically dangerous.

(3) Although the evidence is not completely clearcut, it appears that the psychological stresses resulting from preadolescent competitive sports is in no way excessive, and does not present an emotional health hazard to the young player.

(4) Physical injury (especially the epiphyseal-type) is probably the greatest hazard and concern in preadolescent competitive sports.

(5) There are specific guidelines for competitive preadolescent sports in which all agency-sponsored and interschool-sponsored groups should follow in developing programs of this nature.

Over the years much has been written concerning the pros and cons of exercise and competitive sports on the normal growth and development of the young child. Summaries of animal and human research dealing with the effects of physical activity have been published, and the findings indicate quite clearly that exercise in general not only contributes to the normal growth of bone and muscle tissue, but it also acts as a stimulant in the development of the heart, lungs, and other vital internal organs. Experts in human growth and development claim that it is only when the exercise or physical activity is of the vigorous-type and when it is repeated often enough to cause chronic fatigue or when stressful enough to bring about trauma to a particular part of the body that there is danger of adverse effects on normal bone growth.

While few people would question the positive effects of general exercise on the regular growth and development of the young child, and while few would also argue against competitive sports for young children when they are conducted within the school's physical education classes, much criticism has been directed in recent years at the ever-growing area of agency-sponsored and interschool-sponsored competitive type preadolescent sports (such as Little League baseball, Pop Warner football, and competitive leagues and programs in basketball, soccer, ice-hockey, swimming, and track and field) and their effects on the growth and development of the young participant. It is this area that some authorities have attributed dangers to physical growth and development of young children and to which this chapter will address itself. Thus, the purpose of this chapter is not to elaborate on the benefits or the hazards of physical activity per se, but instead, to report on what is known concerning the effects of competitive sports as previously mentioned on the normal growth and development of the preadolescent.

At the start it should be clearly stated that there is not a sufficient amount of reliable data to make valid and conclusive assessments of the effects of competitive sports on the growth and development of the preadolescent athlete. Before any final evaluation can be made, there must be better agreement among researchers in this area on valid and reliable assessment procedures than have been demonstrated thus far. Furthermore, it is strongly recommended by leaders in this field that the evaluations should be based on not only long-term assessments, but factors such as the type of sport, the intensity and duration of the training program, the nature and frequency of the athletic event, the number of years of participation, and the age at which the sport is started. Although there is still a long way to go in this area before complete evaluation can be made, considerable data are available from which we can start to make reasonably valid decisions concerning the benefits and hazards of agency-sponsored and interschool-sponsored competitive sports for young children.

I. GROWTH AND DEVELOPMENT

A. PHYSICAL GROWTH EFFECTS

Short-Term Research

Short-term research examining the effects of competitive sports on physical growth are somewhat controversial. For example, in a relatively early investigation in which a group of 7th, 8th, and 9th grade male athletes who were taking part in a season of interscholastic sports (football, basketball, track, and baseball) were compared on growth trends with a group of nonparticipants, no differences were noticed between the two groups. When the athletes were compared within themselves, it was found that those who took part in the entire season (17 games) had a greater lag in their growth than those who participated in only 12 games. In another investigation, when height, weight, chest width, bi-acromial width, and bi-cristal width was taken on a group of junior high athletes and nonathletes before and after 6 months of interscholastic sports, the group of athletes showed greater growth in all measurements except height. The nonathletic group measured approximately .37 inches more in height. Evidence has also been published showing no significant differences in height, weight, standing broad jump, motor educability, right and left grips, and lung capacity between a group of male athletes who were participating in 8 months of competitive sports (baseball, basketball, track and field, and touch football) and a group of nonparticipants (ages ranged from 9 to 12 years).

Longitudinal Research

A substantial amount of longitudinal research has been published indicating that there is no solid evidence to show that highly competitive sports or prolonged periods of rigorous training adversely affects the normal physical growth of children. During a period of 4 years, longitudinal growth date was obtained on a group of highly competitive Swedish girl swimmers (ages ranged between 12 and 16 years). During the course of the investigation, periodic checks indicated that physical growth was in no way impaired. Instead, the evidence showed that growth was somewhat acclerated during the period of strenuous training (training program involved spending 6 to 28 hours per week in the water and swimming between 6,000 and 65,000 meters per week). It is interesting to note that two years following the completion of the investigation (at whch time the girls were 18 years of age), the girls were re-examined by doctors and the tests revealed no harmful effects of the swimming competition or of the vigorous training program which had been followed.

In another longitudinal study (5 years) in which height, weight, and skinfold measurements were taken on 10 girl gymnasts (ages 12 to 17 years) and 7 untrained girls of similar age, both groups achieved the same mean for height and weight at the end of the 5 years. While the trained gymnasts had less amounts of subcutaneous fat and greater lean body mass. Similar results have been reported for various groups of young boys (ages ranged from 11 years at the start of the study to 15 years at the conclusion) who were exposed to different degrees of sports participation and training over a period of 4 years.

A number of cross-sectional studies have demonstrated rather convincingly that young participants in interscholastic varsity-type sports are skeletally and physiologically more mature and superior (in body size and build, muscular strength and power, speed, and agility) than youngsters who have similar educational and socioeconomic background, but who are inclined to be nonathletically oriented. For example, of the 112 young boys who took part in a previous Little League Baseball World Series, the majority of them were found to be adolescent and not preadolescent as their chronological ages indicated. In addition, it was noted that although the postpubescent (when based upon the Crampton pubic hair criteria) boys chronological ages did not surpass 12 years, their height and weight were the same as that of the normal 14-year-old-boy. It is noteworthy that not only were all 8 starting pitchers in the World Series postpubescent (except one who was pubescent), but the largest number of postpubescent boys batted in the 3rd, 4th, 5th, or 6th position with the "clean-up" position taken up by only postpubescent boys. Surveys taken have also shown that young boys who participated on Little League baseball teams were on the average about 5 inches taller and weighed 33 pounds more than boys of comparable age who did not play Little League baseball. Young boys and girls (ages 8 to 18 years) taking part in competitive swimming programs have also been found to be taller than nonparticipants of comparable age.

When young athletes (elementary and junior high school levels) are compared to nonathletes of similar chronological age, they are found to be definitely superior in skeletal age and relative maturity (skeletal age as related to chronological age), body size and build, both absolute and relative (to weight and age) strength, explosive muscular power, and speed and agility.

While the literature is scarce concerning the flexibility of preadolescent athletes, information is available to indicate that young children (ages 6 to 13 years) with greater hip and trunk flexibility have an advantage in performing the standing broad jump, softball distance throw, and sprinting. Greater neck rotation and trunk lateral flexion has been shown to be of some value in throwing the softball for distance.

It would appear from the information presented in this section that there is little reason to believe that the physical stress of competitive sports or prolonged periods of rigorous training adversely affect the normal physical growth of the young athlete. As many experts in the field agree, the important question for this age group is not whether the physical activity is competitive in nature, but instead, what is the optimum level of activity that the young participant's body can actually endure without placing it under any unnecessary stress. This, of course, will vary from child to child, depending upon the child's overall health and physical condition, the child's maturation level, and the child's motivational level (in other words, is the child competing because he or she wants to or is it because mother and daddy want them to). In essence, it is quite clear that the important point is not whether the physical activity in which the child is taking part in is considered to be competitive, but rather the caution that is taken to insure that undue stresses are not placed on the young individual. As of this writing, well-documented papers have not been published indicating that undue stress has been placed on young athletes.

B. PHYSIOLOGICAL EFFECTS

Heart Rate Responses

Early research suggested that young children should not be worked at high heart rates for fear of causing permanent damage to the heart. However, more recent and better controlled research in this area has clearly shown that fears expressed by many for children exposed to high stresses of physical activity are unfounded. One of the early claims was that children should refrain from rigorous activity because the child's blood vessel's (primarily the aorta and pulmonary arteries) and heart did not develop at the same rate. This was interpreted to mean that a possible strain would be placed on the circulatory system during vigorous work since the vessels would be unable to conform to the increase blood flow caused by the faster and stronger growing heart. Several years later upon the reevaluation of this work, a mistake in the investigators calculations was discovered. The results actually showed a parallel growth rate and not a contraindication for strenuous exercise.

Another early concern expressed by many involved the difference that exists between pubescent children and older children in terms of the heart/body weight ratio. An analytical study, however, erased this concern when at full speed, it was discovered that the pubescent child's heart actually does less amount of work per unit of heart weight than the older child's heart. In a laboratory-controlled investigation, when young healthy subjects (ages 6 to 15 years) were asked to exercise to exhaustion on a bicycle ergometer, it was noted that they had completely recovered within a matter of a few hours following the work. Although the work load was so strenuous that many of the subjects were actually sick at the end of the work period, none apparently showed symptoms of acute dilatation of the heart. While it is well known that young children have the capability for achieving high heart rates during maximal work (in fact, maximal heart rates of young children exceed those of adults), demands of this nature are seldom, if ever, required of young children in competitive sports. Authorities today generally agree that the human organism is protected by certain safety valves which prevents a healthy child (with a normal heart) from physiologically injuring his or her heart permanently as a result of strenuous exercise. In fact, in most cases during exercise, the skeletal muscles will fatigue early enough so that the child will automatically suspend exercise before the heart is called upon for its very last ounce of energy.

While there have been instances of cardiac arrest and sudden death in young children taking part in competitive sports, autopsies performed on such individuals have generally indicated a family history of cardiac problems or prior cardiac troubles that were either ignored or not diagnosed correctly. It is unfortunate that hazards of this kind have taken place. Problems of this nature could be avoided, however, if a complete and thorough physical examination is given to the child and if the child's complete medical history and background is known prior to being allowed to take part in competitive sports.

A number of studies have been conducted in which heart rate responses of young athletes were studied during or immediately following actual participation in competitive sports. In all of these investigations the electrocardiograms were monitored using biotelemetry equipment. The results, when playing Little League baseball, indicated that batting resulted in the highest mean heart rates (166 beats/min) as compared to playing in the field (128 beats/min). Emotional and not physiological stress was suggested as the probable causes for the increase in rate during batting. The positions of pitcher and catcher were not investigated.

In another investigation in which heart rates were examined of young elementary-aged children while participating in the 200-, 400-, 600- and 800-yd runs, the results indicated that the average heart rates ranged from 190 to 200 beats/min. It is interesting to note that regardless of the length of the run, maximal heart rates were noticed within the first 30 seconds, while recovery was almost complete for all young participants within a period of 90 seconds following the run. The children were apparently not only able to operate at a high steady state (in terms of heart rate) during the running, but in most cases, they were able to maintain rates in excess of 170 beats for the entire period of running.

Oxygen Consumption Responses

The oxygen consumption responses of preadolescents have been reviewed and studied by several investigators. Over a period of 22 months during which time a group of young boys (ages between 10 and 15 years) were engaged in steady running training for the 1- and 2-mile running events, oxygen consumption changes were studied. The results indicated that although mean running performance was improved by 32 seconds in the 1-mile event and 63 seconds in the 2-mile run, the subjects mean maximal oxygen uptake in terms of ml/kg/min did not change significantly from 59.5 due to an increase in mean body weight of 9.2 kg. Average height increased 11.2 cm. In this particular study, 7 of the 14 runners were classified as hard runners because they averaged 1,114 miles per year running while the other 7 runners were declared as easy runners due to the fact that they averaged 336 miles per year. Although the hard runners were slightly younger and smaller, and had a smaller maximal oxygen uptake, they showed a greater increase (13.6%) in maximal oxygen uptake (from 2569 to 2919 ml/min) than the easy runners (8.2% or from 2902 to 3141 ml/min), and they were also able to maintain a higher oxygen consumption per kilogram of body weight throughout the entire year of training. The easy runners showed a decrease from 59.3 to 57.0 ml/kg/min as compared to an increase of 61.9 to 62.2 ml/kg/min for the hard runners. Apparently, the differences between the two groups were due primarily to the easy runners decrease and not to the hard runners increase since the hard runners showed an increase in body weight of 13.5 percent which matched the 13.6 percent maximal oxygen uptake increase, while at the same time, the easy runners body weight increase of 13.1 percent did not parallel their maximal oxygen uptake increase of 8.2 percent. Thus, it is quite clear that the increased body weight for the easy runners played an important part in keeping their maximal oxygen uptake down.

Other Combined Responses

A number of physiological parameters have been combined and examined together during either exercise, training, or competition. In the area of maximal oxygen uptake (ml/kg/min) and maximal ventilation (liters/min, BTPS), track results have demonstrated that maximal oxygen uptake increased somewhere around 18 to 26 percent for young girls and boys (ages 8 to 13 years) following either 6 or 12 weeks of training and competition in running. The greatest increase was found following the 12-week program while the lowest was noticed after training for 6 weeks. The maximal oxygen uptake values varied from a low of 41.1 ml/kg/min for an age group of 10 to 11 years to a high of 78.3 ml/kg/min for an age group of 12 to 13 years. In addition, significant increases in maximal ventilation was also noticed along with significant decreases in submaximal and maximal heart rates. Similar findings have been reported by a number of other investigators working with young children in various track programs.

In addition to the track results reported above, research investigating the physiological effects of swim training and competition upon preadolescents has been studied and reported by a number of researchers. The results have indicated that boys and girls (ages 8 to 18 years) in a 3- to 4-year program of swim training have larger heart and lung volumes as well as higher functional working capacities (as determined by maximal oxygen uptake) and exercise diffusing capacities than healthy untrained boys and girls of similar body size. Also, exercise cardiac output for a given oxygen uptake has been found to be lower in swimmers than in nonathletes. This difference is apparently due to the lower heart rate in the swimmers since no difference was reported between the swimmers and controls in terms of stroke volume.

In another study, one year of competition in swimming and training has also been shown to improve not only the mean work capacity (in terms of the $P.W.C._{170}$ test) of both boys (increase from 851 to 1285 kgm/min) and girls (increase from 683 to 844 kgm/min), but also the mean maximal oxygen uptake (boys = 52.5 to 56.6 ml/kg/min; girls = 40.5 to 46.2 ml/kg/min) and maximal exercise ventilation (boys = 69.1 to 102.2 liters/min — STPD; girls = 60.9 to 70.0 liters/min —STPD). The swimmers were between the ages of 10 and 16 years, and in most cases, took part in more than 5 training sessions per week, with the average swimming distance between 2,118 and 3,194 yards per session.

Reaction and Movement Time

Studies involving total-body and arm reaction, movement, and completion times of preadolescent athletes and nonathletes have found that athletes, in general, are faster on all total body and hand-arm reaction times than nonparticipants. Evidence has also been reported that football athletes, as a group, have faster times than nonparticipants on all total body and arm reaction measures while track athletes, as a group, tend to be faster than nonparticipants in only total-body completion time.

In summary, from the above information, it would appear that there is little reason to believe that the physiological stress and strain placed on young children who are taking part in a highly-organized and well-supervised sports program is likely to be physiologically dangerous.

C. PSYCHOLOGICAL AND EMOTIONAL EFFECTS

Concern has been voiced by many that the preadolescent is not emotionally mature enough to face the psychological stresses that competitive type sports places on an individual. Because there is a lack of valid methods for evaluating psychological and emotional stress, good solid evidence relevant to this problem is rather scarce and somewhat contradictory. Research examining the mental or emotionality responses of Little Leaguers and Middle Leaguers in physical education classes and in Little League and Middle League immediately before competition, immediately after competition, and one and one-half hours following competition has been conducted and published. When using the Galvanic Skin Response test to observe the subjects emotional stress, it was found that children of elementary and junior high school age were no more stimulated by Little League and Middle League baseball competition than they were by physical education softball competition. Emotional stress (as determined by telemetry heart rate), as the result of Little League baseball competition, has also been shown to be minimal.

In another investigation with junior high athletes, it was found, when using the Galvanic Skin Response test, that basketball competition caused the greatest emotional response followed by football and then baseball.

Surveys and questionnaires concerning the attitudes of parents and players toward competitive Little League and Middle League baseball have also indicated that individuals who were participants of such teams were actually better adjusted emotionally as well as socially than individuals who were not participants of such teams. Data is also rather conclusive that young girls and goys who have taken part in competitive swimming over a period of several years are as well balanced psychologically and emotionally as those girls and boys who did not take part.

In one survey in which 1,300 physician-fathers of Little League players were interviewed and questioned, 97 percent indicated that the games in their opinions, did not excite their sons to the point that it affected their health adversely. At the same time, however, it should be pointed out that in one survey reported, it was noted that one-third of the parents interviewed stated that the sleeping and eating habits of their sons following competition were disturbed due to the excitement of the games. Sleep disturbance in young players following highly competitive athletic contests is common and has been found by several investigators.

Specific behavior characteristics of preadolescent participants and nonparticipants in different competitive type sports has been investigated. The results have indicated that there are very few differences in the number of problems evidenced by the two groups. The participants achieved not only higher scores each time on the personality traits, but they also obtained higher social acceptance ratings than the nonplayers. It should be noted, however, that the changes that took place as a result of participation were not statistically significant except for the leadership trait. Although the evidence is not completely clear-cut, it would appear that the psychological stresses resulting from such competitive programs is in no way excessive, and apparently does not present an emotional health hazard to young participants.

III. INJURY

While there has been some concern voiced by parents and outside interest groups that the preadolescent is not physically and emotionally mature enough to face the physiological and psychological stresses that competitive sports places on a person, most authorities agree that a bigger concern should be in preventing physical injuries that occur in competitive sports. In fact, some experts feel that physical injury is probably the greatest hazard for the preadolescent in competitive sports, especially those involving body contact such as football, hockey, wrestling, soccer, etc. At the same time, one also cannot ignore the fact that injuries do sometimes occur even in the so-called non-contact sports. For instance, one study on 100 Little League and Middle

League baseball players reported that there were a total of 146 minor injuries (bruises and cuts). Of the 60 Little Leaguers in the sample, there was a total of 123 injuries reported among 41 players with 19 players having no injuries.

In another investigation involving a 5-year period and more than 5 million Little League baseball players, it was noticed that less than 2 percent of the participants incurred injuries that required medical attention. The primary cause of injury was from the ball being thrown, pitched, or batted, with the batter being injured the most often (40% of the injuries being contusions). With the adjustment of the pitching distance and with the development of the new protective batting helmet, injuries to the batter from pitched balls have been reduced considerably. In this same report, of the 2 percent injured, 41 percent resulted in contusions, 19 percent in fractures (fractures of the fingers resulted in 43%), 10 percent in lacerations, 5 percent in dental injuries, 18 percent in sprains, 2 percent in concussions, 3 percent in abrasions, and 2 percent in various other injuries. The other players (13 to 15 year old) received more sprains, fractures, dislocations, and epiphyseal injuries than the younger ones (8 to 12 year olds). In fact, in the old group there were about twice as many sprains, fractures, and dislocations of the lower leg than among the young participants. The reason for this higher injury rate found in the older group was believed to be due to the wearing of steel spiked shoes since the young players were not permitted to wear steel spikes. It is interesting to note that following this investigation, steel spikes were forbidden to be worn by the older players in Middle League baseball and the injury rate was reduced considerably. These results suggest that the type of shoe worn in Little League and Middle League baseball should be a major consideration by officials and rule makers in developing ways for preventing injuries.

Without a doubt, one of the greatest growth and development concerns the medical profession has had over the years with young children taking part in competitive sports has been the possibility of their gaining permanent damage from epiphyseal type injuries. In 1952, the AAHPER committee on athletic competition for children of elementary and junior high school age took a poll of orthopedic surgeons on what type of athletic competition they felt was appropriate for young children in the 12 to 15 age range. The committee reported that 70 percent of the surgeons recommended that special attention should be given to the hazard of the particular activity in regard to possible injuries of the epiphyseal area of the long bones. The findings of a roentgenographic study in which 162 Little League baseball players (ages 9 to 14 years) elbows of the throwing arm supports the orthopedic surgeons recommendation. Of 80 pitchers examined, 76 had various amounts of epiphysis, osteochondritis, or accelerated growth in the medial humoral epiphysis. At the same time, only 7 of the 47 nonpitchers were found to have similar results. On the basis of these findings and other studies involving the Little Leaguer's elbow and shoulder, it has been recommended by various authorities that pitchers at this level be allowed to pitch only two innings per game and that players under 14 years of age not be permitted to pitch curve balls.

While many physicians regard epiphyseal injuries as a major problem in preadolescent competitive sports, there are also those in the medical field who take a more conservative point of view. For example, in an extensive investigation involving 1,338 athletic injuries witnessed by 4 orthopedists, it was noted that of 371 athletic injuries in participants under 15 years of age, only 1.7 percent were epiphyseal. In another piece of work involving 2,745 athletic injuries of which 673 occurred in children 15 years of age and under, 86 of the injuries occurring in this age group or 12.7 percent were epiphyseal injuries. Thus, some experts feel that most epiphyseal injuries can be lowered and handled without permanent damage provided the physician is alert for symptoms of bone or joint disease. At this point, it should be mentioned in support of competitive sports that some researchers feel that epiphyseal injuries in young children probably occur as often in informal play as in athletics. For example, in a study involving 31 epiphyseal injuries that required hospitalization, it was noted that 77 percent resulted from high falls and vehicular accidents, while only 23 percent were actually from athletically oriented sports.

While the sport of tackle football is one of the most popular participant as well as spectator sports in the United States, it is a contact sport in which the potential for injury is quite high. Data collected on 16,500 athletes taking part in junior high school football in New York indicated that the injury incidents was around 11.2 percent. Injury figures for Pop Warner Tackle Football and Midget Tackle Football are not as high. While several investigators have gathered some excellent local and state-wide data of this nature with high school athletes, data on a national scale involving the various kinds of injuries over a period of several years (especially with preadolescent athletes) are lacking. It is noteworthy that while fatalities have been witnessed in tackle football, there has not been (to this writers knowledge) a single fatality in the Pop Warner Program of tackle football for youngsters during the entire time of its existance. Apparently, because the players are relatively small and matched according to their overall size as well as the fact that they now have good protective equipment all provide a somewhat safe playing environment for the young participants. It is interesting to note that while the fatality record for Pop Warner football is excellent, data from a national poll showed that 43.5 percent of the physicians interviewed were still opposed to body contact sports.

In another interesting report by a group of AAHPER members in which elementary school principals were surveyed, only 2 percent of the schools having interschool sports competition and 8 percent of the communities with agency-sponsored athletic programs reported accidents that were serious enough to require medical attention. While it would appear from the above data that serious injury in interschool and agency-sponsord athletic contests are infrequent, these figures should be viewed with some caution since they do not represent an injury rate, but instead, the observations by the school principal that one or more injuries that were felt to be serious had actually taken place in this school or community during his time in office.

It is well known that provisions for safeguarding the health and safety of the young participant is a top priority to school and health experts. At the same time, it is well known that the universal recommendation is that potential particpants should have a physical examination by a qualified physician before being allowed to play on an athletic team. However, according to the national survey, as reported by the AAHPER Committee, this has not been the general practice. For example, the survey indicated that only 17 percent of the agency-sponsored programs and only 58 percent of the school-sponsored programs required physical examinations. In addition, the report showed that only 28 percent of the coaches in agency-sponsored programs had professional training while 81 percent of the coaches in school-sponsored programs had training as teachers or experience in the particular sport. From the data gathered by the committee, it is quite clear from the health viewpoint that the conditions by which the school-sponsored programs operated were superior to the conditions by which the agency-sponsored programs functioned.

IV. GUIDELINES FOR COMPETITIVE SPORTS FOR THE PREADOLESCENT

In 1968, a Joint Committee made up of members from the American Association for Health, Physical Education and Recreation, the American Medical Association, the American Academy of Pediatrics, and the Society of State Directors of Health, Physical Education and Recreation, developed a policy statement for competitive preadolescent sports. The policy statement places particular emphasis on the following: (1) proper physical conditioning for all children prior to playing competitive sports, (2) good, competent coaching, (3) careful grouping of players according to sex, skill, body size, and physical maturation, (4) good quality, properly fitted equipment, (5) playing area should be properly designed, built, and maintained for the activity involved, (6) rules should be appropriate for the young player in order to make the game safer by adapting the activity to their physical limitations and skills, (7) periodic health appraisals of players, and (8) definite policies for medical care during workouts and contests should be established with each participant checked out and evaluated before being allowed to participate following an injury.

The report recommends a broad program with a variety of activities which includes good sound supervision. It emphasizes that a well-balanced physical education program should precede an interschool athletic program since a sports program by itself provides too narrow a sports experience for the child. The report specifies that local committees representing educational, recreational, medical, and parental interests should be involved in developing and operating preadolescent programs. The document also suggests that the authority and responsibility of the coach, school administrators, physicians, and parents must be well defined.

The report states that each child in the upper elementary grades should have the opportunity to take part in an organized and supervised intramural program. The interschool athletic program should in no way take away from the instructional intramural physical education program in terms of budget or time allotment.

The statement recommends that interschool preadolescent sports competition be restricted to upper elementary grade children, and that games be kept on a neighborhood or community level with playoffs and all-star games prohibited. It further states that special care should be taken to avoid high pressures being placed on the young athlete by charging admission to the games, conducting various commercial promotion gimmicks, having victory celebrations, and conducting excess publicity maneuvers. Exploitation of the young athlete is highly discouraged.

While competitive sports such as basketball, football, baseball, soccer, hockey, wrestling, and softball are recognized by the report as having certain injury risks, these risks, according to the document, are generally associated with the conditions under which these activities are carried out and the level of the supervision which is provided. The sport of boxing, on the other hand, is not recommended for children of this age since its primary purpose is to cause injury. Lifetime competitive sports such as archery, golf, bowling, skating, swimming, tennis, and track are appropriate and are recommended by the report for children of elementary school age. Emphasis is placed on making children more aware of the physiological values of sports and their lifetime recreational value.

In summary, the policy statement, as defined by the Joint Committee, places well-defined restrictions on the type and extent of competitive sports for elementary school age children. The report also stresses the need for sound educational practices under medical supervision, and if the schools and or communities cannot offer this, the report recommends that they should not attempt to have competitive type sport programs for children of elementary school age.

V. SUMMARY

(1) Short-term studies investigating the effects of competitive preadolescent sports on physical growth are controversial, while longitudinal research generally indicates that highly

competitive sports or prolonged periods of hard training adversely affects the normal physical growth of young children.

(2) Evidence is convincing that young athletes of elementary and junior high school age are superior to nonathletes of similar chronological age in the following:

    (a) skeletal age and relative maturity (skeletal age as related to chronological age),
    (b) body size and build,
    (c) muscular strength and power,
    (d) speed and agility,
    (e) total body and hand-arm reaction times.

(3) There is little reason to believe that the physiological stress and strain placed on young participants who are taking part in a competitive sports program that is highly organized and well supervised is likely to be physiologically dangerous.

(4) Evidence indicates that young children involved in 6 weeks or more of vigorous training and competitive running or swimming have greater heart and lung volumes as well as greater lean body mass and functional working capacities (as determined by maximal oxygen uptake and $P.W.C._{170}$ tests) than non-participants of similar age and sex.

(5) Heart rates at submaximal and maximal work loads are decreased in young children following 6 weeks or more of intensive training and competitive running and swimming.

(6) Young swimmers engaged in a long-range swimming program (3 years) have a lower exercise cardiac output for a given oxygen uptake due to a lower heart rate than nonparticipants of similar age and sex.

(7) Although the evidence is not completely clearcut, it would appear that the psychological stresses resulting from competitive preadolescent sports is in no way excessive, and apparently does not present an emotional health hazard to the young athlete.

(8) Physical injury is probably the greatest hazard in preadolescent competitive sports with epiphyseal type injuries being perhaps the greatest growth and development concern to physicians.

(9) While some physicians take a more conservative point of view toward epiphyseal injuries, most are in agreement that they can be handled without further damage provided the physician is alert for symptoms of bone or joint disease.

(10) Data gathered by members of a 1968 AAHPER Committee in which elementary school principals were surveyed indicates quite clearly from the health viewpoint that the conditions by which the school-sponsored athletic programs were operated were superior to the agency-sponsored athletic programs.

(11) Guidelines for competitive preadolescent sports were developed in 1968 by a Joint Committee representing the American Association for Health, Physical Education and Recreation, the American Medical Association, the American Academy of Pediatrics, and the Society of State Directors of Health, Physical Education and Recreation. The policy statement places well-defined restrictions on the type and extent of competitive sports for elementary school age children. The report also stresses the need for sound educational practices under medical supervision and if the schools and communities cannot offer this, they should not attempt to have competitive type sport programs for children of elementary school age.

VI. REVIEW REFERENCES

(1) AAHPER Committee on Desirable Athletic Competition for Children of Elementary School Age. "Desirable Athletic Competition for Children of Elementary School Age," AAHPER, Washington, D.C., 1968.

(2) Adams, J. E. "Bone Injuries in Very Young Athletes," *Clinical Orthopedic,* 58:129-40, 1968.
(3) Adams, J. E. "Injury to the Throwing Arm: A Study of Traumatic Changes in the Elbow Joints of Boy Baseball Players," *California Medical Journal,* 102:127-32, 1965.
(4) Clarke, D. H., and P. Vaccaro. "The Effect of Swimming Training on Muscular Performance and Body Composition in Children," *Research Quarterly,* 50:9-17, 1979.
(5) Cunningham, D. A., and R. B. Eyon. "The Working Capacity of Young Competitive Swimmers, 10-16 Years of Age," *Medicine and Science in Sports,* 5:227-31, 1973.
(6) Cunningham, D. A., P. Telford, and G. T. Swart. "The Cardiopulmonary Capacities of Young Hockey Players: Age 10," *Medicine and Science in Sports,* 8:23-25, 1976.
(7) Godshall, R. W. "Junior League Football: Risks Versus Benefits," *Journal of Sports Medicine,* 3:139-66, 1975.
(8) Gutin, B., A. Trinidad, C. Norton, E. Giles, A. Giles, and K. Stewart. "Morphological and Physiological Factors Related to Endurance Performance of 11- to 12-Year-Old Girls," *Research Quarterly,* 49:44-52, 1978.
(9) Larson, R. L. "Physical Activity and the Growth and Development of Bone and Joint Structures," in *Physical Activity: Human Growth and Development,* (G. L. Rarick, editor), Academic Press, New York, 1973.
(10) Lussier, L., and E. R. Buskirk. "Effects of an Endurance Training Regimen on Assessment of Work Capacity in Prepubertal Children," *Annals New York Academy of Sciences,* 301:734-47, 1977.
(11) Mayers, N., and B. Gutin. "Physiological Characteristics of Elite Prepubertal Cross-Country Runners," *Medicine and Science in Sports,* 11:172-76, 1979.
(12) Rarick, G. L. "Competitive Sports for Young Boys: Controversial issues," *Medicine and Science in Sports,* 1:181, 1969.
(13) Rarick, G. L. "Competitive Sports in Childhood and Early Adolescence," in *Physical Activity: Human Growth and Development,* (G. L. Rarick, editor), Academic Press, New York, 1973.
(14) Rarick, G. L. "Exercise and Growth," in *Science and Medicine of Exercise and Sport,* 2nd edition, W. R. Johnson and E. R. Buskirk, editors), Harper and Row Publishers, New York, 1974.
(15) Roser, L. A., and D. K. Clawson. "Football Injuries in the Very Young Athlete," *Clinical Orthopedic,* 69:212-23, 1970.
(16) Stewart, K., and B. Gutin. "Effects of Physical Training on Cardio-Respiratory Fitness in Children," *Research Quarterly,* 47:110-20, 1976.
(17) v. Dobeln, W., and B. O. Eriksson. "Physical Training, Maximal Oxygen Uptake and Dimensions of the Oxygen Transporting and Metabolizing Organs in Boys 11-13 Years of Age," *Acta Paediatrica Scandinavica,* 61:653-60, 1972.
(18) Wilmore, J. H., and J. J. McNamara. "Prevalence of Coronary Heart Disease Risk Factors in Boys 8 to 12 Years of Age," *Journal of Pediatrics,* 84:527-33, 1974.

13
AGING AND EXERCISE

KEY CONCEPTS TO BE GAINED FROM THIS CHAPTER

(1) It is difficult to separate and define the role of the biological aging process from heredity, increased sedentary living of most average people, and unknown diseases such as atherosclerosis that so often accompany increases in age.

(2) Physiological changes that normally accompany the aging process are also influenced by exercise and physical conditioning.

(3) There are basic principles and guidelines that should be followed in individualized cardiorespiratory exercise programs for the aged.

In the past, most of the attention, recognition, and research in the area of exercise physiology (as it relates to the various physiological effects that accompany the aging process) has been devoted toward the school- and college-age person. The elderly received little or no attention from the researcher. Today, however, this is no longer true. Because of the recent popularity in physical fitness, more and more people of all ages, including the elderly, are now taking part in physical activities of all forms. Researchers are now beginning to flood the market with scientific data for the aged. Age-related research studies and medical technology are now predicting that the average American life expectancy will be 125 years by the year 2020. In some circles, they are even predicting that the average life expectancy will eventually reach an unthinkable 200 years.

With the population trend now moving toward one of older people, and with the popularity of recreation and age-group competition growing by leaps and bounds along with the fact that more and more senior citizens are now being used as subjects in research projects, many vitally and important questions have now been raised. What exactly are the physiological changes that accompany the aging process? How does a 55-year old sedentary female who wants to take part in next years 6-mile Bonnie Bell run train herself so she can compete and join her friends? Are the principles and guidelines for conducting training programs for the elderly the same as it is for the school- and college-age person? Is physical training and athletic competition harmful for the elderly? It is the purpose of this chapter to answer these questions and many others concerning the biological aging process and the effects of physical activity and conditioning.

I. PHYSIOLOGICAL CHANGES ACCOMPANYING THE AGING PROCESS

At the outset, it should be pointed out that there does not appear to be any specific threshold age for which performance deteriorates. Most of the physiological functions apparently have their own individual peaks and declines with age. In fact, some variables such as total blood volume and blood sugars under resting conditions do not appear to show any deterioration with age. In most cases, the various physiological functions reach their peak somewhere between the ages of 20 and 30 years. Research shows that most systems or functions, after reaching their peak, will level off for a period of time before gradually decreasing with age. While some decay in physical performance should be expected with advancing age, it is difficult to separate and define the role of the biological aging process from heredity, increased sedentary living of most average Americans, and even unknown diseases such as hardening of the arteries (atherosclerosis) that so often accompany increases in age. It should be encouraging to know, however, that recent evidence indicates that physical activity may retard or slow down the rate of decline that is associated with aging. Some of the physiological changes accompanying the aging process are shown in Table 13-1.

A. MUSCLE SIZE AND STRENGTH

As an individual gets older, there is a decline in muscle size. It is believed that this decline is due, in part, to a reduced amount of protein as well as a decline in the number and size of muscle

Table 13-1. Physiological Changes Accompanying the Aging Process

Physiological Functions	Age
Muscle size	Decreased
Muscle strength	Decreased
Lean body weight	Decreased
Percent body fat	Increased
Basal metabolic rate	Decreased
Maximal heart rate	Decreased
Overall heart size (Especially the left ventricular cavity)	Decreased
Cardiac muscle strength	Decreased
Maximal Stroke Volume	Decreased
Maximal cardiac output	Decreased
Maximal blood flow	Decreased
Elasticity of blood vessels	Decreased
Blood pressure	Increased
Capillary density of muscle	Unchanged
Maximal oxygen uptake ($\dot{V}_{O_2max}$)	Decreased
Vital capacity	Decreased
Maximal expiratory ventilation ($\dot{V}_{Emax}$)	Decreased
Pulmonary diffusion capacity	Decreased
Ratio of residual volume to the total lung capacity (RV/TLC)	Increased
Reaction time	Decreased
Movement time	Decreased
Bone density	Decreased
Flexibility	Decreased
Elasticity of lung tissue and chest wall	Decreased

fibers. While it is not completely clear, it has been suggested that the decline in the number of muscle fibers may be due to degenerative diseases (that are generally associated with advancing age) affecting the nerve fibers. Recall from earlier discussion that increases in strength are highly related to muscle fiber hypertrophy. In other words, strength increases parallel increases in muscle size. As seen in muscle size, as people get old, there is also a parallel decrease in muscular strength, which probably results from the decline in muscle size. The decline in strength is a gradual one following the age of about 35 to 45 years. However, even at the age of 60, the decline in strength does not appear to exceed 20 percent of an individual's maximum strength.

B. FAT, LEAN BODY WEIGHT, AND BASAL METABOLIC RATE

With advancing age, there is a general trend to accumulate an increase in body fat. This is usually seen in both relative and absolute terms. There are several reasons normally given for this increase in body fat. First of all, with advancing age, there is a decrease in one's ability to release or mobilize stored fatty acids from adipose tissue for energy fuel. This, of course, results in less fatty acids being burned up. Also, as most people get older, they not only generally increase their food intake, but they also become less active. This obviously means that they are more than likely taking in more calories than they are burning up. Besides heredity (which one cannot control), the amount of fat gained (or lost) with increasing age will naturally depend upon one's eating and exercise habits.

Along with the fat increase, as one gets older, their lean body weight decreases. Like muscular strength, changes in lean body weight with age also parallel somewhat the increases and decreases in muscle mass. Therefore, part of the decrease in lean body weight with age is due to the decrease in muscle size along with the decline in calcium and phosphorus content of the bones. The amount of decline in lean body weight as one gets older can also be controlled somewhat by their eating and exercise habits.

Basal metabolic rate (BMR) decreases gradually with increasing age. According to some reports, the rate of decline from the age of 3 through 80 years, is around 3 percent per decade. Others involving longitudinal studies have placed the decline between 1 and 2 percent per decade. Between the ages of 20 and 30, this decline apparently indicates an improved metabolic efficiency, whereas according to Wilmore, a decline for older people past 30 may be due to the decrease in lean body weight that accompanies age. Research is needed to determine the effects of physical activity on BMR in older people.

C. RESPIRATORY SYSTEM

There is good evidence to indicate that pulmonary function is impaired with advancing age. This is evidenced in various pulmonary tests that show a decrease in vital capacity, a decrease in maximal expiratory ventilation ($\dot{V}_{Emax}$), a decrease in pulmonary diffusion capacity, and an increase in the ratio of residual volume to the total lung capacity (RV/TLC). This increase in RV/TLC is the result of a gradual increase in the residual volume with advancing age while total lung capacity remain relatively unchanged. For example, it has been illustrated that residual volume makes up about 20 percent of the total lung capacity for an individual in their late twenties, whereas by the age of fifty, this figure has increased to about 30 percent.

From the evidence reported, these alterations in pulmonary function appear to be due primarily to the lung tissue and chest wall losing their elasticity with age. With a reduced elasticity, it naturally decreases their mobility, and as a result, increases the effort in breathing.

D. CARDIOVASCULAR SYSTEM

A number of studies have shown that as an individual gets older, their overall heart size becomes smaller. The left ventricular cavity may especially decrease in size as a result of reduced activity and in the physical demands of increased age. There is a reduction in the size of the cardiac muscle cell along with a progressive decrease in cardiac muscle strength. Recent research has shown that following the age of 20 years, there is an annual loss of approximately 0.85 percent of heart muscle strength. With advancing age, maximum heart rate decreases gradually. The rule-of-thumb is that maximum heart rate decreases at a rate of not quite one beat per year. A practical way of estimating one's maximum heart rate is to subtract one's age from 220 (this practice is generally followed after one reaches the age of 20).

In addition, maximum stroke volume, cardiac output, and blood flow are all decreased with age. Since the capillary density apparently does not change significantly with age, the reduced blood flow to the working muscles is probably a combination of the smaller size heart (particularly the left ventricular cavity) along with the blood vessels losing their elasticity with age, while at the same time, becoming more and more rigid with gradual increases in blood pressure. It is interesting to note that some researchers, when comparing a 70-year old to a 20-year old, have reported as much as a 50 percent reduction in the elasticity of the large aorta artery of the 70-year old. Note that blood pressures up to 170/90 mmHg in older women and 160/100 mmHg in older men are considered to be in the normal range.

As mentioned in several other places in this text, maximal oxygen uptake ($\dot{V}_{O_2max}$) is the single best measure of physical fitness. Several highly respected studied have illustrated that there is a gradual decline in $\dot{V}_{O_2max}$ with increasing age. Again, it is difficult to determine exactly how much of the decline in $\dot{V}_{O_2max}$ is due to the biological aging process or to inactive sedentary living. deVries mentions 5 physiological variables whose reduced functions with advancing age may contribute to a decline in $\dot{V}_{O_2max}$. They are: (1) heart rate; (2) stroke volume; (3) lung ventilation; (4) lung diffusion capacity for oxygen; and (5) utilization of oxygen by the tissues.

E. NERVOUS SYSTEM

There is some evidence to indicate that reaction time and movement time slow down with increasing age. While the underlying mechanism for this psychomotor decrement is not completely understood, there are those who have done extensive work in this area who feel confident that although a slower conduction time along both the afferent and efferent nerve fibers (in the peripheral nervous system) may account for some of the decrement in reaction time and movement time, the major cause is more directly related to the degeneration of the central nervous system. Recent evidence indicates that excessive activity of nerve cells may have beneficial effects in preventing cognitive (reaction time) decrements in performance with increasing age.

F. BONE DENSITY

Bone density decreases with increasing age which means that elderly people (especially those over 40 years of age) are much more prone for bone injury than young people whose bones have obtained full growth and maturity. This is due to a decrease in minerals (calcium and phosphorus) found in the bone which makes the bones less dense, more porous and harder to heal from an injury. Although everyone is different, the decline in calcium and phosphorus generally starts in the early forties. Studies have shown that extra intake of these minerals may actually slow down or reduce their loss. Studies also indicate that physical activity (endurance type) apparently has a beneficial effect on curbing mineral losses.

II. TRAINING ADAPTATION IN THE AGED

The physiological changes that occur from training school-age children and young- and middle-age adults are now fairly well established. While the training adaptations are not perhaps as well known for the elderly, with the increased research and interest in the aged, it is becoming more and more obvious that the older person can adapt and develop (or improve) their physical working capacity, in some cases, just as much as the young person can. In fact, it appears that the older person can adapt and follow essentially the same sort of conditioning programs that are designed for young adults. While there is no available evidence to indicate that physical exertion, regardless of age and sex, can physiologically harm or injure a normal, healthy person, it should be obvious to the exerciser (young or old) that they should take it relatively easy during the early part of the conditioning program and warm up gradually and slowly with stretching exercises. This is to avoid the possibility of pulled muscles and stiffness of the joints.

Evidence is available to indicate that isometric-type exercises results in uncommonly high blood pressures. Because of this, and its implications, isometric-type exercises are not recommended for older people and especially people with cardiovascular diseases. It should be pointed out that this type of high blood pressure also results from dynamic-type arm work performed above the waist or in work activities around the house such as snow shoveling or digging in the garden. Specific guidelines and principles for prescribing cardiorespiratory-type exercise programs for the aged can be found in the next section.

Table 13-2 illustrates some of the physiological adaptations that have been reported in the literature. While the physiological underlying mechanisms for the various improvements in the elderly are not completely understood, there appears to be no doubt that training can bring about a significantly improved cardiorespiratory system as reflected in: (1) a decrease in heart rate at standard submaximal work loads; (2) an increase in stroke volume at standard submaximal work loads; (3) an increase in blood volume; (4) an increase in total hemoglobin; (5) an increase oxygen

Table 13-2. Summary of the Major Physiological Training Adaptations in the Aged

Variable	Training Effects
Heart rate at standard submaximal* work loads	Decreased
Stroke volume at standard submaximal work loads	Increased
Blood volume	Increased
Total hemoglobin	Increased
Oxygen pulse	Increased
Blood pressure (resting)	Decreased
Vital capacity	Increased
Maximal expiratory ventilation ($\dot{V}_{Emax}$)	Increased
Maximal oxygen uptake ($\dot{V}_{O_2max}$)	Increased
Physical work capacity	Increased
EKG abnormalities	Decreased
Muscle strength	Increased
Lean body weight	Increased
Percent body fat	Decreased
Serum cholesterol and triglyceride levels	Decreased
Flexibility	Increased

*Indicates that the same amount of work was performed before and after training.

pulse; (6) a decrease in resting systolic and diastolic blood pressure; (7) an increase in vital capacity; (8) an increase in maximal expiratory ventilation; (9) an increase in maximal oxygen uptake; (10) an increase in physical work capacity; and (11) a decrease in EKG abnormalities.

In addition to the cardiorespiratory endurance changes, training for older people can also bring about an increase in muscular strength, a decrease in percent body fat, and an increase in lean body weight. Investigators have also found serum cholesterol and triglyceride levels to be reduced as a result of physical conditioning, thus suggesting a possible protective effect against the development of ischemic heart disease (also known as coronary artery disease).

The finding that flexibility of the joints can be increased with training should be an added incentive for developing exercise and training programs for the elderly.

III. BASIC PRINCIPLES AND GUIDELINES FOR CONSTRUCTING AN INDIVIDUALIZED CARDIORESPIRATORY ENDURANCE EXERCISE PROGRAM FOR THE AGED

Although this section is written primarily for the aged, the basic principles and guidelines for constructing an individualized cardiorespiratory exercise program are the same for all ages and sex regardless of their physical condition. Exercise physiology and scientific training methods have advanced so much during the past few years until one single group-training program is no longer applicable or realistic to apply to all people of all ages. The research findings are rather conclusive that exercise and training should be based on individual specific needs, goals, and physical capacities.

It is important to keep in mind that it is essential that before attempting any exercise program, a physical examination is a must. This is especially true for those people who are over 30 years of age and have been living a sedentary life with very little physical activity. In recent years, an important part of the medical examination has been the exercise-stress test. This test is performed on either a bicycle ergometer or a treadmill during which time the individual's electrocardiogram and blood pressure are monitored. Such data are extremely important in prescribing exercise programs for people of all ages (especially middle- and older-aged groups). The importance of this test is obvious since in many cases an abnormal electrocardiogram (an indication of coronary artery disease) will not show up during resting conditions, whereas during exercise, it is more likely to appear.

A. EXERCISE PRESCRIPTION

In prescribing a cardiorespiratory endurance exercise program, four basic factors are involved. They are: (1) intensity; (2) duration; (3) frequency; and (4) mode of activity. Each will be covered separately.

Intensity

This factor is the most critical of all in developing cardiorespiratory endurance fitness. It depends upon an individual's present level of fitness, their present health condition, and the length or duration of the training. The intensity of work can be expressed in several ways including (1) a percentage of maximum heart rate, (2) a percentage of maximal oxygen consumption, (3) number of calories consumed, or (4) in METS. During submaximal or aerobic work, it has been well established that heart rate increases linearly with energy cost (or oxygen uptake) of the work. Because of this and for practical reasons, exercise heart rate has been used by many researchers for determining not only the physiological stress of the work, but also for developing various training programs.

How hard must a person (especially the elderly person) work in order to improve their physical fitness? Evidence now indicates that a sufficient amount of cardiorespiratory endurance can be accomplished by training at somewhere between 60 and 90 percent of maximum heart rate (exhaustive, punishing-type work is not necessary). This represents a maximum oxygen uptake level of 50 to 80 percent. The lower heart rate figure of 60 percent of maximum represents a minimum threshold level for which it must reach in order for improvements to take place. Training at levels below this apparently results in little or no cardiorespiratory improvements. Table 13-3 lists the training heart rates that represent the minimum threshold level of 60 percent of maximum heart rate and the upper level of 90 percent for different middle-age and older age groups. As Figure 13-1 illustrates, cardiorespiratory benefits will be accomplished as long as the exercise heart rate is kept within these levels.

The concept of training at your own individual heart rate threshold level automatically accounts for any improvement that might take place during the training program. For example, as a person's fitness level improves and exercise heart rate for a standard work load decreases, then they automatically must work more in order to reach their minimum threshold level.

Duration

In training for cardiorespiratory endurance, it should be kept in mind that the duration and intensity of the work are interrelated. For example, research shows that improvements in cardiorespiratory endurance (about 15 to 20%) can be noticed with high-intensity (heart rates

Table 13-3. Age-Predicted Maximum Heart Rate and Cardiorespiratory Training Heart Rates That Represent the Minimum and Upper Threshold Levels

Age (yrs)	Age-Predicted (220-Age) Maximal Heart Rate (beats/min)	Training Heart Rates Minimum Threshold Level 60% Heart Rate	Training Heart Rates Upper Threshold Level 90% Heart Rate
20	200	120	180
25	195	117	176
30	190	114	171
35	185	111	167
40	180	108	162
45	175	105	158
50	170	102	153
55	165	99	149
60	160	96	144
65	155	93	140
70	150	90	135
75	145	87	131
80	140	84	126
85	135	81	122
90	130	78	117

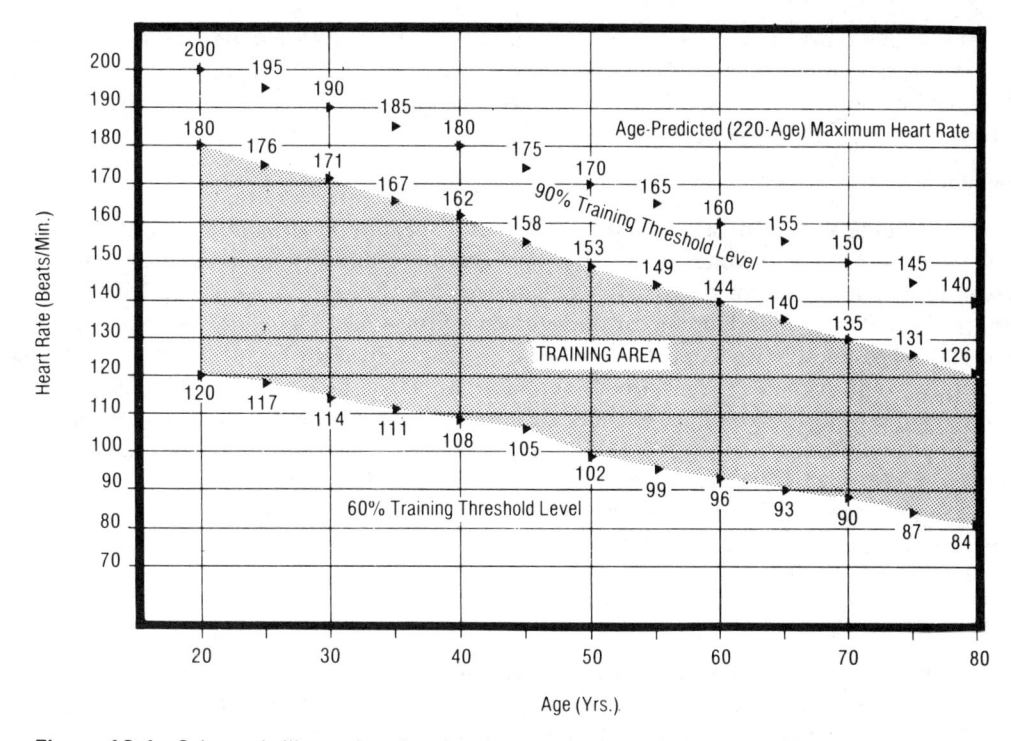

Figure 13-1 Schematic illustration showing the exercise intensity in terms of heart rate needed for developing cardiorespiratory endurance fitness. The minimum threshold level needed is 60 percent of maximum heart rate and the maximum level is 90 percent.

around 85 to 90% of maximum) work lasting for only 5 to 10 minutes per day. However, low-intensity (heart rates around 65 to 75% of maximum) work shows little (about 5%) or no improvement for this period of time. More recent research has shown that continuous training at a low-intensity (heart rates around 65 to 75% of maximum) level for a duration of between 30 to 60 minutes per day will result in significantly greater improvements than training at low-intensity for short periods of time.

Because the general adult population (especially the middle-age and older people) do not really enjoy or tolerate exercise at a high-intensity level and because running requires more energy than leisurely walking (which most elderly people are accustomed to), an often asked question by older people is can one expect to see any improvements by taking part in a walking program (as opposed to a running program) since most elderly people prefer walking to running. The answer to this question is yes provided that the duration and frequency of the training are increased. In other words, to work up for the lower caloric expenditure at the low intensity training level, an individual can merely walk (or run) longer and more often and achieve basically the same results as a person working to near exhaustion for a relatively short period of time.

Before going to the next principle, one important point should be made concerning duration of work. That is, the training duration times mentioned under this principle refers to the length of time that the subjects heart rate is kept within the prescribed training threshold level. For example, if a 65-year old man is training (by walking) at a threshold level of 70 percent of his maximum heart rate, then he would need to get his heart rate up to at least 105 beats/min (Table

13-3) and keep it there for a minimum of 30 minutes in duration. At the same time, if a 40-year old man is training at a threshold level of 90 percent, then he would have to get his heart rate up to 162 beats/min and hold it there for only a period of between 5 and 10 minutes in order to accomplish cardiorespiratory endurance benefits.

Frequency

It may come as a surprise to some people, but a substantial amount of evidence has been found to indicate that in order to develop one's cardiorespiratory endurance capacity, daily exercise and training is not necessary. In fact, studies show that 3 to 5 days per week is an optimal number of workouts for developing cardiorespiratory fitness. Once a regular exercise routine has been established and the workouts have become enjoyable, then the frequency of workouts may be extended to more than 3 to 5 days per week. It is important, however, not to initially start out training everyday of the week since chances are good that the individual, after a couple of weeks, will become completely exhaustive (mentally and physically), and will more than likely quit the program. Since one of the major goals of an exercise program is to make it not only intense enough to see some positive results (in terms of cardiorespiratory endurance), but also to make it enjoyable enough to where it becomes a part of an individual's regular routine. A person should look forward to each workout session and not dread it.

Mode of Activity

In general, it is agreed that activities (of moderate to high energy expenditure) involving the entire body such as walking, jogging, running, swimming, hiking, bicycling, canoeing, cross-country skiing, game-type activities such as basketball, soccer, and aerobic dancing produce the best improvements in cardiorespiratory fitness. On the other hand, activities that are somewhat low in energy cost such as golf, bowling, softball, and most calisthenics do little in way of developing physical fitness. In addition, short, anaerobic-type activities that call for explosive power and speed do little in developing aerobic fitness.

While weight-training programs may improve muscular strength and muscular endurance, they have little or no significant effect on developing one's cardiorespiratory fitness. In addition, as was mentioned earlier in this chapter, because isometric-type weight-training exercises results in uncommonly high blood pressures, they are absolutely not recommended for the elderly and especially people with cardiovascular diseases.

Anyone who has ever worked in an adult-fitness program knows that motivation is probably the most important factor of all in developing a successful program. Because of this, it is extremely important to remember that what ever mode of exercise is selected, it should be one in which the participant enjoys and looks forward to each day. One of the goals in constructing an individualized exercise program is to develop an appreciation for exercise and training to where it eventually becomes a part of your everyday routine and not something that you wake up dreading each day.

deVries and colleagues have developed a progressive exercise program for older men (ages 52 to 88 years) and women (ages 52 to 79 ages) that has been found to be safe and effective in developing physical fitness. An outline of the program is found in Table 13-4. Basically, it is a program that involves calisthenics (for warm-up), a run-walk program for developing the cardiorespiratory fitness, and static stretching for improving joint mobility and preventing soreness. The subjects, in the run-walk phase of the program, work at their own cadence and stride length that is normal and comfortable without any consideration for regulating time.

Table 13-4. A Comprehensive Progressive Exercise Program for the Elderly*

Phase I

Calisthenics (15 to 20 minutes)
1. 5 BX
2. President's Council & Administration on Aging Series (1968)
3. Others

Phase II

Run-Walk Program (15 to 20 minutes)
1. 50 steps run, 50 steps walk
   a. 5 sets the first day
   b. Each day increase the number of sets by one until 10 sets have been completed
   c. Use the same set procedure for each new series of run-walk
2. 50 steps run, 40 steps walk
3. 50 steps run, 30 steps walk
4. 50 steps run, 20 steps walk
5. 50 steps run, 10 steps walk
6. 75 steps run, 10 steps walk
7. 100 steps run, 10 steps walk
8. 125 steps run, 10 steps walk
9. 150 steps run, 10 steps walk
10. 175 steps run, 10 steps walk
11. 200 steps run, 10 steps walk
12. Individual program

Phase III

Static stretching to prevent soreness and to improve joint mobility (15 to 20 minutes)

Source: deVries, H. A. *Physiology of Exercise for Physical Education and Athletics,* 2nd edition, Wm. C. Brown Co., Dubuque, Iowa, 1974, p. 354.
*The exercise program has been shown to be safe and effective when carried out three times per week for normal older men and women in the presence of medical personnel during physiological monitoring.

IV. SUMMARY

(1) There does not appear to be any specific threshold age for which performance deteriorates. Most of the physiological functions have their own individual peaks and declines with age.

(2) There is no available evidence to indicate that strenuous exercise regardless of age and sex can physiologically harm or injure a normal, healthy person.

(3) The observable physiological changes during aging illustrate a decrement in most all functions. These include: a decline in muscle size and strength; decline in basal metabolic rate; decline in lean body weight; an increase in percent body fat; decline in maximal heart rate; decline in blood flow; decline in stroke volume; decline in cardiac output; decline in vital capacity and pulmonary diffusion capacity; a decline in maximal expiratory ventilation; an increase in RV/TLC due to an increase in residual volume with no change in total lung capacity; a decrease in flexibility; slower reaction time and movement time; and a decline in maximal oxygen uptake.

(4) The effects of physical training upon the older person are in direct opposition to the commonly effects of the biological aging process.

(5) Studies show that the older person can adapt and develop their functional capacities by following the same similar conditioning programs as are designed for the young adult, although the achievement level will be somewhat lower for the older person.

(6) Four basic factors are involved in prescribing a cardiorespiratory endurance program for the elderly. They are: intensity, duration, frequency, and mode of activity.

(7) A minimum threshold level of 60% of maximum heart rate is needed to improve cardiorespiratory fitness. Training below 60% results in little or no cardiorespiratory improvements.

(8) The following are recommendations for cardiorespiratory endurance exercise prescription for middle-age and older adults who are considered healthy:

Intensity = 60 to 90% of maximum heart rate
Duration = 5 to 10 minutes of continuous activity at high intensity level
= 30 to 60 minutes of continuous activity at low intensity level
Frequency = 3 to 5 days per week
Mode of Activity = walking, jogging, swimming, bicycling, hiking, cross-country skiing

V. REVIEW REFERENCES

(1) Adams, G. M., and H. A. deVries. "Physiological Effects of an Exercise Training Regimen Upon Women Aged 52-79," *Journal of Gerontology*, 28:50-55, 1973.
(2) Barnard, R. J., G. K. Grimditch, and J. H. Wilmore. "Physiological Characteristics of Sprint and Endurance Masters Runners," *Medicine and Science in Sports*, 11:167-71, 1979.
(3) deVries, H. A. "Physiological Effects of an Exercise Training Regimen Upon Men Aged 52-88," *Journal of Gerontology*, 25:325-36, 1970.
(4) deVries, H. A. *Physiology of Exercise for Physical Education and Athletics,* 2nd edition, Wm. C. Brown Publishers, Dubuque, Iowa, 1974.
(5) Edington, D. W., and V. R. Edgerton, *The Biology of Physical Activity,* Houghton Mifflin Co., Boston, 1976.
(6) Harris, R. "Cardiopathy of Aging: Are the Changes Related to Congestive Heart Failure?", *Geriatrics*, 32:42-46, 1977.
(7) Kart, C. S., E. S. Metress, and J. F. Metress. *Aging and Health: Biological and Social Perspectives,* Addison-Wesley Publishing Co., California, 1978.
(8) Kasch, F. W. "The Effects of Exercise on the Aging Process," *Physician and Sportsmedicine*, 4:64-72, 1976.
(9) Pollock, M. L. "How Much Exercise is Enough," *Physician and Sportsmedicine*, 6:50-64, 1978.
(10) Robinson, S., D. B. Dill, R. D. Robinson, S. P. Tzankoff, and J. A. Wagner. "Physiological Aging of of Champion Runners," *Journal of Applied Physiology*, 41:46-51, 1976.
(11) Sherwood, D. E., and D. J. Selder. "Cardiorespiratory Health, Recreation Time and Aging," *Medicine and Science in Sports*, 11:186-89, 1979.
(12) Sidney, K. H., and R. J. Shephard. "Frequency and Intensity of Exercise Training for Elderly Subjects," *Medicine and Science in Sports*, 10:125-31, 1978.
(13) Sidney, K. H., R. J. Shephard, and J. E. Harrisson. "Endurance Training and Body Composition of the Elderly," *American Journal of Clinical Nutrition*, 30:326-33, 1977.
(14) Wilmore, J. H. *Athletic Training and Physical Fitness: Physiological Principles and Practices of the Conditioning Process,* Allyn and Bacon, Inc., Boston, 1977.

14

PHYSICAL CONDITIONING

KEY CONCEPTS TO BE GAINED FROM THIS CHAPTER

(1) There are specific training programs available for developing strength, local endurance, and cardiorespiratory endurance to their maximum.

(2) There are specific principles and guidelines that must be adhered to in order for optimal training adaptations to take place.

(3) Training programs can be designed to match the specific energy source needed for the athletes specific event or contest.

(4) There are specific factors that affect the development of strength, local endurance, and cardiorespiratory endurance.

(5) The effects of training depend upon the type of exercise involved in the training program, the individual's previous level of training, and how dedicated and motivated the individual is.

(6) Once the optimal training adaptations are obtained, they subside at a relatively slower rate than they were obtained.

(7) Fatigue following long, submaximal type exercise is caused by different factors than fatigue following short, exhaustive type exercise.

A physiology of exercise textbook would not be complete without a chapter on physical conditioning. Over the past few years, interest in fitness and conditioning has grown by leaps and bounds. In fact, it is now becoming more and more a way of life. Some authorities claim that physical activity is probably our most enjoyable, and yet, our most inexpensive form of preventive medicine.

Because of the increased interest and its tremendous importance, this chapter has been written primarily to provide sound information concerning the basic scientific principles and guidelines for constructing an effective general-type physical conditioning program. Another purpose of this chapter is to present the various physiological changes brought about through training that leads to improved performance.

While it is beyond the scope of this book to get into discussion concerning specific training programs for specific sports, it is hoped that the information presented in this chapter can be of some benefit for the interested coach and player in developing an effective conditioning program for their particular sport or event. The author has chosen to organize this chapter into 4 parts. First, some general principles that can be applied to all physical conditioning programs will be discussed. Then, some specific principles and guidelines underlying the development of muscular strength and local endurance as well as aerobic and anaerobic endurance will be covered. Within each of these areas, the physiological adaptations that occur as a result of training will be presented. Finally, the last section of this chapter will be devoted toward discussing fatigue from the point of view of both local as well as general muscular fatigue.

I. GENERAL PRINCIPLES OF PHYSICAL TRAINING

There are 5 general principles that are applicable to all physical conditioning programs: (1) overload principle; (2) specificity of training; (3) individual differences; (4) identifying the major energy system(s) involved; and (5) motivation.

A. OVERLOAD PRINCIPLE

Regardless of which type of conditioning program you select, the overload principle applies. This principle, when applied to weight-training programs, means that a muscle or muscle group will increase in strength and/or local endurance only if it is forced to work for a period of time above the normal maximal strength and endurance capacities. It is important to remember that during a weight-training program when the muscles are gaining in strength and endurance, the work load must be periodically readjusted in order to allow the muscles to continue working above their normal maximal strength and endurance levels. A person should not expect to see any improvements if the training intensity is below the level at which they hope to compete. Figure 14-1 illustrates clearly the importance of the overload training principle for the development of both muscular strength and local endurance.

In order for the overload principle to be successful for training programs involving anaerobic and aerobic type activities such as running, swimming, cycling, hiking, etc., the intensity of the workouts must also be increased periodically. With these types of training programs, the overload is created by either increasing (a) the intensity of the work within each workout; (b) the frequency or number of workouts; or (c) the duration of the workouts at a given intensity. More will be said about the overload principle as each of the various training areas are discussed.

B. SPECIFICITY OF TRAINING

This principle means that conditioning is specific to the overload or resistance used. That is, isotonic resistance will be more effective in developing isotonic strength than it will isometric strength. At the same time, isometric resistance will be better for developing isometric strength than it will for isotonic strength. The same principle applies to eccentric and isokinetic-type muscle contractions.

Another example of how specificity applies to weight-training exercises is that if strength and/or endurance development is wanted for the entire range of joint motion, then it is desirable for the exercises to be performed at all joint angles in the range of motion. This is highly desirable since training a muscle or muscle group at one joint angle does not necessarily mean that there will be an increase in strength and endurance at other angles.

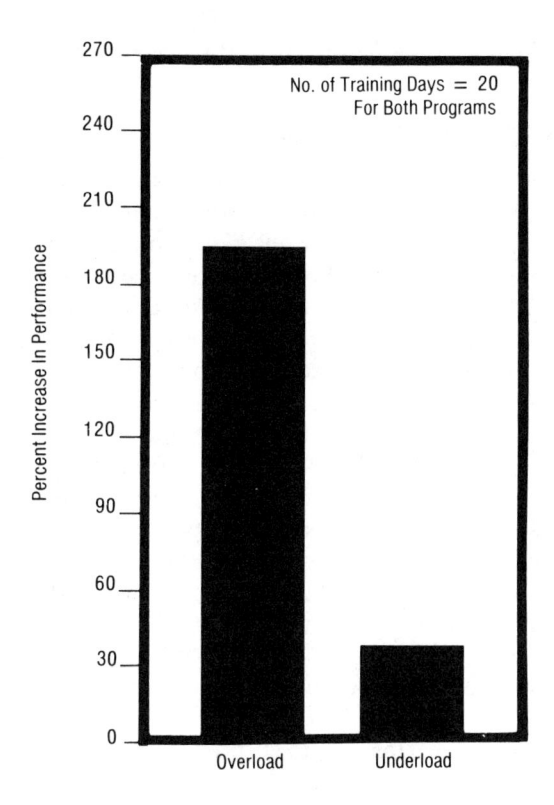

Figure 14-1 Schematic illustration of the overload training principle.

This principle also means that training (whether it is for general overall fitness or for athletic competition) must be specific for not only developing the major energy system(s) involved, but also the specific muscle groups involved along with the exact movement of the skill. For example, weight-training or isokinetic exercises used in developing strength for a baseball pitcher should center primarily around those muscles and their movements that are associated with the overhand baseball throw. The same is true for the outfielder who is trying to develop strength for his throwing arm.

An example of developing the specific energy system(s) involved would be where the recreational jogger would want to concentrate primarily on developing the aerobic (oxygen) system while the intercollegiate sprinter who is training for the 100-yd dash would devote most of his or her time on developing the ATP-CP and lactic acid (anaerobic) systems. At the same time, a person who is training to compete in the middle-distance events would have to devote sufficient time to all three energy systems.

C. INDIVIDUAL DIFFERENCES

It is generally agreed among coaches and exercise physiologists that everybody does not respond to training in the same manner. That is, what may be a significant training intensity for one person may be inadequate for another person. Therefore, the physical educator or coach should not demand that everyone complete the same amount of work at the same rate. Individual differences are real among people and should be anticipated by the coach and physical educator in

256 Essentials of Exercise Physiology

helping them structure their training and conditioning programs to meet the needs of each individual.

D. IDENTIFYING THE MAJOR ENERGY SYSTEM(S) INVOLVED

Recall from Chapter 2 that the ATP-CP energy system is the immediate source of energy for muscle contraction and that there are two metabolic pathways by which it is formed: namely, the anaerobic pathway and the aerobic pathway. The anaerobic route does not require oxygen and uses only carbohydrates (glycogen and glucose) in its production of ATP, whereas the aerobic pathway requires the presence of oxygen and it can use not only carbohydrates, but also fat and protein in its production of ATP. Figure 2-5 illustrates the relative contribution of each metabolic pathway during physical performance of difference durations. One of the most important training principles for any sport or recreational activity is to identify the major energy system that is required for that particular activity or event and then devote time and effort by way of training for the development and/or improvement of that system. Figure 14-2 illustrates the various energy systems that are predominantly needed for some selected sports and recreational activities. Once the predominant energy systems have been identified, an important question that most people will need to know is just how much time should be spent in the training program toward developing that particular energy system(s). To help answer this question, Table 14-1 has been included. The table illustrates the relative contribution of the three major energy systems during various track running events. The information in Table 14-1 has been published in several other books and it may serve as an excellent guide for helping to determine exactly how much time should be spent in developing a particular energy source.

In looking at the data in Table 14-1, it can be clearly seen that an athlete training for the 100-yd dash should devote only about 2 percent of the time to development of the anaerobic (lactic acid) system, whereas 98 percent of the time should be spent on developing the speed (ATP-CP) system. Although the table was developed for various track running events, it can also be applied to other activities. In other words, because the relative contribution of the various energy sources is directly related to the length of time and intensity that a specific activity can be performed, an activity such as a gymnastic routine that requires 3 minutes can be analyzed with regard to the amount of time that should be placed on training the specific energy sources needed for that

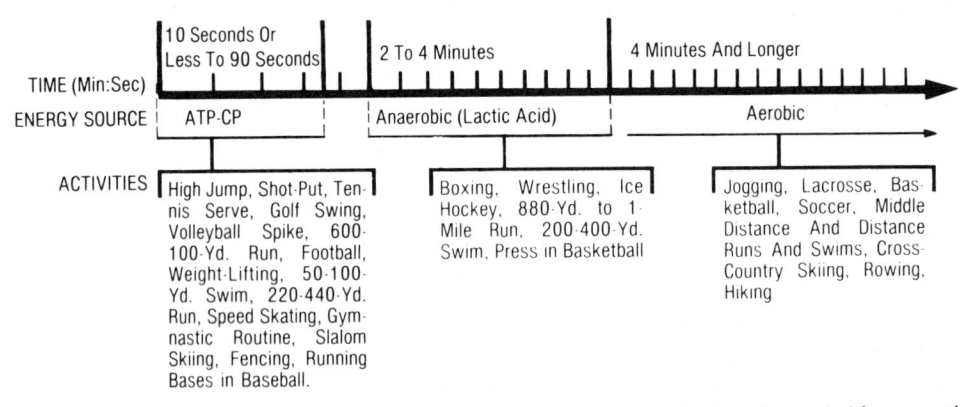

Figure 14-2 Illustration of the various energy systems that are predominantly needed for several sports and recreational activities.

TIME (Min:Sec)	10 Seconds Or Less To 90 Seconds	2 To 4 Minutes	4 Minutes And Longer
ENERGY SOURCE	ATP-CP	Anaerobic (Lactic Acid)	Aerobic
ACTIVITIES	High Jump, Shot-Put, Tennis Serve, Golf Swing, Volleyball Spike, 60-100-Yd. Run, Football, Weight-Lifting, 50-100-Yd. Swim, 220-440-Yd. Run, Speed Skating, Gymnastic Routine, Slalom Skiing, Fencing, Running Bases in Baseball.	Boxing, Wrestling, Ice Hockey, 880-Yd. to 1-Mile Run, 200-400-Yd. Swim, Press in Basketball.	Jogging, Lacrosse, Basketball, Soccer, Middle Distance And Distance Runs And Swims, Cross-Country Skiing, Rowing, Hiking.

Table 14-1. Percentage of Training Time Spent in Developing the Energy Sources for Various Track Running Events

Event	Performance Time (minutes:seconds)	Speed (ATP-CP) (%)	Aerobic Capacity (Oxygen) (%)	Anaerobic Capacity (Lactic Acid) (%)
Marathon	135:00 to 180:00	—	95	5
6 mile	30:00 to 50:00	5	80	15
3 mile	15:00 to 25:00	10	70	20
2 mile	10:00 to 16:00	20	40	40
1 mile	4:00 to 6:00	20	25	55
880 yards	2:00 to 3:00	30	5	65
440 yards	1:00 to 1:30	80	5	15
220 yards	0:22 to 0:35	98	—	2
100 yards	0:10 to 0:15	98	—	2

Source: Wilt, F. "Training for Competitive Running," in *Exercise Physiology*, (H. B. Falls, editor), Academic Press, New York, 1968, p. 411.

particular event. For instance, the table shows that 30 percent of the time should be geared toward developing speed while 65 percent should be spent on developing the anaerobic system and 5 percent on the aerobic system.

It is important to remember that all three energy systems are actually involved during physical activity, however, their relative contributions during work will vary, depending upon the time and intensity to perform.

Fox and Mathews have studied and compiled an extensive list of sports involving the amount of time that should be devoted toward developing the various energy systems for each sport. Their results are found in Table 14-2. By using the information in this table as a general guideline, training programs can be developed for specific sports and recreational activities. More will be said about this later in the chapter.

E. MOTIVATION

It is well known among coaches and physical educators that motivation is one of the most (if not "the" most) important principles of physical conditioning. Whether the training is to prepare an individual for intercollegiate athletic competition or whether it's to trim off a few pounds of ugly fat in order to fit into a new dress, proper motivation is absolutely essential if the goal that the coach or housewife has set for themselves is to be obtained. While motivation, in some cases, can be obtained through the coach, media, friends, husband, wife, or outside interest groups, in most instances, it must come from within the individual person. Because conditioning requires so much self-discipline and effort, the person must be totally dedicated and "want" to do it bad enough.

II. DEVELOPMENT OF MUSCULAR STRENGTH AND LOCAL ENDURANCE

Muscular strength is generally defined as the maximum amount of force that a particular muscle or muscle group can exert against a resistance. *Local endurance,* on the other hand, is the ability of a muscle or a group of muscles to perform work either by isometric, isotonic, eccentric, or isokinetic contractions over a given period of time. It has been pretty well established over the

Table 14-2. The Predominant Energy System(s) of Different Sports

| | % Emphasis According to Energy Systems |||
Sports or Sport Activity	Speed (ATP-CP)	Anaerobic (Lactic Acid)	Aerobic (Oxygen)
1. Baseball	80	20	—
2. Basketball	85	15	—
3. Fencing	90	10	—
4. Field Hockey	60	20	20
5. Football	90	10	—
6. Golf	95	5	—
7. Gymnastics	90	10	—
8. Ice Hockey			
a. forwards, defense	80	20	—
b. goalie	95	5	—
9. Lacrosse			
a. goalie, defense, attack men	80	20	—
b. midfielders, man-down	60	20	20
10. Rowing	20	30	50
11. Skiing			
a. slalom, jumping, downhill	80	20	—
b. cross-country	—	5	95
c. pleasure skiing	34	33	33
12. Soccer			
a. goalie, wings, strikers	80	20	—
b. halfbacks, or link men	60	20	20
13. Swimming and diving			
a. 50 yds, diving	98	2	—
b. 100 yds.	80	15	5
c. 200 yds.	30	65	5
d. 400, 500 yds.	20	40	40
e. 1500, 1650 yds.	10	20	70
14. Tennis	70	20	10
15. Track and field			
a. 100, 220 yds.	98	2	—
b. field events	90	10	—
c. 440 yds.	80	15	5
d. 880 yds.	30	65	5
e. 1 mile	20	55	25
f. 2 miles	20	40	40
g. 3 miles	10	20	70
h. 6 miles (cross-country)	5	15	80
i. Marathon	—	5	95
16. Volleyball	90	10	—
17. Wrestling	90	10	—

Source: Fox, E. L., and D. Mathews. *Interval Training: Conditioning for Sports and General Fitness,* W. B. Saunders Co., Philadelphia, 1974, p. 184.

Physical Conditioning   259

years that the development of muscular strength is the result of an increase in the size (and not the number) of the individual muscle fibers (hypertrophy), whereas the development of local endurance is more closely associated with an increase in the number of capillaries in the trained muscle. Although it is not completely clear, it is believed as Figure 14-3 illustrates that the increase in fiber size is due to one or more of the following:

(1) An increase in the total amount of myosin, actin, and other myofibrillar proteins.
(2) An increase in the number of the contractile element, the myofibril per muscle fiber.

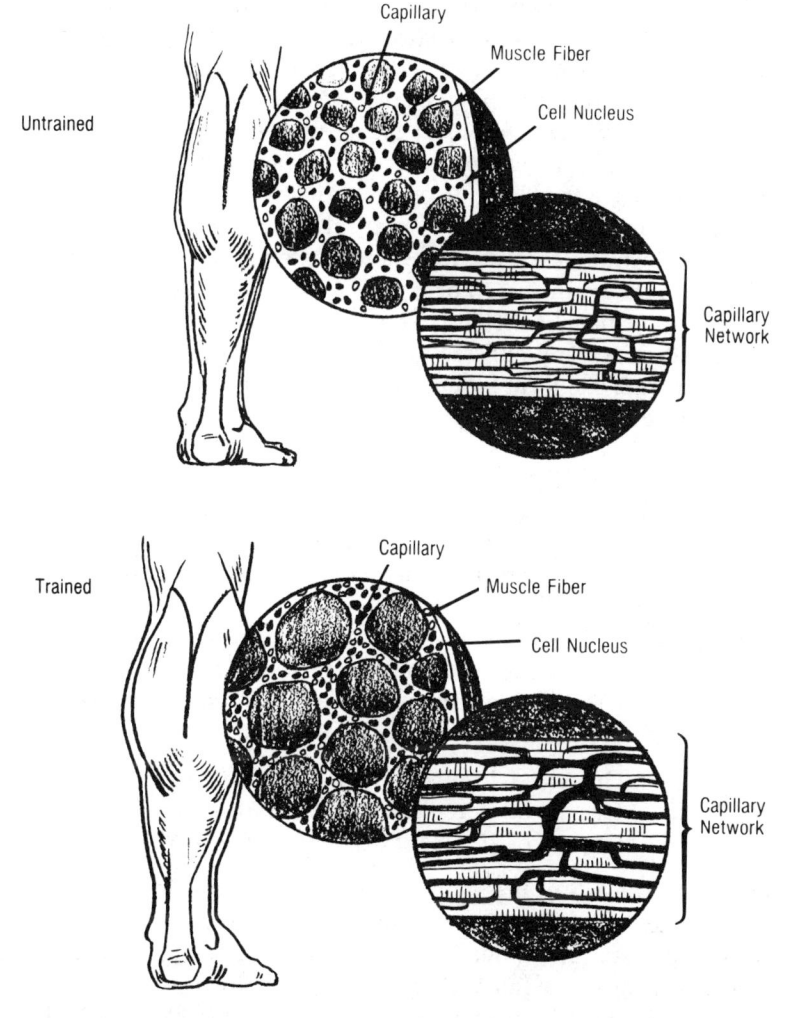

Figure 14-3 Schematic illustration showing the development of muscular strength as the result of increasing the individual muscle fibers (hypertrophy).

(3) An increase in thickness as well as in strength of the connective tissue, the tendons, and the ligaments.
(4) An increase in vascular tissue (capillaries and venules) per fiber.
(5) An increase in myoglobin concentration as well as other biochemical changes such as an increase in the number as well as the size of the mitochondria, an increase in ATP, CP, glycogen, and an increase in several enzymes (especially *creatine kinase* which facilitates the breakdown of CP and *phosphofructokinase* which facilitates glycolytic activity).

The first three above are more closely related to the development of strength whereas the bottom two are more likely to be associated with local endurance development.

Anyone who has been around a weight-training room or an athletic fitness club knows that there are as many different weight-training methods for developing strength and endurance as there are people working out. The problem facing most people is whether to use isotonic, isometric, or the popular isokinetic-type exercises in their strength and endurance training program. In fact, research is available to suggest that a weight training program utilizing eccentric-type contractions (negative work) may also be effective in developing muscular strength. Figure 14-4 illustrates each of these exercises. Since all of these methods have certain advantages and disadvantages, the coach or trainee must choose the one that best fits his or her specific needs. At the same time, it should be stated again that regardless of the training method chosen, if the overload principle is adhered to, strength and local endurance can be developed. Each of the specific strength and local endurance training methods (isotonic, isometric, eccentric, and isokinetics) will be discussed separately.

A. ISOTONIC

Isotonic (dynamic and concentric are terms used synonymously with isotonic) work is when a muscle contracts and shortens under a constant load throughout the entire joint range. That is, the force being exerted by the muscle is greater than the external force which opposes the muscle, and therefore, movement occurs.

Although there is lack of agreement among experts concerning the best isotonic training program for building strength and local endurance, the work of DeLorme and Watkins appears to be one of the most effective techniques used today. They recommend the following progressive resistance program to be carried out on 4 consecutive days per week:

> One set of 10 repetitions with $\frac{1}{2}$ 10 RM's
> One set of 10 repetitions with Δ 10 RM's
> One set of 10 repetitions with full 10 RM's

The initial program consists of determining by trial and error the most weight that can be lifted 10 consecutive times but no more than 10. This is then called the 10 repetitions maximum (10 RM's). The exercises are then carried out in 3 sets of 10 reptitions each. For example, the first set incorporates ½ or 50 percent of the full 10 RM; the second set incorporates ¾ or 75 percent of the full 10 RM; and finally the third set includes the full or 100 percent of the 10 RM. The third set is considered the most important part of the program since this represents the greatest maximum resistance for the muscle. Note that the first and second sets are considered as warm-up repetitions. When more than 10 repetitions are possible during the third set, a new full 10 RPM load is established.

Just the opposite of DeLorme's method is the Oxford technique. This procedure utilizes a total of 100 repetitions divided up equally into 10 sets. The first set incorporates the full (or 100

Isometric Exercise

Isotonic Exercise

Isokinetic Exercise

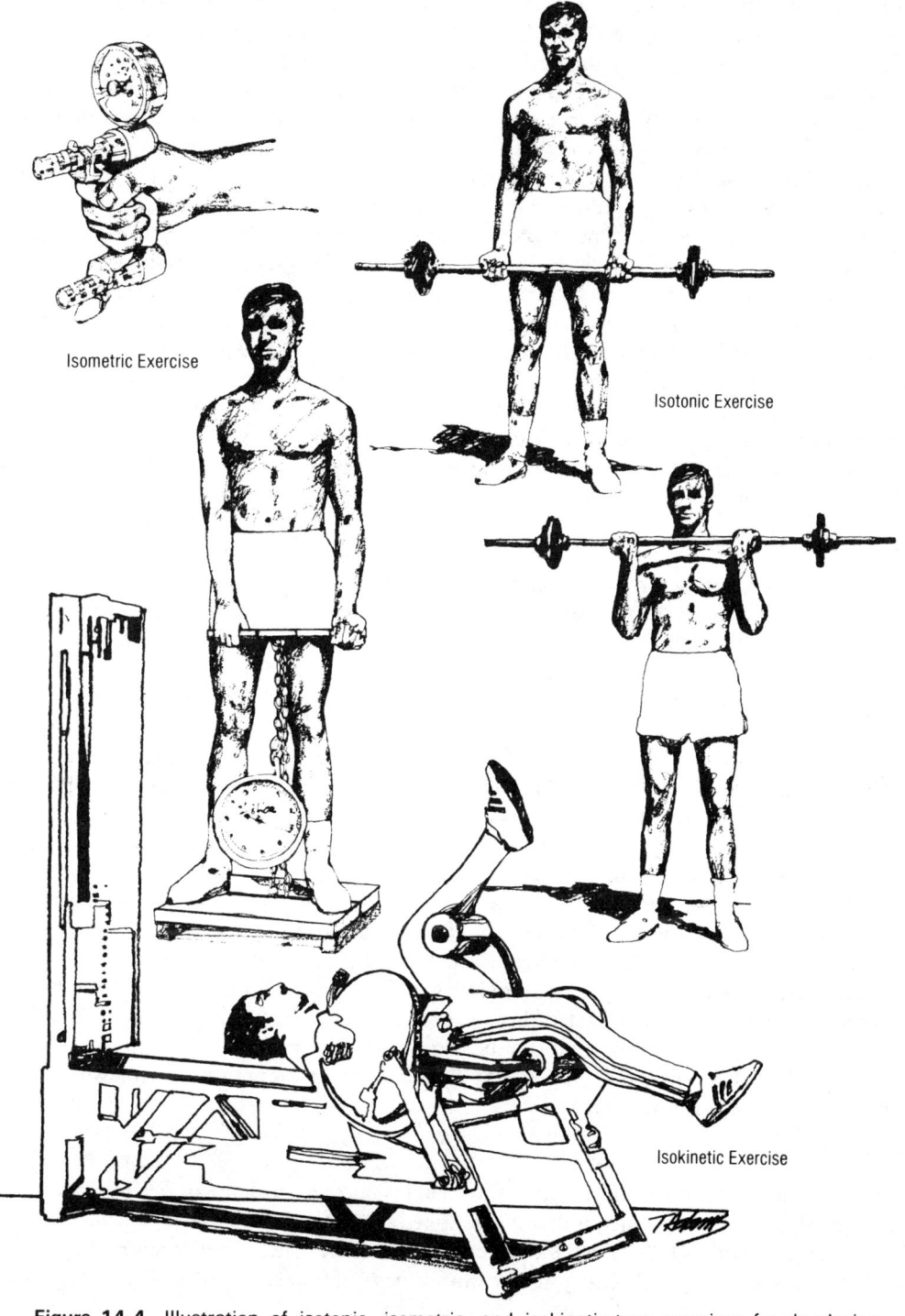

Figure 14-4 Illustration of isotonic, isometric, and isokinetic-type exercises for developing muscular strength and endurance.

percent) 10 RM with each succeeding 10 RM set performed at reduced resistance to theoretically match the decrease in strength which is brought about by fatigue. This technique is also very popular and it supposedly allows the person to perform all sets at 10 RM.

Although the DeLorme and Oxford methods are considered to be effective isotonic programs for developing muscle hypertrophy, recent work has shown that a weight training program utilizing fewer repetitions maximum is just as effective. For example, it has been found that isotonic strength gains are maximized by incorporating between 5 and 7 RM's into 3 sets each training session. While training frequency should be a minimum of 3 times per week (every other day), if the muscles are already somewhat conditioned and can tolerate the work, the number of times may be increased to 5 per week. For sedentary people who are just starting out, 3 times per week is recommended for optimal results. In summary, it appears from the available research that the greatest improvements in isotonic strength is probably obtained from 3 sets each training day with each set performed somewhere between 5 and 7 RM's, 3 to 5 times per week. One final note, while it is clear that strength and local endurance can be increased simultaneously as a result of overload training, if endurance development is the objective and not strength, then the load should be lightened and the number of repetitions increased. Research shows that the most effective way to increase local endurance is to incorporate between 20 and 30 RM's into 3 sets each training session. Training frequency should be between 3 and 5 times per week.

B. ISOMETRIC

In recent years, a popular fad among movie stars, business executives and even athletes has been isometric exercises. Isometric (static is a term used synonymous with isometric) contraction is when a muscle contracts but does not shorten. Muscle contraction during maintenance of posture and equilibrium as well as in holding an object is one of isometrics. Since isometric contraction opposes the force of gravity, its function is fixation. In addition, since no movement is involved during isometric contraction, no work (according to the physicist's equation of $W = F \times D$) is performed. Instead, all of the energy goes into the development of heat.

The development of strength and local endurance by isometric techniques was popularized by Hettinger and Muller of Germany in 1953. Their program involved static contractions of 2/3 maximum held for 6 seconds once a day for 5 days/week. They hypothesized that their method would yield strength gains of approximately 5 percent per week above the starting level. Other investigators failed to find such increases. On the basis of more recent research, the best results appear to be obtained by training 5 days per week, with each training session involving maximal contractions of 6 seconds in length and repeated 5 to 10 times daily.

It should be pointed out that because strength gains have been found to be specific to the joint angle trained, it is highly recommended that if isometric contractions are utilized, that at least 3 angles within the full range of joint motion be trained with the previously mentioned isometric training program. Otherwise, the trainee may find his or her strength gain somewhat limited within the joint range of movement.

C. ECCENTRIC

Eccentric contraction is a third type of muscular contraction that can occur. This type of contraction results when the tension that is developed is less than the opposing outside force, so the muscle is stretched or lengthened during contraction. The function of eccentric contraction muscles is deceleration, as in checking the forward velocity of the arm in various throwing actions of the arm such as in throwing a baseball, shotput, football, etc., or of the leg as the extremity reaches its limit in the forward phase of walking or running. Another example of eccentric contraction is the use of the biceps brachii during the down phase of a chin-up.

Although weight-training programs utilizing only eccentric-type contractions are not common and have not been incorporated by coaches in their training programs, a few studies have been published indicating that eccentric contractions may be beneficial in developing strength and local endurance (especially in terms of physical therapy and rehabilitation). When compared to other programs, however, they apparently are not as effective, and in fact, they appear to bring about greater degrees of residual soreness. For example, some researchers have found, when comparing static, concentric, and eccentric type contractions, eccentric contractions where found to subjectively bring about much greater levels of pain several hours after exercise. In fact, the greatest pain was reported to be 48 hours following exercise. Causative factors are, as of yet, unknown and more research is needed in this area.

D. ISOKINETICS

Isokinetic contraction (also called accommodating resistance exercise) combines both isometric and isotonic features in that it not only involves a maximum effort (similar to isometric) at all joint angles, but it is also carried out through a complete range of motion (similar to isotonic). This type of muscular contraction is generally carried out with specific types of equipment called the Cybex, the Mini-Gym, and the Nautilus. Because the specially designed apparatus fluctuates according to the amount of muscle exertion that is applied to it, maximal resistive effort is permitted throughout the entire range of joint motion. Note that the Mini-Gym and the Cybex fluctuate by controlling the speed of contraction, whereas the Nautilus fluctuates by changing the moment arm through specially shaped cams. Through this controlled acceleration, the resistance becomes proportional to the muscular effort applied to it. For example, when the subject's arm or leg is in position to exert strong effort against the handle or pedal of the device, it does so. At the same time, when the limb is in a position of relatively weak leverage, the subject receives proportionately less resistance. Thus, the user actually makes his or her own resistance with the amount of effort that is exerted at each angle and with each repetition. The device can accommodate anything from fingertip pressure to hundreds of pounds. By permitting the individual to work at high levels in those positions where the body is structured to do so, and to slack off in those positions where the skeletal musculature is weak, isokinetic exercise appears to provide a safe and effective training stimulus for both sexes of all ages.

Isokinetic traning techniques are the newest, and as Figure 14-5 illustrates, they have been found to be comparable (at both slow- and fast-speed training) to or even better than the traditional methods previously mentioned for developing strength and local endurance. Theoretically, this should be expected since this type of exercise permits development of a maximum effort at whatever speed of contraction the tester wants throughut the complete range of joint movement. By being able to exert a continuous maximum effort, this allows for a greater number of motor units to be brought into play during the actual contractile process. Thus, with this technique, a greater overload can be placed on the exercised muscles than was previously possible.

Although the purchasing of the specially designed isokinetic equipment is probably a handicap for some schools, numerous coaches and athletic trainers at this writing, have already developed their entire weight-training and rehabilitation programs around isokinetic

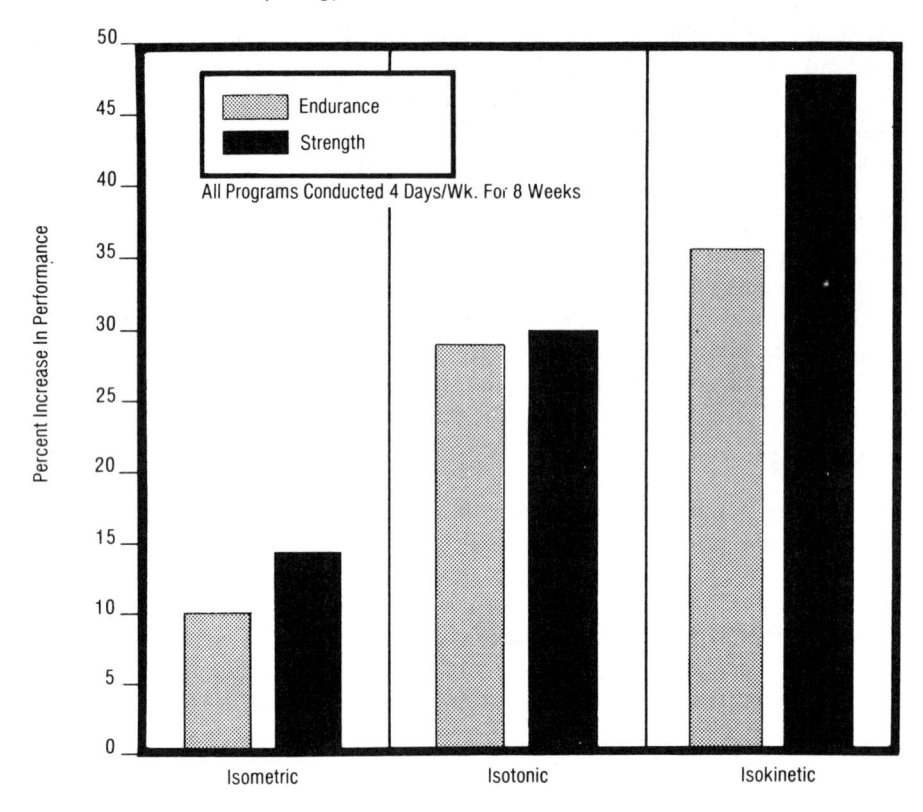

Figure 14-5 Schematic comparison of isotonic, isometric, and isokinetic-type exercises in developing muscular strength and local endurance.

contractions. In fact, all of the isokinetic companies have designed and developed several isokinetic pieces of apparatus for specific purpose of developing strength and local endurance in areas such as football, swimming, running, kicking, volleyball, throwing, and shot putting.

Although isotonic and isokinetic exercises produces strength and local endurance that is more applicable to motor performance, causes more muscle hypertrophy, produces better neuromuscular coordination, causes strength to be developed more uniformly throughout the range of motion, isometric exercise is an important supplement to other exercises because of its simplicity and rapid results. For instance, it requires less time, less energy, less space, and little or no equipment. In addition, isometrics can be used in places such as the home or office whereas isotonic and isokinetic programs are not feasible. Also, because isometric exercise involves no joint movements, it can be incorporated during a time of recovery from a bone or joint injury in order to prevent a significant loss of muscular function and coordination.

In addition, as was pointed out in Chapter 13, isometric-type exercises are not recommended for older people or people with cardiovascular disease because of their potential danger. For example, isometric exercise causes a much greater increase in blood pressure than the other types of contractions, and it is believed that this increase in pressure is due, in part, to an increase in intrathoracic pressure. This is commonly caused from making an expiratory effort with a typically closed glottis; thereby, creating a higher than normal pressure within the thoracic cavity.

By doing this, it restricts the return of blood from the lower limbs and thus results in a high blood pressure and a decreased blood flow to the heart and brain.

III. FACTORS AFFECTING STRENGTH AND LOCAL ENDURANCE

A. NERVOUS SYSTEM

There is a substantial amount of evidence that indicates that strength training may be influenced by the nervous system. Although not totally clear, it appears that the nervous system may influence strength gains by two ways. First, by calling more motor units into play per contraction, and second, by increasing the actual rate of impulses to each individual motor unit. The rapid increase in strength that is commonly experienced during the first few weeks of training may be due, in part, to the nervous system learning and adapting to the strength training. This neural influence on human strength may help to explain the great feats of strength that is often observed in weightlifters, shot putters, karate experts, and even the small, skinny person who lifts the corner of a car off of a person during a time of emergency.

B. AGE AND SEX

It is well known that regardless of the type of training program selected, the amount and rate of muscular strength and local endurance improvement is limited to a certain degree by an individual's age and sex. Figure 11-1 illustrates clearly the variation in muscular strength in relations to age and sex under normal living conditions. In essence, it shows that boys reach their peak strength in their middle-to-late twenties, after which it gradually declines the rest of their life. It appears that men generally lose around 1 percent of their strength per year following their late twenties. Of course the rate of decline is influenced by one's level of activity.

Figure 11-1 also indicates that girls' strength increases at about the same rate as boys' until they reach between the ages of 8 and 12 years. Afterwards, the rate of increase steadily declines. The female reaches her peak in the early-to-middle twenties, after which it declines at about the same rate as in men. Evidence indicates that men are normally about 30 to 40 percent stronger than females in terms of absolute strength.

While local endurance generally follows the same age and sex trend as strength, it should be mentioned that most authorities generally agree that if the strength factor is ruled out, there is no significant differences in local endurance between men and women.

It should be pointed out that since the strength curve in Figure 11-1 represents normal living conditions, an effective strength training program can change the shape of the curve at any point in time. For a more complete sex comparison of strength, the reader is referred to Chapter 11.

C. BODY BUILD

Briefly, body build is related to an individual's body form and structure. An individual's body build is usually assessed by determining his or her somatotype. While there are several somatotyping procedures, they typically rate the body on three separate components; namely, mesomorphy (reflects muscularity), ectomorphy (reflects linearity), and endomorphy (reflects adiposity). An individual's somatotype is apparentlyl a genetic trait which is established early in life. While physical training only has a somewhat slight influence on an individual's body build, research does show that those individuals who are classified as mesomorphy respond more effectively to strength developing exercises than those with a high degree of either ectomorphy or endomorphy.

D. MUSCLE LENGTH

It has been well illustrated that a muscle can generate a considerable amount of more tension when it is put under stretch. This simply means that a muscle has its strongest contractile force when it is fully extended or stretched slightly beyond its normal resting length. At the same time, as the muscle shortens during contraction, its contractile force decreases steadily until finally the muscle is unable to generate any additional force beyond the fully contracted position. It should be noted that by placing the muscle on sudden stretch, initial contractile force can be increased. As Jensen and Fisher pointed out, this sudden stretch activates the stretch reflex system, thus resulting in an additional number of impulses to be added to those received from the central nervous system. In physical education, there are several skills in which the stretch reflex system is used quite effectively. For example, in the vertical jump just before the actual movement, the participant squats placing the jumping muscles on sudden stretch and alerting the stretch reflex system. This apparently causes the jumping muscles to receive impulses from their own spindles along with the impulses initiated in the central nervous system. This results in a stronger contraction than if there had been no impulses from the stretch reflex. If the squat is eliminated, the height of the jump is generally lower. Other examples of where the stretch reflex system is used in making stronger contractions is the sprinter getting set in the starting blocks to run his race or the baseball pitcher at the top of his windup getting ready to release the ball. Or also, the basketball player in a squat position under the goal preparing himself to jump up and get the rebound. In all of the above examples, if the stretch reflex system was not brought into play by placing the muscles under sudden stretch, then the contractile force of the muscle would not be near as strong to allow the sprinter to have a more explosive start, the pitcher to throw the ball faster, or the basketball player to jump as high.

E. STRENGTH (AFFECTING LOCAL ENDURANCE)

There is no doubt that strength plays an important role in local endurance. Stronger subjects are generally able to exercise longer than weaker ones when the work is performed against a given resistance without regard to strength. On the other hand, the majority of research reports that if strength is not a variable, then the weaker subjects show as much endurance as the stronger ones. It is also well documented that strength contributes to the development of local endurance. For instance, suppose an individual has sufficient strength to perform 50 concentric-eccentric elbow flexion curls with a given amount of weight. If this individual's strength were improved 80 percent, he would apparently be strong enough to perform the exercise a great deal more than 50 times.

F. CIRCULATION (AFFECTING LOCAL ENDURANCE)

Research has reported significant improvement in localized circulation as the result of local endurance training. Hence, improved blood flow increases the ability of the transport system to deliver nutrients to the muscle and waste products such as carbon dioxide, lactic acid and water from the working muscles. Therefore, it seems highly probable that increased circulation within the local area is one of the most important functions in the development of local endurance.

IV. RETENTION OF MUSCULAR STRENGTH AND LOCAL ENDURANCE

It is generally felt among researchers working in this area that the most difficult part of a strength and local endurance weight-training program is their development and not so much their retention. In fact, once improvements have been made, it appears that they are relatively easy to keep. While evidence involving complete immobilization following training is scarce, evidence is available involving subjects who have refrained from exercise and training for a given period of time following a period of training. The available evidence shows that strength when gained from a 3-week isotonic training program, was still retained following a 6-week period of detraining. The weight-training program consisted of 3 sets at a 6 maximum resistance load, 3 times weekly. In the same investigation, it was also reported that strength was further improved during a subsequent 6-week training regime in which the subjects performed only one set of exercises one time per week. The work load consisted of one maximum resistance. Similar results have been found and reported in the literature involving muscular strength when trained and tested by way of isometric techniques.

In studies investigating the retention of local endurance, it has been noted that local endurance gained during a period of 8 weeks of isotonic training consisting of elbow flexion curls was lost much faster during the initial few weeks of a detraining period. The training consisted of working with an arm-lever ergometer at a rate of 40 times each minute with a resistance of 11 pounds. The work was performed to exhaustion. After 12 weeks of detraining, the subjects were retested and it was found that they had retained approximately 70 percent of the endurance that they had originally gained.

In summary, the available evidence in this area appears to indicate that strength and local endurance gains can be retained if maximum exertions are used at least once every week or even once every other week. It has been suggested by authorities in this area that the retention of strength and local endurance of this type is probably due to changes of the nervous system brought about by the training program.

V. DEVELOPMENT OF AEROBIC AND ANAEROBIC ENDURANCE

Aerobic (with oxygen) endurance is generally characterized by moderate contractions of large muscle groups for an extended period of time, during which maximum cardiorespiratory adjustments are necessary, as in swimming, bicycling, and distance running. Since aerobic endurance refers to the ability of the heart, vascular system, and lungs to provide oxygen and nutrients to the working tissues and to remove the waste products of metabolism, it is quite clear that the primary goal of aerobic endurance training is to improve and/or increase the capacity and efficiency of these three systems in order that a greater amount of oxygen can be supplied to the cells. This type of training is often referred to as cardiorespiratory or cardiovascular training.

Anaerobic (without oxygen) endurance is generally characterized by strong contractions from activities that require energy at such rates from the breakdown of the ATP-CP and glycolysis systems that aerobic metabolism cannot possibly provide. Such athletic activities include stop-and-go sprints in basketball, tennis, ice-hockey, soccer, lacrosse, field hockey, and football, sprint events in track and swimming as well as in cycling, weight-lifting, boxing, and wrestling, and other everyday activities such as a lumber-jack cutting wood or shoveling snow rapidly to clear your driveway. Because the ATP-CP and glycolysis energy systems are tremendously important to anaerobic endurance, the development of them to their fullest is the major goal of anaerobic endurance.

A. PHYSIOLOGICAL ADAPTATIONS WHICH ACCOMPANY AEROBIC AND ANAEROBIC ENDURANCE TRAINING

The physiological adaptations which accompany anaerobic endurance training will be mentioned first since they include primarily the cellular effects, whereas the aerobic changes are noticed at both the tissue as well as the oxygen transport system. The anaerobic changes involve the ATP-CP and the lactic acid systems.

Anaerobic Endurance Changes

Evidence is clear that following anaerobic endurance training, one of the significant changes that is generally experienced is an increase in the capacity of the ATP-CP system. This is tremendously important for those activities requiring short bouts of vigorous movement in which aerobic metabolism cannot possibly provide. The increased capacity for ATP-CP is due to the increased storage of both ATP and CP that is found in the muscles following training. Also, there is an increase in the level of enzyme activity in the ATP-CP system. This enzyme is called *creatine kinase* and it is responsible for the oxidation of CP which, when it is broken down, releases energy for the resynthesis of ATP. Both of these combined obviously allow for an increased capacity of the ATP-CP energy system.

In addition to the ATP-CP system, anaerobic endurance training also increases the glycolytic capacity (lactic acid system). This is illustrated quite clearly by trained subjects who are able to demonstrate much higher levels of lactic acid following a maximal work out. This enlarged capacity is apparently due to an increase in the activity level of several glycolytic enzymes following training. For example, *phosphofructokinase,* an important enzyme in anaerobic glycolysis has been shown to increase by more than 50 percent in some studies. This, and other important enzymes, by increasing their level of activity, bring about a faster and greater amount of glycogen broken down to lactic acid. This results in more ATP energy being produced from the lactic acid energy system. This increased capacity for lactic acid and ATP-CP should obviously enhance the performance of those anaerobic activities that rely so much on these systems.

Aerobic Endurance Changes

It is generally agreed among researchers that the following physiological changes accompany aerobic endurance training.

Heart Rate and Heart Size. With endurance training, while the thickness of the ventricular wall remains normal, the size (volume) of the ventricular cavity of the heart becomes large which means that it is able to hold more blood during the resting or diastolic period. The opposite is true for anaerobic training. The thickness of the ventricular wall increases while the size remains normal. As training progresses, this results not only in a slower heart rate for a standard submaximal work load, but also in a slower resting heart rate (bradycardia) and a slight decrease in maximal heart rate. The increased size of the heart causes stroke volume and cardiac output to be increased. This greater efficiency of the heart (circulating more blood while beating less frequently) allows a larger blood flow to reach the muscles with less stress imposed on the heart, lungs, and vascular systems. For stroke volume, there is not only an increase in the resting value, but also submaximal and maximal exercise values are increased. In the case of cardiac output, maximal cardiac output is increased, however, for rest and a standard submaximal work load, cardiac output is not significantly changed. Since cardiac output for the trained and untrained person are about the same during rest and submaximal work, it is obvious that the trained person is able to accomplish his or her cardiac output at a much lower heart rate.

Finally, aerobic training also improves the heart rate recovery process once exercise has been terminated: the better trained the individual, the faster his heart rate returns to the pre-exercise level.

Blood Pressure. Although there is very little change for a normal, healthy person in resting blood pressure as a result of aerobic training, the blood pressure recovery process following exercise is improved. For example, the better trained the individual, the quicker his blood pressure returns to the pre-exercise level. In addition, during heavy work the untrained subject experiences a progressive fall in systolic pressure (which indicates the person is approaching exhaustion), whereas training retards the appearance of this phenomenon so that heavy work can be continued for a relatively longer period of time without any significant changes in blood pressure. Also, people who have hypertension (high blood pressure) have been shown to be able to lower their resting blood pressure with endurance training.

Blood Distribution. During training there is a modification of blood distribution which lowers the amount of oxygen required by the active muscles during a standard submaximal exercise, and consequently the necessary blood flow (per kilogram of working muscle) to these muscles is lowered. The trained subject is able to compensate for this reduced blood flow to the working muscles by extracting more oxygen. In other words, endurance training brings about a greater arterial-venous oxygen difference (a-$\bar{v}_{O_2}$ diff). When trained, for the same cardiac output, more blood stays available for the other organs of the body. For instance, training improves the ability to exercise in hot weather because so long as less blood is required by the active muscles to perform a given amount of work more blood is available for heat dissipation in the skin and thus body temperature remains lower.

Blood. Total blood volume and hemoglobin is also influenced by endurance training. The additional blood volume plays an important role in heat dissipation (especially during work in hot temperature) since the blood transports heat from the deep core of the body to the outer peripheral areas. At the same time, the additional hemoglobin increases the capacity of the circulatory system to carry substances to and from the active muscles. In addition to the blood volume and hemoglobin changing as a result of training, blood composition also changes. For example, more red blood cells and less water content are found following training. This tends to increase the blood viscosity and its oxygen carrying capacity, thus resulting in greater work performance.

Capillaries. There is an increase in the number of capillaries and an increase in the use of latent capillaries (in the lungs and in the trained muscles) as a result of extensive endurance training. This increase in total capillaries causes the exchange between the blood and the tissue cells and between the lungs and the blood to become more efficient (since resistance is lowered), thus permitting greater exchange of gases and other by-products between the tissue cells and the blood and between the lungs and the blood.

Lungs. Extensive training brings about certain changes in the respiratory system also. These changes are progressive and they take place in 4 to 6 weeks resulting in more efficient respiration. Because of the normal physiological changes due to training, such as large oxygen consumption and decreased carbon dioxide production, pulmonary ventilation for a standard submaximal exercise bout is reduced (however, pulmonary ventilation for maximal work is increased), the work of breathing decreases, the amount of oxygen needed by the respiratory muscles is decreased, and blood flow to the respiratory muscles is smaller (due to increased efficiency). These changes in pulmonary ventilation are associated with a decrease in rate and an increase in depth of breathing. In the trained athlete even at rest the depth of breathing is greater and the respiratory rate may decrease from around 20 to about 8 breaths per minute. Also the trained endurance athlete with the larger lung capacity tends to have a greater alveolar-capillary surface area which provides for a greater diffusion capacity during both rest and exercise conditions.

Maximal Oxygen Uptake. There is no doubt that maximal oxygen uptake (defined as the greatest oxygen uptake attained by an individual while breathing air at sea level during the performance of physical work) can be increased with endurance training. In fact, it is generally agreed that, depending upon age and fitness, it can be increased by about 5 to 20 percent. Maximal oxygen uptake has been accepted as the best single measure of an individual's cardiorespiratory capacity. This measurement depends upon the functional dimension of the oxygen transporting system which includes the lungs, the heart, the size of the capillary bed of the skeletal muscles, and the capacity of the blood to carry oxygen. Since maximal oxygen uptake is related to body size, it is usually expressed in terms of milliliters (ml) of oxygen per kilogram (kg) of body weight per unit of time. A maximal oxygen uptake above 50 ml/kg/min is considered to indicate a good level of circulatory-respiratory fitness for young men, and above 40 ml/kg/min for young women. However, it is not unusual to find values around 75 to 94 ml/kg/min and 55 to 74 ml/kg/min for highly trained male and female endurance athletes, respectively. This is illustrated in Figure 11-4 where untrained sedentary males and females are compared to olympic-caliber athletes.

Lactic Acid. Endurance training brings about a decrease in the level of lactic acid for a standard submaximal exercise. This adaptation is extremely important for those athletes (such as distance runners, swimmers, and cyclists) who compete mainly in distance events which require a high level of aerobic endurance. If these athletes have the capacity to pace themselves throughout the race at a high level without necessarily building up a high lactic acid level at the beginning of the race, then they will be able to have a greater capacity at the end for a strong finish without having been fatigued earlier in the race. The causative factor for the lower lactic acid levels at submaximal work is not entirely known, however, it may be due, in part, to a more efficient oxidation of glycogen and fatty acids. During maximal work, training also brings about an increase capacity for lactic acid. This means that more ATP can be produced through anaerobic metabolism and therefore improve performance in activities that call upon the ATP-CP and lactic acid systems for energy.

Increased Neuromuscular Efficiency. Training also results in improved neuromuscular efficiency (which means less energy or oxygen is needed to accomplish a standard amount of work). According to Jensen and Fisher, this is brought about by several factors. They are: (1) more efficient transmission of nerve impulses, (2) less resistance from antagonistic muscles, (3) less wasted (non-contributing) motion, (4) less fatty tissue in the muscles, and (5) more efficiency in the contractile processes of the muscle fibers.

Slow (ST) and Fast (FT) Twitch Muscle Fibers. Training for ST and FT muscle hypertrophy appears to be very specific to the activity and sport. Recall from Chapter 1 that with endurance training, both fiber types become better suited for producing ATP for aerobic work, while at the same time, fiber type can still be clearly identified and separated on the basis of twitch contraction times since FT fibers remain FT fibers and are not changed into ST fibers. While training may cause an increase in size and capacities, in short, it does not bring about changes in the proportion of ST and FT fibers in a muscle. Studies show that increases in glycolytic capacity of a muscle is greater in the FT fibers than in the ST fibers. A substantial amount of evidence is available to show that world class sprinters are characterized by high percentages (up to around 74%) of FT fibers in their leg muscles, while world class distance runners possess a much higher level of ST fibers (up to around 75%) in their leg muscles than normal proportions for untrained subjects. Swimmers and canoeists have been shown to have between 60 and 70 percent of ST fibers in their shoulder muscles. For a more detail discussion on muscle fiber type, the reader is referred to Chapter 1.

Myoglobin. The development of aerobic endurance is also the result of an increase in the concentration of myoglobin in the sarcoplasm. Since myoglobin has the ability to combine with oxygen as well as being able to store oxygen in the muscle, its major role in cardiorespiratory endurance is performed by releasing this stored oxygen to the mitochondria when the intracellular oxygen tension drops to a certain level. Myoglobin may also serve as a means for the rapid delivery of oxygen within the cell during high levels of muscular activity.

Oxidation of Carbohydrates and Fats. With endurance training, the capacity of the skeletal muscles to oxidize both carbohydrates (glycogen) and fats is increased. This obviously gives an advantage to the trained person during endurance activities. Two causative factors are generally recognized for the increased muscles capacity to oxidize carbohydrates. First of all, there is a substantial amount of evidence that shows that the mitochondria in the skeletal muscle fiber increases not only in size, but also in number following endurance training. Secondly, studies have illustrated that following training, there is an increase in the level of enzyme activity in the Krebs cycle and in the electron transport system. This means that, in the presence of oxygen, a high amount of ATP can be manufactured. In addition, it appears that capacity for glycogen storage in the muscles following training is also increased. This increased storage capacity for glycogen has been related to an increase in the level of enzyme activity; specifically, glycogen synthetase. The function of this enzyme is to synthesize glycogen in the skeletal muscles.

Like carbohydrates, the increased capacity of the skeletal muscles for oxidizing fats is related to two very important factors. First, there appears to be an increase in the amount of fatty acids that are released from adipose tissue following training. This means that there will be more fats available for fuel, and secondly, there is also an apparent increase in the level of enzyme activity (prior to as well as in the Krebs cycle and electron transport system) for not only the oxidation process, but also for the activation and transportation of the fats.

Other Changes. Aerobic endurance training will bring about a decrease in percent body fat and an increase in lean body weight (note that both of these items are discussed in detail in Chapter 9). It has also been shown with a considerable amount of evidence that regular endurance training (aerobic-type) will lower cholesterol and triglyceride levels in the blood, of which both have been associated with cardiovascular disease. A summary of these aerobic changes is shown in Table 14-3.

B. AEROBIC AND ANAEROBIC TRAINING METHODS

Recall earlier in this chapter that the general principles of training such as specificity and overload apply to all physical conditioning programs. In other words, for any training program to be effective, it must develop not only the specific energy system(s) involved, but it must also develop the specific muscle or muscle group as well as the specific movement patterns involved in the activity. In addition, it was learned earlier that in order for any training program to be successful, it should follow the progressive overload principle. In the development of aerobic and anaerobic endurance, this means that as the person becomes endurance trained, any additional gains in endurance will only be experienced if he or she accomplishes more work during each of the training sessions than can be normally accomplished.

Once it has been established which specific energy system(s) is involved in training as well as the specific movement patterns and muscle or muscle groups involved, selecting the proper

Table 14-3. Summary of the Major Physiological Changes Brought about by Aerobic Endurance Training

Variable	Rest	Submaximal Exercise*	Maximal Exercise
Heart rate	Reduced	Reduced	Reduced
Cardiac hypertrophy	Increased	—	—
Stroke volume	Increased	Increased	Increased
Cardiac output	Unchanged	Unchanged	Increased
Blood pressure (normal person)	Unchanged	Unchanged	Unchanged
Blood volume, total hemoglobin & red blood cells	Increased	—	—
Blood flow (per kilogram of working muscle)	—	Reduced	Unchanged
Capillarization	Increased	—	—
Oxygen consumption	Unchanged	Reduced	Increased
Lactic acid levels in muscle & blood	Unchanged	Reduced	Increased
Pulmonary ventilation	Increased	Reduced	Increased
Respiratory efficiency	Increased	Increased	Increased
a-$\bar{v}O_2$ diff	—	Increased	Increased
Pulmonary diffusion capacity	Increased	Increased	Increased
Neuromuscular efficiency	—	Increased	Increased
Myoglobin concentration	Increased	—	—
Blood distribution for work in heat	—	Increased	Increased
Percent body fat	Reduced	—	—
Lean body mass	Increased	—	—
Serum lipids (cholesterol and triglycerides)	Reduced	—	—
Oxygen extraction by muscles	Unchanged	Increased	Increased
Mitochondria (size and number)	Increased	—	—
Blood pressure (hypertensives)	Reduced	Reduced	Reduced
Oxidation of carbohydrates	Increased	—	—
Oxidation of fats	Increased	—	—
Muscular storage of ATP-CP	Increased	—	—

*Indicates that the same amount of work was performed before and after training.

training method that will bring about the desired changes is the next logical step. Table 14-4 illustrates some of the more popular training regimes. Within this table are the approximate development percentages of the three energy systems for each of the various training programs.

While it can be seen in Table 14-4 that aerobic endurance can be developed by several methods such as jogging, continuous slow and fast running, or swimming, it is generally agreed among coaches and exercise physiologists that interval training is probably the most popular aerobic and aerobic type training program used today. Certainly, it is probably the most highly studied of all training programs. A substantial amount of sound evidence has been collected on interval training. In fact, entire books have been written on it. This training technique includes a number of work bouts with short rest intervals between bouts.

As any coach or physical educator knows, one of the primary objectives of a training program is to obtain the greatest possible workload with the smallest physiological strain. The fact that this can best be achieved through the methods of interval training is well supported on heart rate and blood lactate data. One of the advantages that interval training has is that it is very flexible and can be adapted for developing not only aerobic endurance, but also anaerobic endurance as well as the ATP-CP system (or all three systems equally as well).

The interval training method is based upon the overload principle. In order for the overload principle to be successful for interval training over a period of time, the intensity of the workouts must also be progressively increased as endurance is gained. In interval training, it has been well documented that the intensity of the workouts can be adjusted by the manipulation of 5 different variables of which they are:

(1) Rate and distance,
(2) Number of repetitions during each workout,
(3) Time of rest interval between the work intervals,
(4) Type of activity during rest interval, and
(5) Number of training periods per week.

It has been suggested that in order for optimal changes in the effectiveness of the oxygen transport system to be accomplished through interval training, the work bouts should be between 3 and 5 minutes in length, with light activity or short rest intervals between the bouts. The level of conditioning of the individual and the purpose of the training should determine the number of training periods per week, the number of repetitions during each workout, the intensity of each repetition, and the amount of rest between each bout.

In training for endurance, heart rate should be used as the criterion for determining the optimal training intensity. For example, heart rate during interval training should be kept at a rate between 60 and 90 percent of maximum during each of the 3 to 5 minute work periods. For healthy, sedentary people, the lower figure (60%) is sufficient for increases in endurance to be noticed, while a trained athlete should use the upper level (90%). Note that because maximal heart

Table 14-4. Several Training Methods and the Approximate Development Percentages of the Various Energy Systems

Training Method	Speed (ATP-CP)	Aerobic System (Oxygen)	Anaerobic System (Lactic Acid)
Repetitions of sprints	90	4	6
Continuous slow running	2	93	5
Continuous fast running	2	90	8
Slow interval training	10	60	30
Fast interval training	30	20	50
Repetition running	10	40	50
Speed play (fartlek)	20	40	40
Interval sprinting	20	70	10
Acceleration sprinting	90	5	5
Hollow sprints	85	5	10
Jogging	—	100	—

Source: Wilt, F. "Training for Competitive Running," in *Exercise Physiology*, (H. B. Falls, editor), Academic Press, New York, 1968, p. 407.

rate is sometimes difficult to determine directly (due to expensive laboratory equipment and expertise needed), estimates using the following equation can be used for both males and females with a relatively high degree of accuracy:

$$\text{Maximal heart rate} = 220 - \text{age}$$

Normally, the rest interval between exercise intervals should be equal to or less than the time of the actual work bouts. Also, it may be determined by the recovery heart rate. Generally, when the heart rate reaches 120 beats per minute, the individual starts the next exercise bout. Figure 13-1 illustrates the maximal heart rate for various ages and their training target zone for aerobic endurance training.

As stated earlier, the level of conditioning of the person and the purpose of the training should determine the number of training periods per week. For example, the competitive endurance athlete will need to train between 5 and 7 days per week, whereas the team sports athlete who is supplementing his regular training program with aerobic endurance training can benefit from working out 2 to 4 times per week. At the same time, the sedentary person who is training for general endurance fitness can also benefit by working out between 2 and 4 days per week. Once the training benefits have been developed, they can be expected to be retained for several months with a weekly maintenance training program of only one workout.

Recall from earlier discussion that the anaerobic process comes into play when sufficient oxygen is not available to produce enough energy aerobically and that this process is very important in explosive-type activities such as sprinting, football, weight-lifting, ice-hockey, basketball, etc. It is generally agreed that anaerobic endurance training for the development of the ATP-CP energy system is developed best by working the specific muscles maximal for a period of less than 30 seconds. Because it is believed that energy for short work intervals is supplied from myoglobin-bound oxygen, it is strongly recommended that the length of the recovery interval should be limited to slightly less than that of the work interval in order that myoglobin cannot have time to be completely restored with oxygen during each recovery period. For example, if the work interval is 20 seconds, then the recovery period should be about 10 to 15 seconds.

Table 14-4 illustrates that repetitions of sprints, accleration of sprints, and interval training is excellent for developing this system. As the work extends beyond about 20 to 30 seconds, the anaerobic energy demand placed on the ATP-CP system decreases while the demand on the breakdown of glycogen to lactic acid increases. Training for the development of the lactic acid energy system calls for maximum efforts of no more than 1 to 2 minutes in length followed by recovery periods of between 1 and 15 minutes, depending upon the already existing anaerobic level of the subject. Subjects with poor anaerobic capacities will need longer recovery periods than those athletes with already fairly high anaerobic levels. This should be repeated several times (4 or 5 times). Evidence shows extremely high levels of lactic acid in the blood following this type of training, thus indicating tremendous overload of the lactic acid energy system. Again, interval training appears to be the best method for developing the lactic acid energy system while at the same time, repetitions of sprints could be used with fairly good results.

Research shows that work efforts longer than 1 to 2 minutes do not really overload the lactic acid anaerobic system, but instead, it starts to rely more upon the aerobic system. Evidence shows that highly trained subjects are generally able to tolerate significantly higher lactate levels than untrained subjects. It should be pointed out that because in the development of the lactic acid energy system, the levels of lactic acid may be so high and the time for recovery may be so long that complete recovery may not be possible. Therefore, to avoid the possibility of fatigue interfering with aerobic training, the anaerobic conditioning should come at the end of the training session.

Table 14-4, when combined with Tables 14-1 and 14-2, can be very useful to the coach and athlete. For example, once the coach or athlete has obtained from Table 14-1 or 14-2 the amount (or percentage) of training time needed for developing the specific energy sources for the athlete's particular event, they should then attempt to match as close as possible these percentages to one of the training regimes listed in Table 14-4. For example, because the 3-miler (5,000 meters) in track and the 1500 meter swimmer, as obtained from Table 14-2, should devote about 10 percent of the training time to development of speed, 70 percent to aerobic development, and 20 percent to anaerobic lactic acid development, interval sprinting is the type of training most closely matched to the requirements of these performers (Table 14-4). The only difference, of course, is that the mode of exercise for the runner would have to be running and for the swimmer, it would have to be swimming. Remember, in adopting one of the training methods in Table 14-4, it is important to keep in mind that for activities such as rowing, skiing, ice-hockey, and swimming, the mode of exercise for each of the training sessions should be rowing, skiing, skating, and swimming, respectively, instead of running.

Below is a brief description of the various types of training methods found in Table 14-4.

Repetitions of Sprints. This type of training involves several repetitions of sprints over distances between 60 and 220 yards at absolute maximum speed. Because the heart beats so fast (around 200 beats/min or higher) during this type of training, a heart expansion stimulus does not normally take place since the heart does not fill to its maximum during the diastolic or resting period. As a result, an increased stroke volume of the heart is not generally produced. Instead, the primary effect of sprint training is the development of the ATP-CP energy system.

Continuous Slow Running. Continuous slow running is a form of training that develops almost totally aerobic endurance. Some authorities also refer to this type of running as LSD (long, slow distance). It involves running over long distances (somewhere between 3 and 20 miles and even further) at slow speeds (7 minute miles and slower). The amount of distance covered in this type of training is generally determined by the individual's competitive distance. For instance, a 6-miler might run between 12 and 18 miles, while a miler might run between 3 and 5 miles. This type of training is performed at a relatively low intensity (about 60 to 80 percent of the maximum heart rate), and is generally considered to be the best method for developing stroke volume and capillarization. Note that when this type of training is being used, the speed by which it takes to bring the heart rate up to between 60 and 80 percent of maximum heart rate will depend upon the ability of the individual athlete. For example, a 7-minute mile pace might be the appropriate speed for an inexperienced high school miler, while at the same time, a 6-minute mile pace might be adequate for a world-class marathon runner.

Continuous Fast Running. While this type of training is more intense than the slow continuous running, it also develops mainly aerobic endurance. The distances covered in this type of training are often in excess of the competitive distance; however, they are usually not as long as those performed in the slow continuous running. For instance, a 6-miler, instead, of running 12 to 18 miles as ws suggested under continuous slow running training might run 8 to 10 miles at a steady, but faster pace, while a miler might run 1½ to 2½ miles, and repeat the distance 2 to 3 times, alternately walking and jogging for 5 minutes after each run. This type of training is performed at a relatively high intensity (about 85 to 90 percent of maximum heart rate).

Slow Interval Training. This type of training causes the heart to beat approximately 180 times per minute during the work phase, and develops mostly aerobic endurance. It is generally restricted to distances up to 880 yards. Note that these would include repetitions of either 110, 220, 440, and 880 yards. The speed by which this type of training is carried out is somewhat faster than in continuous fast running training, but at the same time, slower than the athlete's normal competitive speed. An example for an athlete who is capable of running the mile in 4 minutes might be as follows: running twenty 220-yd intervals in a time of 33 seconds each with each run followed by jogging 110 yards in 30 to 45 seconds each. Complete recovery is usually not experienced by the athlete during the between runs. Generally, when the recovery heart rate reaches 120 beats per minute, the athlete starts the next work bout.

Fast Interval Training. During the work or "effort" phase of the fast interval training, the heart beats in excess of 180 beats per minute. It develops primarily anaerobic endurance or speed. This type of training is much more intense in terms of speed than continuous slow running, continuous fast running, or slow interval. It is usually restricted to distances between 110 and 440 yards. An example for a 4-minute miler might be as follows: running several 440-yd intervals in 56 to 59 seconds each, with each run followed by jogging 440 yards in 2 to 3 minutes each. Again, like the slow interval training, complete recovery is not normally witnessed by the athlete during the between runs (when the recovery heart rate reaches 120 beats per minute, the athlete generally starts the next work bout). Fast interval training is generally not undertaken until a good overall background of aerobic or general endurance has been developed.

Repetition Running. When compared to interval training, repetition running generally involves longer distances (somewhere between 880 yards and 2 miles) with a more complete heart rate recovery (by way of walking) following each run. Normally, the heart rate will drop well-below 120 beats per minute between each run. When using this type of training, the speed determines whether an aerobic or anaerobic training benefit takes place. For instance, when the repetitions are run at speeds near racing conditions, anaerobic endurance is developed. On the other hand, when the pace is slower than racing speed, aerobic endurance is usually developed. When repetitions of running beyond competitive distance are undertaken, the speed by which they are run should be significantly slower than the racing speed. At the same time, when repetition running reaches competitive speed, the distance of the fast run should not surpass half the racing distance for which the individual is training.

Speed Play. This type of training (also known as "fartlek" training) involves informal fast and slow-running (as compared to the formal fast-slow running in interval training) alternately at various speeds and distances over unmarked terrains such as golf courses, forests, country roads, etc. All of the aforementioned types of training may be combined in various ways in speed play. While the lack of control by the coach is a major criticism of speed play (note that the athlete must be conscientious and responsible before embarking on this type of training), when carried out properly, this type of training should develop not only aerobic and anaerobic endurance, but also speed.

Interval Sprinting. This form of training consists of sprinting for 50 yards and jogging for 60 yards after each for distances up to 3 miles. In other words, for each 440 yards, the athlete would combine four 50-yd sprints with four 60-yd jogs. Because of early fatigue (generally after the first several sprints), this type of training not only keeps the athlete from running at his or her maximal sprint speed, but it also causes the athlete to gradually extend his or her recovery jogging time. Therefore, the major training effect is primarily aerobic endurance.

Acceleration Sprinting. This type of training develops almost exclusively speed and strength. It involves 50 to 110 yards of jogging, followed by 50 to 110 yards of fast striding, and finally 50 to 110 yards of sprinting. Following a recovery (via walking) distance of 50 to 110 yards, the procedure should be repeated (note that several repetitions should be conducted). As Wilt points out, this type of training is excellent when running outside in cold weather, since the athlete, instead of suddenly reaching his or her top sprint speed, gradually obtains it, and therefore avoids the possibility of muscle injury as so often occurs in conditions of low atmospheric temperatures.

Hollow Sprints. Hollow sprints involves sprinting, jogging, sprinting, walking, and repeating. An example may be: sprint 50 to 110 yards, jog 50 to 110 yards, sprint 50 to 110 yards for recovery prior to the next repetition. This type of training, provided adequate recovery takes place during the walking phase, mainly develops speed and muscular strength.

Jogging. Jogging has gained a tremendous amount of popularity in recent years, especially with older adults who are not training for competitive purposes, but instead, to lose a few pounds of fat and for health reasons. For example, it is well known that jogging is one of the best ways of improving the cardiovascular system for fighting coronary heart disease. Jogging, especially recreational jogging, generally consist of long, slow running. While there are several jogging programs available, Table 14-5 illustrates one for both men and women that is very simple to understand and follow. The frequency of this program is 3 days per week with a distance of 2 miles to be covered in each session. The progression is from step one to step 18. It is important to remember that regardless of how long it takes, step two should not be attempted until step one has been accomplished in the prescribed time. This holds true for all steps. None is to be attempted until the previous step time has been accomplished. The interested reader is referred to Chapter 13 for another illustration of a progressive exercise program for older men and women for the purpose of developing cardiorespiratory endurance.

Note that most of the information from the previous discussion dealing with the various training methods was taken from the excellent work of Wilt, Fox and Mathews.

Table 14-5. A Basic Jogging Program for Both Men and Women

Basic Steps	1 Mile Check Time (min:sec)	Total Target Time for 2 Miles (min:sec)
1. Slow walk	20:00	40:00
2. Alternate ¼ mile slow walk & ¼ mile fast walk	18:00	36:00
3. Fast walk	16:00	32:00
4. Alternate 330 yd fast walk & 110 yd slow jog	14:30	29:00
5. Alternate 220 yd fast walk & 220 yd slow jog	13:00	26:00
6. Alternate ¼ mile fast walk & ¼ mile slow jog	13:00	26:00
7. Alternate ½ mile slow jog & ¼ mile fast walk	11:30	23:00
8. Alternate ¾ mile slow jog & ¼ mile fast walk	11:30	23:00
9. Slow jog	10:00	20:00
10. Alternate ¼ mile fast jog & ¼ mile slow jog	9:30	19:00
11. Alternte ¼ mile slow jog & ¼ mile fast jog	9:00	18:00
12. Alternate ½ mile slow jog & ½ mile slow jog	9:00	18:00
13. Alternate ½ mile fast jog & ¼ mile slow jog	8:30	17:00
14. Alternate ¼ mile slow jog & ¾ mile fast jog	8:30	17:00
15. Fast jog	8:00	16:00
16. Alternate ¼ mile fast jog & ¼ mile faster jog	7:30	15:00
17. Alternate ½ mile fast jog & ½ mile faster jog	7:30	15:00
18. Faster jog	7:00	14:00

Source: Roby, F., and R. Davis. *Jogging for Fitness and Weight Control*, W. B. Saunders Co., Philadelphia, 1970.

C. FACTORS AFFECTING AEROBIC AND ANAEROBIC ENDURANCE

Numerous factors relate to and influence aerobic and anaerobic endurance. It is important to know what has been found through research and observation concerning these factors.

Age and Sex

The effects of age and sex on aerobic endurance have been studied repeatedly. The results indicate that up to the beginning of puberty, girls are approximately equal to boys, however, women tend to obtain their maximum capacity at ages 12 to 14 years, whereas men continue to increase until around 25 to 30. On the whole, the evidence, although far from complete, indicates that after maximum aerobic endurance is reached, it remains fairly constant for 3 to 5 years, then begins to decline gradually as a result of several changes that take place in the cardiorespiratory system with increased age. For example, as people get older, they gradually decrease their capacity for transforming energy aerobically. In addition, the ability to transport blood to active muscles has decreased, and skeletal muscles have become weaker. At the same time, however, it appears that many older people who keep active, can carry on work with a lower heart rate and less evidence of fatigue than certain young people. The well-known marathon runner, Mr. Clarence DeMar, for instance, is a good example of this fact. It was found that DeMar, even after the age of 60, had a significantly greater work capacity than most men of 20 years of age. At the "young" age of 49, he had a maximum oxygen uptake of around 58 ml/kg/min.

When comparing aerobic endurance between men and women, there is only a small difference in light submaximal exercise, but considerable differences in heavy, maximal work. The maximum aerobic capacity (maximum oxygen uptake) is about 20 to 25 percent lower in women while the maximal pulmonary ventilation, stroke volume, cardiac output, a-$\bar{v}_{O_2}$ diff, and oxygen intakes are also higher in men. As Jensen and Fisher point out, there are several reasons why the female is limited in their cardiorespiratory endurance capacity when compared to the male. They are: (1) a more rapid heart rate, (2) a small heart with a smaller capacity to deliver blood, (3) smaller chest cavity resulting in inferior lung capacity, and (4) the blood of women is limited in its oxygen-carrying capacity due to fewer red blood cells.

Body Build

Physique studies show quite clearly that most individuals who experience success in aerobic endurance activities such as long-distance running have a high degree of ectomorphy with some degree of mesomorphy. At the same time, sprinters and field event athletes with explosive ATP-CP and lactic acid anaerobic power tend to be more toward the mesomorphy body build. On the other hand, individuals favoring the endomorphy classification, are more inclined to be successful in aerobic endurance activities such as long-distance channel swimming, rather than in those involving running. These findings are apparently due, in part, to the fact that in swimming the body weight is supported by the water and not carried horizontally and vertically by the muscles as it is in running and jumping in track and field.

Fat

It is generally known that high percentages of fat in relation to total body weight are detrimental and lead to obesity. Research has indicated that the relative degree of "fat-free" (lean body weight) body weight is not only important from the point of view of health, but it also apparently plays an important role in obtaining high levels of human performance in activities where the body weight must be actually moved from one place to another. It is generally well known that high percentages of body fat actually decreases the ability of the cardiorespiratory system to supply oxygen to the various parts of the body, thereby lowering one's cardiorespiratory endurance capacity. It has been suggested by some authorities in the field that fat causes poor performance in the area of cardiorespiratory endurance because it not only places an overload on the circulatory system and heart to have to pump more blood to a larger vascular system, but fat also acts as dead weight in the body (thus raising resistance to movement) while contributing nothing to muscle contraction (since it lacks the ability to do so). Note as was pointed out in the previous discussion, while fat may be detrimental to most physical activities that require either horizontal or vertical-type movements on land, it is apparently an asset to swimmers who need the fat for insulation purposes (especially channel swimmers) and for buoyancy purposes. The increased buoyancy and decreased heat loss due to the subcutaneous fat more than offsets the disadvantage of the greater weight to be moved.

Muscular Strength

There is no doubt that the strength of the working muscles is a limiting factor in endurance activities. For example, a resistance that is easily moved by strong muscles may quickly fatigue weak ones. This is obviously true because as Morehouse and Miller point out, when a strong muscle lifts a relatively light load, very few muscles are actually called into play. As these same fibers become tired and exhausted, their threshold of irritability is apparently raised, and they fail to respond to the stimuli. As a result, fresh fibers are then stimulated and thus brought into play while the fatigued fibers, meanwhile, recover and resume the work later on if necessary.

Skill

It is quite clear that during physical performance a skilled person uses less energy and works at a higher efficiency level than the unskilled. For example, studies have shown that unskilled swimmers may require more than twice as much energy as a skilled swimmer to swim the same distance even though they are both swimming at the same speed. It is well known that training improves the skill and the efficiency of any motion or sequence of motions involved in muscular activity. In fact, some studies show that training may result in as much as a 25 percent savings in energy expenditure of the total energy needed before training. This obviously has a tremendous influence on endurance performance.

Pacing

Although it is generally agreed tht work is performed at a higher efficiency level if it is carried out at an even pace over the entire period of time, there has been some interesting research published in the literature against the even pace. While the even pace may be advocated by the physiologists in the laboratory, to the athlete in competition, it probably has very little meaning since there are obviously other factors involved in athletic competition besides maintaining an even pace over the entire distance. In fact, if an athlete kept an even pace throughout the entire distance of a track event, he probably would lose the race. Investigators working in this area has shown that when subjects were tested over three different pace plans for middle-distance running events, they perform better if they run the initial part of the distance a little slower than their average speed and then run the last portion as fast as they can. Starting out fast results in an earlier accumulation of lactic acid which means that more of the race is run with a high lactic acid level, thus lowering the efficiency level. Authorities recommend that it is better to perform endurance type activities (such as running and swimming) on a pace pattern that delays the build-up of lactic acid until the end of the race. Note that the three pace plans mentioned above were as follows: one plan called for each subject to run one trial at constant speed, one trial with a fast first minute and slower remainder, and one trial with a slow first minute and faster remainder.

Evidence in this area also indicate that quick changes in an individual's pace can also be very costly in terms of energy cost. In other words, an individual should avoid quick changes while running, swimming, bicycling, etc. when endurance is the major factor of the performance. If a change is to be made during the event, the individual should do it gradually in order to allow the cardiorespiratory system to make adjustments accordingly. The exception to this of course is in the final sprint to the finish line when endurance is not the major concern, but instead, speed and beating the opponent across the finish line.

Circulation

Evidence indicates significant improvement in blood flow as the result of aerobic endurance training. Thus, improved blood flow increases the ability of the vascular system to deliver oxygen and carbon dioxide to and from the working muscles, respectively. Increased blood flow is also a vital improvement for heat dissipation during work in hot climates, where maintaining normal body temperature plays a tremendously important part for the performer. It should be obvious that by virtue of an improved vascularization of the active muscle tissue that this is probably one of the most important functions in the development of an improved cardiorespiratory endurance.

Hyperventilation

Hyperventilation (when lung ventilation rate is greater than is needed for the existing metabolic rate) has no appreciable effect on oxygen values in the blood because blood is already fully saturated with oxygen when it leaves the lungs. However, since carbon dioxide is "blown off" faster than it is produced during hyperventilation, it does result in a lowering of the carbon dioxide level in the cardiorespiratory system. Hyperventilation has been found to nearly double the breath-holding time. Thus, in anaerobic-type activities such as underwater swimming, crawl-stroke sprinting, or even short track sprint events where breath holding is perhaps important, hyperventilation may be of some value. However, in other types of activities where breath holding is not necessarily important, its value is questionable. For example, although hyperventilation may increase breath holding time, extensive hyperventilation prior to an athletic event (especially underwater swimming) may have severe consequences and should be used with caution. The combination of hyperventilation, breath holding, and exercise produce hypoxia (lack of oxygen) under unusual conditions. For instance, research shows that hyperventilation causes a fall in alveolar partial pressure of carbon dioxide from 40 mmHg to 15 mmHg and increases alveolar partial pressure of oxygen tension from 100 mmHg to 140 mmHg. At the same time, the increased metabolism brought about by swimming quickly lowers the arterial partial pressure of oxygen while raising the arterial partial pressure of carbon dioxide. It is possible under these conditions to lose consciousness and perhaps drown due to a decreased cerebral oxygen tension. Studies show that a drop in partial pressure of oxygen below approximately 19 mmHg will result in unconsciousness before a person reaches this "breaking point" (an increase in alveolar partial pressure of carbon dioxide to around 50 mmHg) which means they can no longer hold their breath. Since a person's urge to breathe is primarily controlled by the amount of carbon dioxide accumulated in the lungs and arterial blood, and not necessarily by the partial pressure of oxygen, it is highly possible, as experts agree, to incur hypoxia without even feeling an urge to breathe if the hyperventilation prior to the event is severe and extensive. Highly competitive underwater swimmers should be informed of the factors contributing to anoxia and the danger of ignoring the urge to breathe. Every physical educator and coach should also be aware of these potential hazards that are associated with hyperventilation in order that they might inform their participants.

Oxygen Debt

Although the oxygen debt is not a major limiting factor in aerobic endurance, it is vitally important in anaerobic endurance. Anaerobic endurance for activities requiring short bursts of vigorous movement from 1 to 3 minutes is generally limited by the size of an oxygen debt that can be tolerated. The untrained person will generally stop work when an oxygen debt of about 10 liters has been reached, while a trained person can tolerate an oxygen debt of somewhere around 17 to 18 liters. This obviously plays an important part in anaerobic endurance.

Environmental Factors

Since a complete discussion on the environmental factors can be found in Chapters 7 and 8, they will only be mentioned briefly here. There is no doubt that a hot, humid environment as well as a hot, dry environment places great demands upon the cardiorespiratory system. For example, heart rates are higher, sweat rates are higher, respiratory rates are faster, pulmonary ventilation is higher, and oxygen consumption is higher. Because of the added strain on the circulatory system to provide sufficient blood to the working muscles and to the skin for heat dissipation, it is quite obvious that activities involving the cardiorespiratory system will be somewhat affected when performing in hot climates. Short activities involving the anaerobic energy system will not be nearly as affected as the long distance-type activities. Trained people are known to be able to tolerate the heat much better than untrained people. As pointed out in Chapter 7, cold weather apparently poses very few problems for the individual during maximal performance because increased metabolic heat due to the activity soon warms him or her to a normal operating temperature. Prior to the body warming up, heat is lost mainly to the atmosphere by way of radiation and convection. Once the individual starts to sweat, heat is also lost by evaporation.

As was mentioned in Chapter 8, as one ascends to high altitude, the decreased barometric pressure causes the partial pressure of oxygen to be reduced. This decreased oxygen pressure decreases the arterial oxygen saturation of the blood which, in turn, decreases the amount of oxygen available to the working muscles. Consequently, there is no doubt that activities lasting more than 2 minutes in which aerobic energy is essential will be hampered by high altitude. At the same time, anaerobic activities lasting a few seconds to 2 minutes will not be adversely affected except following exercise in which it will generally take longer than normal to recovery.

VI. MUSCULAR FATIGUE

Fatigue comes in all shapes, forms, and degrees. General overall body fatigue simply means that the body is unable to cope with the everyday stresses, whereas local fatigue in one muscle or in one functional muscle group means that the muscle or muscle group is simply unable to continue

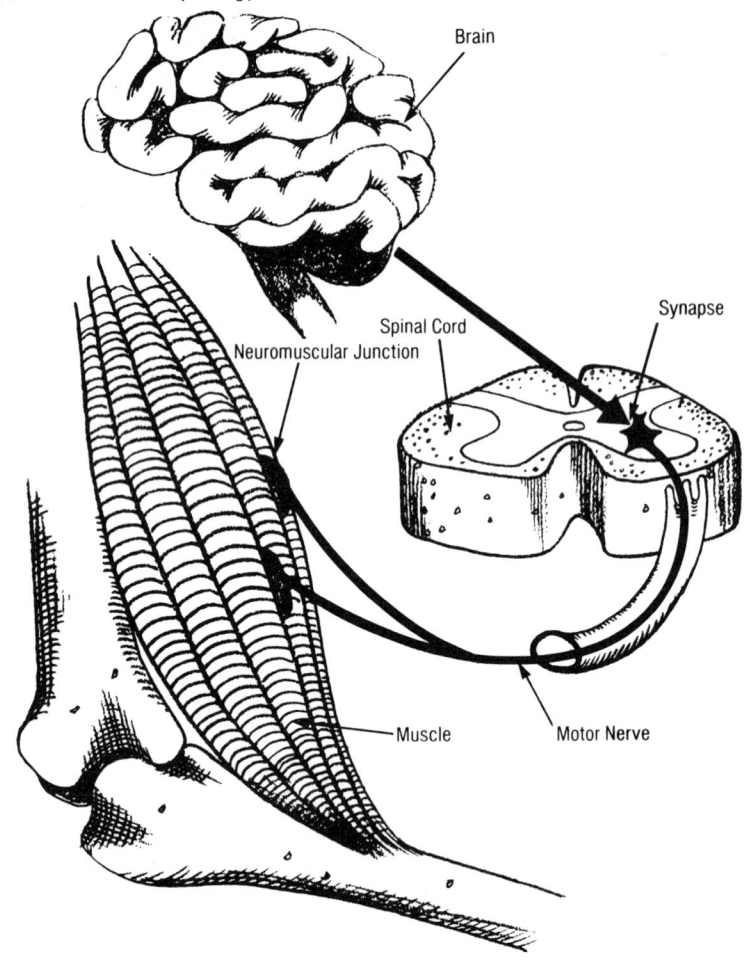

Figure 14-6 Schematic illustration of the possible sites of muscular fatigue.

contracting at the same rate of energy expenditure over a given period of time. While there are other forms of fatigue such as emotional and boredom, we are concerned primarily with local muscular fatigue in this text.

A question that has been raised many, many times over the years is what causes fatigue and where is the actual site of fatigue. The possible sites of muscular fatigue are shown in Figure 14-6. They range from the brain all the way down to the muscle itself. With physical activity, the site of local muscular fatigue appears to be peripheral (in other words, in the muscles themselves), and more than likely involves the contractile mechanism. Evidence shows that the FT fibers of the contractile process have a greater fatiguability than that of ST fibers. This is apparently due to the fact that FT fibers have a rather high glycolytic capacity, but a low aerobic capacity. Studies show that exercises of severe intensity results in high levels of lactic acid produced by the FT fibers. Therefore, evidence seems to indicate that local muscular fatigue that is brought about by exercises of anaerobic nature (such as short, explosive type of high intensity) is due to lactic acid build-up.

At the same time, fatigue that is associated with long, submaximal type activities is not necessarily due to lactic acid, but instead, it appears to be brought about by several factors; namely, (1) depletion of muscle glycogen in ST and FT fibers; (2) dehydration (a loss of body fluids); (3) a loss in body electrolytes such as potassium and salts; (4) hypoglycemia (results from a low blood glucose level); (5) depletion of liver glycogen; (6) hyperthermia (results from high increase in body temperature); and finally, plain old boredom.

VII. SUMMARY

(1) The basic principles of any physical training program are:
  (a) *Overload principle.* Demands that the work intensity be maximal and that it be gradually increased as the individual's fitness level improves during the course of the conditioning program.
  (b) *Specificity of training.* Requires that the training program be specific to develop not only the predominant energy system(s) involved, but also the specific muscle groups involved as well as the specific movement patterns involved.
  (c) *Individual differences.* Because individuals respond in different ways to identical stimuli, the coach should not insist that every individual on the team perform the same workout at the same rate. Individual differences must be expected and training programs structured to meet these differences.
  (d) *Determining the major energy system(s) involved.* The primary energy systems for any given sport or activity can be decided on the basis of its intensity and performance time.
  (e) *Motivation.* Proper motivation is essential for optimal training to take place.

(2) Four types of muscle contraction are identified: (a) isotonic (dynamic and concentric) is when a muscle contracts and shortens under a given load; (b) isometric (static) is when a muscle contracts but does not shorten; (c) eccentric results when the tension that is developed is less than the opposing outside force and thus, the muscle is stretched or lengthened during contraction; and (d) isokinetics or accommodating resistance exercises (conducted with specific types of equipment such as the Cybex, the Mini-Gym, and the Nautilus) involves a maximum effort throughout the entire range of joint motion.

(3) The development of strength and local endurance can be accomplished by way of the overload principle using progressive resistance exercises. Whe the muscle increases its strength and endurance, its individual fibers get larger. While it is not completely clear, it is believed that the increase in fiber size is due to the following:
  (a) increase in total amount of myosin, actin, and other myofibillar proteins,
  (b) increase in vascular tissue (capillaries and venules) per fiber,
  (c) increase in the thickening of the connective tissue, tendons, and ligaments,
  (d) increase in the number of myofibrils per muscle fiber,
  (e) increase in myoglobin concentration as well as the number and size of mitochondria,
  (f) increase in ATP-CP, glycogen, and enzymes.

(4) Factors such as age, sex, nervous system, body build, length of muscle, circulation, and strength (affecting endurance) have an influence upon the development of strength and local endurance.

(5) Once strength and local endurance are developed, they are relatively easy to retain. In fact, they may be retained with as little exercise as once each week or even once every other week provided that maximum resistance contractions are used.

284 Essentials of Exercise Physiology

(6) Physiological changes brought about by anaerobic endurance training include: (a) increased amount of both ATP and CP stored in the muscles and (b) increased lactic acid or glycolytic capacity.

(7) Physiological changes brought about by aerobic endurance training are as follows:
- (a) reduced heart rate (for rest, submaximal, and maximal work),
- (b) quicker heart rate recovery following work,
- (c) cardiac hypertrophy,
- (d) increased stroke volume (for rest, submaximal, and maximal work),
- (e) increased cardiac output (for maximal work with little or no change during submaximal work),
- (f) reduced blood pressure during rest and exercise as well as quicker recovery following work,
- (g) increased blood volume, hemoglobin and red blood cells,
- (h) reduced blood flow per kilogram of working muscle,
- (i) increase in number of capillaries,
- (j) increased maximal oxygen uptake per minute,
- (k) lactic acid is decreased for a standard submaximal work load while there is an increased capacity for lactic acid during maximal work,
- (l) pulmonary ventilation is decreased for a standard submaximal work load and increased for a maximal work load,
- (m) increased respiratory efficiency,
- (n) increased lung volume and diffusion capacity,
- (o) increased neuromuscular efficiency,
- (p) increased myoglobin concentration,
- (q) ST and FT fibers are better suited for producing ATP for aerobic work,
- (r) improved blood distribution for work in heat,
- (s) reduced body fat with an increased muscle mass (lean body mass),
- (t) reduced serum lipids (cholesterol and triglycerides), and
- (u) increased skeletal muscle capacity for oxidizing carbohydrates and fats.

(8) There are specific factors that affect the development of aerobic and anaerobic endurance. They are: (a) age and sex, (b) body build, (c) fat, (d) strength, (e) skill, (f) pacing, (g) circulation, (h) hyperventilation, (i) oxygen debt, and (j) environmental factors.

(9) The most popular and scientifically studied aerobic and anaerobic training methods used today is interval training. The overload principle when applied to interval training can be accomplished through the manipulation of the following variables:
- (a) rate and distance,
- (b) number of repetitions during each workout,
- (c) time of rest interval between the work intervals,
- (d) type of activity during rest interval, and
- (e) number of training periods per week.

(10) the various training methods and their areas of development are:
- (a) repetitions of sprints—speed and strength,
- (b) continuous slow running—aerobic endurance,
- (c) continuous fast running—aerobic endurance,
- (d) slow interval training—aerobic endurance,
- (e) fast interval training—anaerobic endurance or speed,

(f) repetition running—aerobic and anaerobic endurance,
  (g) speed play (fartlek)—aerobic and anaerobic endurance,
  (h) interval sprinting—aerobic endurance,
  (i) acceleration sprinting—speed and strength,
  (j) hollow sprints—speed and strength,
  (k) jogging—aerobic endurance.

(11) The site of local muscular fatigue appears to be peripheral (in the muscle itself) and more than likely involves the contractile mechanism.

(12) Evidence indicates that local muscular fatigue that is brought about by anaerobic-type work (short and high-intensity) is due to lactic acid build-up, whereas fatigue that is associated with long, submaximal type work (aerobic) is due to several factors; namely, (a) depletion of muscle glycogen in ST and FT fibers; (b) dehydration; (c) loss of body electrolytes; (d) hypoglycemia; (e) depletion of liver glycogen; (f) hyperthermia; and (g) boredom.

(13) Proper intensity level for aerobic endurance training can be determined from the heart rate. The intensity of the work should be high enough to get the heart rate between 60 and 90 percent of its maximum. Maximum heart rate may be determined by subtracting the person's age from 220.

(14) The ATP-CP system is best developed by working maximum for a period of less than 30 seconds. This should be repeated several times with recovery periods of about 1 minute between the work bouts. Training for the development of lactic acid should be no longer than 1 to 2 minutes. Rest periods between work should be between 1 and 15 minutes, depending upon the already existing anaerobic level of the subject.

VII. REVIEW REFERENCES

(1) American College of Sports Medicine. *Guidelines for Graded Exercise Testing and Exercise Prescription.* Lea and Febiger, Philadelphia, 1979.
(2) Astrand, P. O., and K. Rodahl, *Textbook of Work Physiology,* 2nd edition, McGraw-Hill, Co., New York, 1977.
(3) Berger, R. "Optimum Repetitions for the Development of Strength," *Research Quarterly,* 33:334-38, 1962.
(4) Clarke, D. H. "Adaptations in Strength and Muscular Endurance Resulting from Exercise," in *Exercise and Sport Sciences Reviews,* (J. H. Wilmore, editor), Vol. 1, Academic Press, New York, 1973.
(5) Craig, A. B. "Underwater Swimming and Drowning," *Journal of Sports Medicine and Physical fitness,* 2:23-26, 1962.
(6) DeLorme, T. L., and A. L. Watkins. "Techniques of Progressive Resistance Exercise," *Archives of Physical Medicine and Rehabilitation,* 29:263-73, 1948.
(7) deVries, H. A. *Physiology of Exercise for Physical Education and Athletics.* Wm. C. Brown, Publishers, Dubuque, Iowa, 1974.
(8) Fox, E. L. *Sports Physiology,* W. B. Saunders Co., Philadelphia, 1979.
(9) Fox, E. L., and D. Mathews. *Interval Training: Conditioning for Sports and General Fitness,* W. B. Saunders Co., Philadelphia, 1974.
(10) Getchell, B. *Physical Fitness: A Way of Life,* 2nd edition, John Wiley & Sons, Inc., New York, 1979.
(11) Jensen, C. R., and A. G. Fisher. *Scientific Basis of Athletic Conditioning,* Lea & Febiger, Philadelphia, 1972.
(12) Lamb, D. R. *Physiology of Exercise: Responses and Adaptations,* Macmillan Publishing Co., Inc., New York, 1978.
(13) Lesmes, G. R., D. L. Costill, E. F. Coyle, and W. J. Fink. "Muscle Strength and Power Changes During Maximal Isokinetic Training," *Medicine and Science in Sports,* 10:266-69, 1978.
(14) Mathews, D. K., and E. L. Fox. *The Physiological basis of Physical Education and Athletics,* 2nd edition, W. B. Saunders Co., Philadelphia, 1976.

(15) O'Shea, J. P. *Scientific Principles and Methods of Strength Fitness,* Addison-Wesley Co., Reading, Mass. 1975.
(16) Pollock, M. L. "How Much Exercise Is Enough," *The Physician and Sportsmedicine,* 6:50-64, 1978
(17) Roby, F., and R. Davis. *Jogging for Fitness and Weight Control,* W. B. Saunders Co., Philadelphia, 1970.
(18) Sheehan, G. *Running and Being,* Simon and Schuster, New York, 1978.
(19) Sysler, B., and G. Stull. "Muscular Endurance Retention as a Function of Length of Detraining," *Research Quarterly,* 41:105-09, 1970.
(20) Ullyot, J. *Women's Running,* World Publications, Mountain View, California, 1977.
(21) Waldman, R., and G. Stull. "Effects of Various Periods of Inactivity on Retention of Newly Acquired Levels of Muscular Endurance," *Research Quarterly,* 40:396-401, 1969.
(22) Wilmore, J. H. *Athletic Training and Physical Fitness: Physiological Principles and Practices of the Conditioning Process,* Allyn and Bacon, Boston, 1976.
(23) Wilmore, J. H. "Individual Exercise Prescription," *The American Journal of Cardiology,* 33:757-59, 1974.
(24) Wilt, F. "Conditioning of Runners for Championship Competition," *Journal of American Medical Association,* 221:1017-21, 1972.
(25) Wilt, F. "Training for Competitive Running," in *Exercise Physiology,* (H. B. Falls, editor), Academic Press, New York, 1968.

APPENDIX A
UNITS OF MEASURE

WORK/ENERGY

1 kilocalorie = 3087 foot-pounds = 426.4 kilograms-meters* = 426.4 kilopond+-meters = 4,186 joules = 3,9680 British Thermal Units (B.T.U.)
1 foot-pound = 0.13825 kilogram-meters = 0.00032389 kilocalories = 1.3558 joules
1 kilogram-meter = 1 kilopond-meter = 7.23 foot-pounds = 0.0023427 kilocalories = 9.8066 joules
1 MET = approximately 0.25 liters of oxygen = approximately 1.25 kilocalories

POWER (WORK/TIME)

1 horsepower = 4.564 kilogram-meter/minute = 33,000 foot-pounds/minute = 10,694 kilocalories/minute = 550 foot-pounds/second = 746 watts = 75 kilopond-meters/minute
1 kilocalorie/minute = 51.457 foot-pounds/second = 3.9685 B.T.U. = 0.093557 horsepower = 69.767 watts = 426.78 kilopond-meters/minute = 426.4 kilogram-meter/minute = 3087 foot-pounds/minute
1 watt = 0.73756 foot-pounds/second = 0.001341 horsepower = 6.12 kilopond-meters/minute = 0.01433 kilocalories/minute = 1 joule/second = 3.41304 B.T.U./hour = 44.22 foot-pounds/minute
1 liter O_2 consumed/minute = 15,575 foot-pounds/minute = 2153 kilogram-meter/minute = 5.05 kilocalorie/minute
1 foot-pound/minute = 0.1383 kilogram-meter/minute = 0.00003 horsepower = 0.0226 watt
1 kilogram-meter/minute = 7.23 foot-pounds/minute = 0.00022 horsepower = 0.1635 watt

WEIGHT

1 pound = 16 ounces = 454 grams = 0.454 kilogram
1 kilogram = 35.27 ounces = 1,000 grams = 2.2 pounds
1 gram = 0.035 ounces = 0.0022 pounds = 0.001 kilogram

*A kilogram-meter is the distance through which 1 kilogram moves 1 meter.
†A kilopond is the force acting upon a mass of 1 kilogram at normal acceleration of gravity.

DISTANCES

1 inch = 2.54 centimeters = 25.4 millimeters = 0.0254 meters
1 kilometer = 1,000 meters = 0.62137 miles
1 meter = 100 centimeters = 1,000 millimeters = 39.37 inches = 3.28 feet = 1.09 yards
1 foot = 30.48 centimeters = 304.8 millimeters = 0.304 meters
1 mile = 5280 feet = 1760 yards = 1609.35 meters = 1.61 kilometers
1 centimeter = 0.3937 inch

VOLUME

1 liter = 1.0567 U.S. quarts = 1,000 milliliters
1 milliliter = 0.03381 fluid ounces
1 pint = 0.473 liter = 0.5 quart
1 quart = 0.946 liters = 2 pints

VELOCITY

1 mile/hour = 88 feet/minute = 1.47 feet/second = 0.45 meters/second = 26.8 meters/minute = 1.61 kilometers/hour
1 kilometer/hour = 0.62137 miles/hour = 16.7 meters/minute = 0.28 meters/second = 0.91 feet/second
1 feet/second = 0.3048 meters/second = 18.3 meters/minute = 1.1 kilometers/hour = 0.68 miles/hour

TEMPERATURE

°F = (9/5 × °C) + 32
0°C = 32°F
100°C = 212°F
273°K = 32°F = 0°C
°C = (°F — 32) × 5/9

APPENDIX B
STPD CORRECTION FACTORS

Standard temperature and pressure, dry (STPD) correction factors are used for reducing volume of moist gas to volume occupied by dry gas at 0°, 760 mmHg. Corrections to STPD are necessary when determining the amount of gas molecules in your sample such as the oxygen consumed and the carbon dioxide produced. Such corrections will usually result in a reduction in your sample volumes.

Observed Barometric Reading, Uncorrected for Temperature	15°	16°	17°	18°	19°	20°	21°	22°	23°	24°	25°	26°	27°	28°	29°	30°	31°	32°
700	0.855	851	847	842	838	834	829	825	821	816	812	807	802	797	793	788	783	778
702	857	853	849	845	840	836	832	827	823	818	814	809	805	800	795	790	785	780
704	860	856	852	847	843	839	834	830	825	821	816	812	807	802	797	792	787	783
706	862	858	854	850	845	841	837	832	828	823	819	814	810	804	800	795	790	785
708	865	861	856	852	848	843	839	834	830	825	821	816	812	807	802	797	792	787
710	867	863	859	855	850	846	842	837	833	828	824	819	814	809	804	799	795	790
712	870	866	861	857	853	848	844	839	836	830	826	821	817	812	807	802	797	792
714	872	868	864	859	855	851	846	842	837	833	828	824	819	814	809	804	799	794
716	875	871	866	862	858	853	849	844	840	835	831	826	822	816	812	807	802	797
718	877	873	869	864	860	856	851	847	842	838	833	828	824	819	814	809	804	799
720	880	876	871	867	863	858	854	849	845	840	836	831	826	821	816	812	807	802
722	882	878	874	869	865	861	856	852	847	843	838	833	829	824	819	814	809	804
724	885	880	876	872	867	863	858	854	849	845	840	835	831	826	821	816	811	806

Appendix B

726	887	883	879	874	870	866	861	856	852	847	843	838	833	829	824	818	813	808
728	890	886	881	877	872	868	863	859	854	850	845	840	836	831	826	821	816	811
730	892	888	884	879	875	871	866	861	857	852	847	843	838	833	828	823	818	813
732	895	890	886	882	877	873	868	864	859	854	850	845	840	836	831	825	820	815
734	897	893	889	884	880	875	871	866	862	857	852	847	843	838	833	828	823	818
736	900	895	891	887	882	878	873	869	864	859	855	850	845	840	835	830	825	820
738	902	898	894	889	885	880	876	871	866	862	857	852	848	843	838	833	828	822
740	905	900	896	892	887	883	878	874	869	864	860	855	850	845	840	835	830	825
742	907	903	898	894	890	885	881	876	871	867	862	857	852	848	843	837	832	827
744	910	906	901	897	892	888	883	878	874	869	864	860	855	850	845	840	834	829
746	912	908	903	899	895	890	886	881	876	872	867	862	857	852	847	842	837	832
748	915	910	906	901	897	892	888	883	879	874	869	864	860	854	850	845	839	834
750	917	913	908	904	900	895	890	886	881	876	872	867	862	857	852	847	842	837
752	920	915	911	906	902	897	893	888	883	879	874	869	864	859	854	849	844	839
754	922	918	913	909	904	900	895	891	886	881	876	872	867	862	857	852	846	841
756	925	920	916	911	907	902	898	893	888	883	879	874	869	864	859	854	849	844
758	927	923	918	914	909	905	900	896	891	886	881	876	872	867	861	856	851	846
760	930	925	921	916	912	907	902	898	893	888	883	879	874	869	864	859	854	848
762	932	928	923	919	914	910	905	900	896	891	886	881	876	872	866	861	856	851
764	935	930	926	921	916	912	907	903	898	893	888	884	879	874	869	864	858	853
766	937	933	928	924	919	915	910	905	900	896	891	886	881	876	871	866	861	855
768	940	935	931	926	922	917	912	908	903	898	893	888	883	879	874	868	863	858
770	942	938	933	928	924	919	915	910	905	901	896	891	886	881	876	871	865	860
772	945	940	936	931	926	922	917	912	908	903	898	893	888	883	878	873	868	862
774	947	943	938	933	929	924	920	915	910	905	901	896	891	886	880	875	870	865
776	950	945	941	936	931	927	922	917	912	908	903	898	893	888	883	878	872	867
778	952	948	943	938	934	929	924	920	915	910	905	900	895	890	885	880	875	869
780	955	950	945	941	936	932	927	922	917	912	908	903	898	892	887	882	877	872

Source: Peters, J. P., and D. D. Van Slyke: *Quantitative Clinical Chemistry.* Vol. II. (Methods), The Williams and Wilkins Co., Baltimore, 1932, reprinted 1956, p. 129.

APPENDIX C
BTPS CORRECTION FACTORS

Body temperature and ambient pressure, saturated (BTPS) correction factors are used for correcting volumes of air moved by the lungs to volumes occupied at body temperature of 37°C, saturated with water vapor. Unlike STPD corrections, BTPS corrections are not necessary when determining the amount or number of gas molecules (such as oxygen and carbon dioxide), but instead, they are made when only volumes taken up by the gas molecules are determined such as the various lung volume measurements (vital capacity, maximal breathing capacity, tital volume, etc.).

BTPS Exhaled Gas t°C	Factors to Convert Gas Volume to 37°C Saturated P_B mmHg		
	750	760	770
20	1.102	1.102	1.101
20.5	1.100	1.099	1.099
21	1.097	1.096	1.096
21.5	1.094	1.093	1.093
22	1.091	1.091	1.090
22.5	1.089	1.089	1.088
23	1.086	1.085	1.085
23.5	1.083	1.082	1.082
24	1.080	1.079	1.079
24.5	1.077	1.077	1.076
25	1.074	1.074	1.073
25.5	1.071	1.071	1.070
26	1.069	1.069	1.068
26.5	1.066	1.065	1.065
27	1.063	1.062	1.062
27.5	1.061	1.060	1.060

Source: Lamb, D. R. *Physiology of Exercise: Responses and Adaptations,* Macmillan Publishing Co., Inc., New York, 1978, p. 415.

GLOSSARY

Acclimatization: Refers to the body becoming physiologically adjusted through continued exposure to environmental stresses such as heat, cold, altitude.

Acetylcholine(Ach): Chemical substance released at synapses causing transmission of an impulse from one nerve fiber to another.

Acetylcholinesterase: Enzyme that breaks down acetylcholine into acetic acid and choline.

Acidosis: Condition in which the acid-base balance shifts to the acid side due to below normal blood bicarbonates or increased levels of unbuffered acids.

Actin: Thin protein filament of the muscle which combines with the myosin cross bridge to produce shortening tension.

Action Potential: Change in electrical activity across a nerve or muscle membrane.

Active Transport: Expenditure of metabolic energy to move substances across a membrane.

Actomyosin: Refers to the interaction of actin and myosin protein filaments during muscle contraction.

Acute: Severe intensification of an event of short duration.

Adenosine Diphosphate (ADP): Chemical compound resulting from the breakdown of ATP for energy during muscle contraction.

Adenosine Triphosphate (ATP): Chemical compound split into ADP and phosphate to produce needed body energy.

Adipose Tissue: Tissue characterized by large fat storage.

Aerobic: Refers to the utilization of oxygen.

Aerobic Power: Physiological index expression of total body endurance, same as maximal oxygen uptake, maximal oxygen consumption, cardiovascular endurance capacity.

Afferent Nerve: Sensory nerve that conducts impulses from the senses to the central nervous system.

Alactacid Oxygen Debt: Oxygen used to restore ATP and CP in muscles during recovery period.

Alkalosis: Condition in which the acid-base balance shifts to the alkaline side.

All-or-None Law: Refers to a motor unit that either fires or does not fire.

Alveolar Air: Air in the alveoli involved in the exchange of gases with the blood in the pulmonary capillaries.

Alveolar Ventilation: Rate at which the alveolar air is renewed each minute by atmospheric air.

Alveoli: Small air sacs in lungs where exchange of gases takes place with the blood found in nearby capillaries.

Amino Acids: Nitrogen-containing substances that are the basic structures of proteins.

Amphetamines: Drugs that are synthesized to produce central nervous system stimulation similar to epinephrine.

Anabolic-Androgenic Steroids: Group of synthetic drugs having an effect on the body to produce male characteristics.

Anabolic Steroid: Drugs that are synthesized to produce the anabolic or growth-stimulating characteristics of the male androgen, testosterone.

Anaerobic: Refers to the absence of oxygen.

Anaerobic Threshold: Situation where metabolic demands of exercise cannot be covered completely by aerobic sources and anaerobic metabolism increases.

Androgenic Hormones: Hormones that affect and increase male sex characteristics.

Androgens: Steroid hormones that affect the male sex characteristics.

Anemia: Low count of red blood cells which limits oxygen transport or reduced hemoglobin concentration.

Angina Pectoris: Severe pain in chest caused by a lack of blood to the heart.

Arteriole: Small artery that controls the flow of blood from the arteries to the tiny capillaries.

Arteriosclerosis: Thickening and hardening of the arteries caused by a loss of elasticity in the arteries.

Arteriovenous Anastomoses: Channels located in the skin that are used for shunting arterial blood directly into the venous system when necessary without passing through the capilliary bed.

Arteriovenous Oxygen Difference (a-$\bar{v}_{O_2}$ diff): Difference in the oxygen content of arterial mixed venous blood.

Artery: Branching tube which carries blood from the heart.

Aspartates: Potassium and magnesium salts of the amino acid called aspartic acid.

ATPase: Enzyme that hydrolyzes ATP.

Atrium: One of the two chambers of the heart which receives blood.

ATP-CP System: Anaerobic energy system which provides the quickest source of ATP for use by muscles when CP is broken down to manufacture ATP.

Axons: Fiber extension from the nerve cell which conducts nerve impulses away from the nerve cell body.

Barometric (Atmospheric) Pressure: Refers to the force per unit area exerted by the earth's atmosphere.

Basal Metabolic Rate (BMR): Refers to the minimal muscle activity and other basic functions necessary for life of an organism.

Beta Oxidation: ATP production from fatty acids that takes place in the mitochondria of the cells.

Biopsy: Process involving the removal and examination of body tissues.

Blood Doping: Injection of either whole blood or packed red blood cells into a participant the day prior to competition in hopes of increasing blood volume and its oxygen-carrying capacity, thus improving endurance performance.

Blood Pressure: Force that moves blood into arteries and drains blood from the arteries as blood moves through the circulatory system.

Body Density: Mass per unit volume determined by dividing body weight measured in the air by the weight of the water displaced.

Bradycardia: Decreased or slower heart rate.

Bradykinin: Substance believed to excite pain nerve endings.

BTPS: Abbreviation for body temperature and pressure, saturated with water vapor used as a reference point for making gas volume corrections.

Buffer: Any compound that lessens the change in pH of a fluid when acids or bases are added.

Calorie: Refers to the amount of heat required to raise the temperature of water 1 degree centigrade.

Calorimeter: Device used to measure the amount of heat a body liberates.

Capillary: Network of small blood vessels located between arteries and veins where materials exchange between blood and tissues.

Carbamino Compound: Products formed from the chemical combination of plasma proteins and/or hemoglobin and carbon dioxide.

Carbohydrate: Basic foodstuff composed of hydrogen, oxygen and carbon which makes up sugars, starches, and cellulose.

Carbohydrate Loading: Diet becomes predominantly carbohydrates three to four days prior to competition.

Carbonic Anhydrase: Enzyme which increases the reaction of carbon dioxide with water.

Cardiac: Relating to the heart.

Cardiac Output: Refers to the amount of blood pumped by the heart in one minute; product of heart rate and stroke volume.

Cardiorespiratory Endurance: Ability of body to take in and distribute adequate amounts of oxygen to working muscles during physical activities.

Cardiovascular: Relating to the heart and blood vessels.

Central Nervous System: The brain and spinal chord.

Cerebellum: Part of brain located near the base of the skull which controls movement.

Cerebral Cortex: Grey matter of the brain which makes up the outer layer of the cerebrum.

Cerebum: Largest part of the brain composed of right and left hemispheres.

Chemoreceptors: Nerve cells that are sensitive to chemicals carried in the blood.

Chloride Shift: Movement of chloride ions to preserve the ionic equilibrium between plasma and red blood cells.

Cholesterol: Fatlike chemical found in all animal tissues.

Cholinesterase: Chemical that breaks down acetycholine.

Chronic: Refers to lasting a long time, even after the immediate stimulus has stopped.

Ciliated Cells: Cells with beating cilia found making up large surfaces of the nasal passages.

Citric Acid Cycle (Krebs Cycle): Metabolic pathway found in mitochondria in which carbon dioxide is produced and hydrogen ions and electrons are removed from carbon atoms.

Collagen: Fibrous protein that makes up a large part of ligaments and tendons.

Concentric Contraction: Shortening of muscle due to muscle contraction.

Conduction: Transfer of heat between objects of different temperatures that are in contact.

Convection: Refers to air blowing over the skin surface which removes air warmed by the body and replaces it with cooler air.

Core Temperature: Body temperature monitored by the hypothalamus and insulated from environmental temperature.

Coronary Arteries: Blood vessels that carry blood away from the heart.

Cortex: Outer covering of the brain.

Cortisol: Hormone produced by the adrenal cortex which causes the conservation of stored carbohydrates.

Creatine Phosphate (Phosphocreatine): Chemical that can give phosphate to ADP to quickly restore ATP in the tissues.

Cristae: Refers to the folding of the inner membrane of the mitochondria.

Cross Bridges: Myosin extensions.

Cross Education: Training of the muscles of one limb causes a significant improvement in the opposite limb.

Cytochromes: Proteins involved in the electron transport system of the mitochondria.

Dehydration: Excessive loss of body water.

Dendrites: Cell body projections which pick up impulse and transmit toward the cell body.

Depolarization: Reduction of the electrical charge across the resting cell membrane.

Diastasis: Period of cardiac cycle when the entire heart is completely relaxed.

Diastole: Resting period of the cardiac cycle.

Diastole Pressure: Minimum level arterial blood pressure falls in the time between successive heartbeats.

Diffusion: Movement of molecules due to their kinetic energy.

Disaccharide: Compound made up of two simple sugars.

Dry Bulb Thermometer: Instrument used to record air temperature.

Dynamic Contraction: Alternation of contracting and relaxing of muscles.

Dysmenorrhea: Painful menstruation.

Eccentric Contraction: During contraction the muscle lengths.

Ectomorphy: Body type having characteristics of linearity and fragility.

Efferent Nerve: Nerve cell that carries motor impulses away from the central nervous system to a response organ.

Efficiency: Expression written as a per cent of total energy used which may be expressed as either gross or net efficiency.
(Gross)—total energy used divided into the total measurable work.
(Net)—total energy used minus the basal requirements divided into the measurable work.

Electrocardiogram (EKG, ECG): Recording on graphic paper showing the spread of the cardiac impulse through the heart.

Electron Transport Chain or System (ETS): Series of chemical reactions in the mitochondria where hydrogen ions and electrons combine with oxygen to form water and ATP is resynthesized.

Endomorphy: Body type having characteristics of roundness and softness.

Enzyme: Protein compound that speeds up a chemical reaction.

Epimysium: Sheath of connective tissue which holds the muscle fibers in bundles.

Epinephrine: Hormone produced by the adrenal gland which stimulates body structures that are not innervated by direct sympathetic fibers.

Ergogenic Aid: Factor that improves work performance.

Estrogen: Female sex hormone responsible for growth of sex organs and secondary sex characteristics as well as cellular proliferation.

Evaporation: Loss of heat due to the conversion of water in sweat to a vapor.

Excitatory Postsynaptic Potential (EPSP): Postsynaptic neuron shows a transient increase in electrical potential from its resting membrane potential.

Exercise Prescription: Advised and directed training program designed to strengthen and condition the body in a safe manner.

Expiratory Reserve Volume (ERV): Amount of air that can be expired after normal expiration.

Extrafusal Fiber: Normal muscle cell.

Extrapyramidal Tracts: All the tracts besides the pyramidal tract itself which transmit motor signals from the cortex to the spinal cord.

Free Fatty-Acid (FFA): Fatty acids that are carried in the blood and are not esterfied to glycerol but combined with proteins in the albumin fraction.

Fatigue: State of decreased capacity for work due to previous work load.

Fast-Twitch Fibers: Muscle fibers with fast contractile characteristics and a low capacity to use oxygen that are used in short burst of activities.

Fat-Soluble Vitamins: Vitamins soluble in solution only when attached to fatty acids.

Functional Residual Capacity (FRC): Amount of air remaining in lungs after an unforced expiration.

Gamma Motor Neuron: Efferent nerve cell that stimulates the ends of an intrafusal muscle fiber.

Glucose: Blood sugar.

Glycerol: Compound composed of three atoms of carbon combined with three hydroxyl groups that combines with fatty acids to form fat.

Glycogen: Common storage form of carbohydrate in muscle and liver.

Glycogen Phosphorylase: enzyme that determines the rate of glycogen breakdown during the early stages.

Glycolysis: Metabolic breakdown of glycogen.

Golgi Tendon Organ: Proprioceptor found within a muscular tendon.

Heat Cramp: Severe pain due to muscular contractions caused by prolonged exposure to environmental heat.

Heat Exhaustion: Extreme fatigue due to prolonged exposure to environmental heat.

Heat Stroke: Serious heat disorder due to overexposure to heat causing high body temperature, dry skin, delerium, or unconsciousness, and sometimes death.

Hematocrit: Percent of blood volume that is made up of red blood cells.

Hemodynamics: Study of the physical laws influencing blood flow.

Hemoglobin: Protein of the red blood cell containing iron and capable of combining with oxygen.

Hering-Breuer Deflation Reflex: Stretch receptors are relieved of stretch and expiration begins.

Hering-Breuer Inflation Reflex: Lungs are protected from overdistention by nerve impulses which inhibit inspiration.

Homeostasis: Striving of the body to maintain physiological stability.

Hormone: Chemical substance secreted by endocrine glands into the blood stream to effect other tissues or organs.

Hypertension: Increased blood pressure.

Hyperthermia: Increased body temperature.

Hypertrophy: Increase in the size of an organ or cell.

Hyperventilation: Increased depth and frequency of breathing resulting in elimination of carbon dioxide.

Hypotension: Decreased blood pressure.

Hypothalamus: Part of the brain that controls many of the pituitary gland hormones.

Hypoxia: Deficiency of oxygen in the blood or tissues.

Inspiratory Capacity: Maximum amount of air inspired from a resting expiratory level.

Inhibitory Postsynaptic Potential (IPSP): Decrease in electrical potential of a post-synaptic neuron from its resting membrane potential.

Inspiratory Reserve Volume (IRV): Amount of air that can be inspired after a normal inspiration.

Intercoastal Muscle: Muscles found between the ribs.

Interneuron (Internuncial Neuron): Nerve cell found between sensory and motor nerve cells.

Intrafusal Fibers: Muscle fibers found within the muscle spindles.

Ion: Electrically charged atom.

Ischemia: Lack of blood flow (thus oxygen) to parts of the body.

Isokinetic Contraction: Muscular contraction in which a muscle puts force against a variable resistance.

Isometric (Static) Contraction: Muscular contraction in which a muscle creates force with no observable movement.

Isotonic Contraction: Muscular contraction in which a muscle creates force against a constant resistance causing either shortening or lengthening movement.

Kilocalorie (kcal): Amount of heat required to raise the temperature of one kilogram of water one degree centigrade.

Kilopond Meter (kpm): Amount of force required to accelerate a mass of one kilogram one meter per second.

Kinase: Enzymes that use ATP as a substrate.

Kinesthesis: Body position awareness.

Krebs Cycle: Enzyme-catalyzed reactions in the mitochondria of cells which causes catabolism of fats, carbohydrates, and proteins to carbon dioxide and water.

Lactate Dehydrogenase (LDH): Enzyme upon which pyruvate is changed to lactate and NADH to NAD^+.

Lactacid Oxygen Debt: Part of the recovery oxygen used to remove accumulated lactic acid from the blood following exercise.

Lactic Acid (Lactate): Final product of anaerobic glycolysis.

Lean body Weight (LBW): Body weight that does not include fat tissue.

Lipid: Fat, triglycerides.

Lipoprotein: Proteins with fatty acid chains attached.

Maximal Oxygen Uptake (Maximal Oxygen Consumption; Maximal Oxygen Intake; Maximal Aerobic Power; V_{O_2} Max.): Maximum amount oxygen that can be consumed per minute.

Maximal Voluntary Ventilation (MVV); Maximal Breathing Capacity (MBC): Maximum volume of air inspired or expired per unit time.

Menstruation: Periodic cycle in the female uterus involving the discharge of the menses.

Mesomorphy: Body type characterized by a square, hard, rugged and prominent muscles.

Metabolism: Total of all the chemical changes in the body that make it possible for cellular function.

METS: (Metabolic Equivalents): Expression used to describe the energy cost of work. One MET represents the net energy cost during rest; two METS corresponds to two times the resting value.

Minerals: Twenty-two metallic elements necessary for cell functioning.

Mitochondria: Structures found in cell cytoplasm that contains the respiratory enzyme systems responsible for ATP formation.

Monosaccharides: Final product of digestion in the form of six carbon atom sugars, glucose, fructose, galactose.

Motor Neuron: Nerve cell which affects muscular contraction.

Monounsaturated: Fat molecule in which the carbon chain contains one double bond

Motor Cortex or Motor Area: Area of cerebral cortex that controls the nerve impulses causing contractions of skeletal muscles.

Motor Endplate: Neuromuscular junction where the motor nerve ending makes contact with the muscular fiber.

Motor Unit: Motor neuron and all the muscle fibers innervated by the motor unit.

Muscle Spindle: Receptor found among the fibers of a skeletal muscle that is stimulated by changes in muscle tension.

Myelinated Nerves: Nerves wrapped by myelin sheaths (Schwann cells) that conduct faster than nonmyelinated in nerves.

Myocardium: Heart muscle.

Myofibril: Active subunit of muscle contraction that is a subdivision of the muscle fiber embedded in the sarcoplasm of a muscle fiber.

Myoglobin: Iron-containing protein responsible for oxygen transport and storage in muscles.

Myoneural (Neuromuscular) Junction: Union of a muscle and its nerve cell, also called motor end plate.

Myosin: Protein that forms the thick filament of the myofibril involved in muscular contraction.

Myosin ATPase: Name given to the part myosin plays in catalyzing the breakdown of ADP and ATP during muscular contraction.

Nicotinamide Adenine Dinucleotide (NAD): Coenzyme that acts as an electron acceptor in many oxidation reactions of energy metabolism and electron donor in reduction reactions.

Noradrenaline (Norepinephine): Hormone secreted by sympathetic nerve endings and the adrenal medulla which increases cardiac function.

Obesity: Excessive amount of body fat.

Osmosis: Diffusion of a solvent through a solvent membrane from a lower to a greater concentration area.

Ossification: Hardening of bone.

Overload Principle: Loading a cell or tissue with more than the usual amount of stress.

Oxidation: Removal of an electron or addition of a proton.

Oxygen Debt: Volume of oxygen used during exercise recovery above what is consumed at rest in the same period.

Oxygen Deficit: Period during exercising when oxygen consumption is below what is needed to supply the ATP required for the exercises.

Oxygen System: Aerobic energy system that produces ATP when food is broken down and provides most of the energy needed for endurance activities.

Oxyhemoglobin (HbO_2): Substance formed when oxygen loosely connects with hemoglobin.

Pacinian Corpuscles: Sense organs whose function is to record pressure on the skin.

Parasympathetic Nervous System: Portion of the autonomic nervous system which functions to maintain homeostatic body conditions.

Partial Pressure: Gas pressure exerted in relation to its concentration in a gas volume.

Perimysium: Connective tissue surrounding a muscle bundle or fasciculus.

Pheripheral Nervous System: Portion of the nervous system outside the brain or spinal cord.

pH: Notation used to indicate the power of the hydrogen ion by giving the degree of acidity or alkalinity of a solution using 7 as neutrality.

Phosopholyphids: Fat found in the body which plays an important role in blood clotting and maintaining the membrane structure of all cells.

Phosphagen: Chemical compounds which refers collectively to ATP and CP.

Phosphocreatine: Compound stored in muscles whose breakdown aids in producing ATP.

Phosphofructokinase: Enzyme causing the conversion of fructose-6-phosphate and ATP to fructose, 1; 6 phosphate and ADP.

Polyunsaturated: Fat molecule in which the carbon chain contains two or more double bonds.

Postsynaptic Membrane: Cell membrane which receives a synaptic input from a membrane.

Power: Amount of work force used per unit of time.

Precapillary Sphincter: Band of smooth muscle that controls the blood flow into the true capillaries.

Pressure Gradient: Process by which gases move from a point of high pressure to one of low pressure.

Presynaptic Membrane: Membrane that covers the terminal housing the neurotransmitter.

Presynaptic Terminal: Nerve ending that has the neurotransmitter.

Proprioceptors: Sensory receptors in muscles, joints, and tendons which send information concerning body position and movements.

Proteins: Compounds composed of chains of amino acids which makes one of the basic foodstuffs.

Pulse: Arterial wall distention which travels as a wave down the arteries.

Pulse Pressure: Difference in the systolic and diastolic blood pressure.

Purkinje Fibers: Excitable heart fibers that conduct impulses along the heart surface from the SA node to the ventricles.

Pyramidal (Corticospinal) Tract: Tract area where impulses from the motor area are sent down to the anterior neurons of the spinal cord.

Pyruvate (Pyruvic Acid): End product of aerobic glycolysis.

Radiation: Transfer of heat by electromagnetic waves.

Reaction Time: Amount of time required to react to a stimulus.

Red Blood Cells: Blood cells that carry hemoglobin and get oxygen from the lungs to the tissues.

Reflex: Response produced automatically by receptor stimulation.

Renshaw Cell: Internunical neuron in the spinal cord which has the ability of synapsing with and inhibiting other motorneurons from coming into play.

Repetition Maximum (RM): Greatest load that can be lifted over a given number of repetitions before fatiguing.

Repolarization: Process of reforming the charged state across a membrane after depolarization has occurred.

Residual Volume (RV): Amount of air that remains in the lungs after the maximum expiration.

Respiratory Exchange Ratio (R, R.Q.): Ratio of the amount of CO_2 produced and the amount of O_2 used for the oxidation of glucose, fatty acids, and proteins.

Respiratory Quotient: See Respiratory Exchange Ratio.

Resting Membrane Potential: Electrical difference across the cell membrane at rest.

Sarcolemma: Membrane of the muscle cell.

Sarcomere: Distance between the functional contractile unit that extends from Z line to Z line.

Sarcoplasm: Protoplasm in the muscle cell.

Sarcoplasmic Reticulum: Endoplasmic reticulum in the muscle cells that deal with calcium release, protein synthesis, glycogen metabolism.

Sarcotubular System: System composed of tubules that aid in transmission of the electrical signal and provides an activating substance for muscle contractile process.

Schwann Cells: Cells that make up the myelin sheath of a nerve cell.

Semipermeable Membrane: Membrane selectively permeable to some but not all substances.

Sensory Nerve: Nerve cells that send impulses from a receptor to the central nervous system.

Sino-Atrial Node (SA Node): Specialized muscle mass known as the "pacemaker" which initiates each heart beat.

Skeletal Muscle: Muscle that attaches to the skeletal system and cause body movement by a shortening or pulling action of muscle on its bony attachment.

Slow-Twitch Fibers: Muscle fibers with slow contractile characteristics and high oxidative capacity associated with endurance-type activities.

Smooth Muscle: Involuntary muscle found in the walls of almost every organ of the body.

Somatotype: Physical classification of the human body.

Spatial Summation: Nerve responsiveness increases due to the additive effect of numerous stimuli.

Specific Gravity: Ratio of the density of an object to the density of water.

Specific Heat: Amount of heat required to raise the temperature of a unit of substance one degree centigrade.

Sphygmomanometer: Instrument designed to measure indirectly the arterial blood pressure.

Starling's Law of the Heart: States the greater the initial length of the cardiac muscle fiber, the stronger the myocardium contraction.

Static Contraction: Muscle tension during contraction is sustained throughout a period of activity.

Steady State: State during which a physiological function remains at a constant value.

Steroid: Substance derived from the male hormone, testosterone which has masculinizing properties.

STPD: Standard temperature, pressure, dry.

Strength: Capacity of a muscle to exert force in one maximum effort.

Stretch Receptors: Refers to the muscle spindle and tendon organ.

Stretch Reflex: Basic neural mechanism for maintenance of muscle tonus.

Stroke Volume: Volume of blood pumped by the left ventricle during one heart beat.

ST Segment: Refers to the repolarization of the ventricles after contraction.

Submaximal Exercise: Rate of exercise that is less than maximum and is expressed as a percentage of maximal rate of oxygen uptake.

Summation: Minimum number of stimuli received from presynaptic terminals to elicit a post-synaptic neuronal discharge.

Sympathetic Nervous System: Thoracolumbar part of the autonomic nervous system.

Synapse: Point at which two neurons are connected.

Systole: Contractile phase of the cardiac cycle.

Systolic Pressure: Highest level of arterial blood pressure during the systolic ejection of blood from the ventricle.

Temporal Summation: Successive discharges from the same presynaptic terminal that are strong enough to cause a neuronal discharge.

Terminal Cisternae: Channels located in the sarcoplasmic reticulum which, along with the T-tubule, make up a structure called a triad.

Testosterone: Male sex hormone having masculinizing properties.

Tidal Volume (TV): Amount of air expired or inspired with each breath.

Total Lung Capacity (TLC): Amount of air in the lungs after maximal inspiration.

Triad: Structure formed where two portions of the sarcoplasmic reticulum come together with a transverse tubule, and it carries the action potential into the myofibrils.

Triglycerides: Three fatty acids on a glycerol molecule.

Tropomyosin: Protein in the muscle associated with muscular contraction by producing an inhibiting effect upon actin-myosin interaction.

Troponin: Protein in the muscle associated with muscle contraction by producing a calcium interaction that releases the inhibition on actin-myosin interaction.

T-Tubules: Sarcolemma tubular invaginations that form a transverse network throughout the muscle fiber.

Unmyelinated Nerves: Nerves where the Schwann cells were present, but did not form multiple wrapping and remain not myelinated.

Valsalva Maneuver: Making a forced expiratory effort against a closed glottis.

Vasoconstriction: Decrease in the diameter of a blood vessel usually resulting in a blood flow reduction.

Vasodilation (Vasodilatation): Increase in the diameter of a blood vessel usually resulting in a blood flow increase.

Vasomotor: Referring to vasoconstriction and vasodilation.

Vein: Vessel of the circulatory system that carries blood toward the heart.

Ventilatory Efficiency: Amount of ventilation necessary per liter of oxygen consumed.

Viscera: Internal organs of the body.

Vital Capacity (VC): Maximum amount of air forced to be expired after a maximal inspiration.

Water-Soluble Vitamins: Vitamins that are soluble in water.

Water Bulb Thermometer: Thermometer with a wetted wick wrapped around the wick that measures temperature by the amount of moisture in the air.

Work: Product of the application of a force through a distance.

INDEX

A-band, 2
Acclimatization
    to altitude, 161-164
    to cold, 150-151
    to heat, 144-146
Acetazolamide, 164
Acetyl molecule, 21
Acetylcholine (Ach), 113-117
Acid-base balance, 70-71
Acids, 70
Actin, 2, 8-12
Actomyosin, 8
Adenosine diphosphate (ADP), 11-12
Adenosine monophosphate (cAMP), 206
Adenosine triphosphate (ATP), 5, 9-12
Adrenergic vasoconstrictor fibers, 101
Aerobic (oxygen) endurance development, 267-282
Aging, 242-252
    cardio-respiratory endurance training program, 247-251
    physiological changes, 243-245
    training adaptation, 246-247
Alcohol, 201
Alkalies, 201
Altitude, 155-166
    acclimatization to, 161
    effects of physical performance on, 156-157
    physiological adaptations to, 157-161
    sickness, 164-165
    training and conditioning, 161-164
Alveolar ventilation, 60
Amino acids, 23, 170
Amphetamines, 202-203
Anabolic steroids, 203-204
Anaerobic endurance development, 267-282
Anaerobic glycolysis, 20
Angina pectoris, 79
Arteriovenous (A-V) anastomoses, 97-98
Arteriovenous oxygen difference (a-$\bar{v}_{O_2}$ diff.), 66, 269
Atrioventricular (A-V) node, 75-76
Aspartic acid salts, 204-205

Barbiturates, 202
Basal metabolic rate (BMR), 42-45, 220-221, 244
Bases, 70-71
Bench-stepping, 28
Benzolamide, 164
Beta oxidation, 22
Bicarbonate ions, 68-71
Bicycle ergometer, 31-32
Blood ammonia, 204-205
Blood doping, 205
Blood flow, 94-109, 281
Blood pressure, 99-100, 102-108
    aerobic training effects on, 269
    and aging, 245-247
    definition of, 99
    factors affecting, 106-107
    of females, 216
    measurement of, 102-104
    responses to exercise, 104-106
    values of arteries, 99
Blood volume, 160, 216, 269
    aerobic training effects, 269
    and altitude, 160
    of females, 216
    values for men and women, 216
Body composition, 185-195
    anthropometric measurements, 194-195
    effects of training on, 272,279
    methods for assessing, 188-195
Body density, 188
Bohr effects, 68
Bone density, 245
Bradykinin, 101
BTPS, 36, 291

Caffeine, 205-206
Calcium, 3, 8-11
Calorimetry, 32-36
    direct, 32
    indirect, 32-36
Capillaries, 97-98, 269

305

Carbaminohemoglobin, 69-70
Carbohydrate, 168, 175, 178-181, 271-272
Carbohydrate loading, 180
Carbon dioxide, 68-70
Carbonic anhydrase enzyme, 69
Cardiac output, 81-83, 160, 217-218, 268-269
Central nervous system (CNS), 110-131
    basal ganglia, 119-120
    cerebellum, 117
    cerebral cortex, 117-118
    cerebrum, 118
    excitation of contraction, 112-113
    motor cortex, 117-118
    motor units, 115-117
    premotor cortex, 117-118
    proprioceptors, 120-124
    reflexes, 124-126, 266
    Renshaw cells, 124
    reticular formation, 120
    sensory cortex, 117-118
    synapse, 113-115
    substantia nigra, 120
    thalamus, 118
Chloride shift, 69
Cholesterol, 272
Cholinergic vasodilator fibers, 101
Cholinesterase, 117
Circulation, 94-109, 281
Citric acid cycle (Krebs cycle or tricarboxylic acid cycle), 21
Coefficient of oxygen utilization, 68
Coenzyme A (CoA), 21-22
Cold acclimatization, 150-151
Countercurrent heat exchange, 148
Creatine phosphate (CP), 17-18
Cross bridges, 2, 8-11
Cross education, 128-129
Cytochromes, 21

Dead space, 60
Diet, see Nutrition
Direct calorimetry, 32
Disaccharides, 168
Dysmenorrhea, 222

Efficiency, 15-17
Electrocardiogram (ECG), 81, 91-92
Electron transport system (respiratory chain), 21
Endurance
    aerobic and anaerobic, 267-283
    local, 257-267
Energy, 14, 17-36, 39-45
    ATP-CP, 17-18
    defined, 14
    and metabolism 18-23
    indirect methods of determining, 39-42
Epimysium, 2
Epinephrine, 136
Ergogenic aids, 200-210
Excitatory post-synaptic potential (EPSP), 115

Fast twitch (FT) muscle fibers, 4-8, 270-271
Fat-soluble vitamins, 171-173
Fatigue, muscular, 281-283
Fats, 21-22, 168-170, 178-181, 244, 271-272
Fatty acids, 169-170
Females, 211-229
    physiological characteristics of, 216-222
        basal metabolic rate, 220
        cardiovascular system, 216-218
        femininity, 224-225
        gynecological factors, 222-223
        heat adaptation, 221-222
        injuries, 225
        male vs female world performance comparisons, 226-228
        respiratory system, 218-220
        response to stress, 225
        trainability of, 226
        training and athletic competition effects on pregnancy, childbirth, and the postpartum period, 223-224
    structural characteristics, 211-216
Flavoprotein, 21
Fructose, 168

Galactose, 168
Gas laws, 62-65
Gas transport, 65-70
Gases, exchange, 62
Glucose, 18-21, 168
Glycerol, 169
Glycogen, 18-21, 168
Glycogen phosphorylase, 5, 20
Glycogenolysis, 20
Glycolysis, 18-21

Heart, 74-93
    aerobic training effects, 268, 273
    cardiac cycle, 79-81
    cardiac hypertrophy, 90
    cardiac output, 81-83
    coronary circulatory system, 78-79
    effects of the aging process, 243-245
    electrocardiogram (ECG), 91-93
    heart volume of men and women, 216
    Starling's law of the heart, 87-88
    stroke volume, 87-90
    structural properties of, 74-79
Heart rate, 83-87
    aerobic training effects, 268, 272-276
    and aging, 245-251
    altitude, 159-160
    factors affecting, 86-87
    female, 216-217
    preadolescent, 233-234
    regulation of, 83-84
    response to exercise, 84-86
Heat acclimatization, 144-146
Hemodynamics, 99-101
Hemoglobin (Hb), 158-159, 216, 269, 273

aerobic training effects, 269, 273
altitude, 158-159
female, 216
values for men and women, 216
Hering-Breuer deflation reflex, 55
Hering-Breuer inflation reflex, 55
Hydrogen atoms, 21
Hypercapnia, 56
Hyperventilation, 38, 281
Hypoxemia, 56
Hypoxia, 160
H-zone, 2-3

I-band, 2-3
Indirect calorimetry, 32-36
closed circuit, 32-34
open circuit, 32-36
Inhibitory post-synaptic potential (IPSP), 115
Intrathoracic pressure, 106, 264-265

Kilocalorie (kcal), 14, 137
Kilopond, 31-32
Krebs cycle (tricarboxylic acid cycle or citric acid cycle), 21
Kymogram, 34

Lactic acid, 38, 270
Lactose, 168
Lean body weight (or "fat-free"), 185-195, 244, 272, 279
Lipase, 21-22
Lung diffusion capacity, 159, 245
Lung ventilation, response to exercise, 58-65
Lungs, 50-73
aerobic training effects, 269
altitude, 157-159
dead space, 60
regulation of, 54-58
respiratory muscles, 52-54
structural properties of, 51-52
volumes and capacities, 60-61

Maltose, 168
Maximal oxygen uptake
aerobic training effects, 270-278
altitude, 159-160
definition of, 219
effects of aging on, 245-246
female, 219-220
preadolescent, 234-235
values for men and women of various sports, 221
Maximal voluntary ventilation (MVV), 219, 235, 244, 246
Menstruation, 222-223
Metabolism, 13-49
definition of, 14
during exercise, 23-28
during recovery, 25-26
during rest, 23
METS, 17
Minerals, 171-174

Mitochondrial, 6, 260
Monosaccharides, 168
Motor units, 115-117
"all-or-none" law, 115-116
definition of, 115
structural properties of, 115-117
Movement time, 126-128, 235
Muscle-biopsy, 179
Muscles
A-band, 2
actin, 2, 8-12, 259-260
actomyosin, 8
adenosine diphosphate (ADP), 11-12
adenosine triphosphase (ATP), 5, 9-12, 260
cardiac, 1
contraction, 9-11
creatine kinase, 260
cross bridges, 2, 8-11
epimysium, 2
fast twitch (FT) muscle fibers, 4-8
fatigue, 281-283
glycogen phosphorylase, 5, 20
glycolytic, 5
hypertrophy, 259, 264
H-zone, 2-3
I-band, 2-3
mitochondrial, 6, 260
muscle-biopsy, 179
myofibrils, 2, 260
myoglobin, 6, 260, 271
myosin, 2, 8-12, 259-260
myosin ATPase, 5
perimysium, 2
phosphofructokinase, 5, 260, 268
respiratory muscles, 52-54
sarcolemma, 2
sarcomere, 2
sarcoplasm, 2
sarcoplasmic recticular tubules (or longitudinal), 2
sarcotubular system, 2
size and strength of during aging, 243-244
skeletal, 1
slow twitch (ST) muscle fibers, 4-8
smooth, 1
strength, 214-216, 257-267, 280
terminal cisternae, 3
triad, 3
tropomyosin, 2
troponin, 2
T-tubules (or transverse), 2-3
Z-line, 2-3
Muscular Fatigue (see muscle fatigue)
Myofibrils, 2, 260
Myoglobin, 6, 260, 271
Myosin, 2, 8-12, 259-260
Myosin ATPase, 5

Neuron (nerve cell), 111-112
Nicotonamide adenine dinucleotide (NAD), 20

Norepinephrine, 136
Nutrition, 167-199
   carbohydrate loading, 180
   carbohydrates, 168
   daily food requirements, 174-175
   diet and performance, 178-183
   essential food groups, 176-177
   fats, 168-170
   minerals, 171, 173-174
   pre-game meal, 177-178
   proteins, 170, 181
   spacing and number of meals, 177
   vitamins, 171-173
   water, 172-174

Oxygen
   aerobic endurance development, 270
   altitude, 159-160
   as an ergogenic aid, 206-207
   coefficient of oxygen utilization, 68
   dissociation curves of hemoglobin, 66-68
   gross oxygen cost of exercise, 39-40
   maximal oxygen uptake, 219, 221, 234-235,
      245-246, 270-278
   net oxygen cost of exercise, 39-40
   oxyhemoglobin, 65-66
   preadolescent oxygen consumption
      responses, 234-235
   pulse, 218
Oxygen debt, 25-28, 281-282
   alactacid, 26-28
   definition of, 25-26
   lactacid, 26-28
   limiting factor in anaerobic endurance,
      281-282

Pacing, 280
Percent Body Fat (see Body Composition)
Perimysium, 2
Peripheral circulatory system, 94-109
pH, 70-71
Phosphodiesterase, 206
Phosphofructokinase, 5, 260, 268
Phosphoric acid, 11
Physical conditioning, see Training
Physical work capacity (P.W.C.), 235
Pneumotaxic reflex, 55
Polysaccharides, 168
Power, 15
Preadolescence, 230-241
   guidelines for competitive sports, 238-239
   injuries, 236-238
   physical growth effects, 231-233
   physiological effects, 233-235
   psychological and emotional effects, 235-236
Proprioceptors, 120-126
   kinesthesis or kinesthetic muscle sense, 121
      Golgi tendon organs, 122
      muscle spindles, 121-122
      Pacinian corpuscle, 122-123
   vestibular apparatus, 123-124
Proteins, 170, 181

Pulmonary ventilation, 58-59
   aerobic training effects, 269, 273
   altitude, 157-158
   definition of and response to exercise, 58-59
Purkinje system, 75-76

Reaction time, 126-128, 235
Reflexes, 124-126, 266
Renshaw cells, 124
Respiration, 50-73
   external or pulmonary ventilation, 50-51
   internal or cellular respiration, 50-51
   regulation of, 54-58
Respiratory chain (electron transport system), 21
Respiratory quotient (R.Q.) or respiratory
      exchange ratio, 36-42

Salt (sodium chloride), 207-208
Sarcolemma, 2
Sarcomere, 2
Sarcoplasm, 2
Sarcoplasmic reticulum tubules (or longitudinal), 2
Sarcotubular system, 2
Saturated fats, see Fatty Acids
Sino-atrial (S-A) node, 75-76
Skill, 280
Skinfold, measurements, 192-194
Sliding filament theory, 8-10
Slow twitch (ST) muscle fibers, 4-8
Somatotyping, 265, 279
Starches, 168
Starling's law of the heart, 87
Steady state, 25
STPD, 36, 289-290
Strength
   development of, 257-265
   effects of aging process on, 243-244, 246
   factors affecting strength and local endurance,
      265-266
   female, 214-216
   retention of, 266-267
   training effects, 280
Stroke volume, 87-89
   aerobic training effects, 268
   altitude, 159-160
   effects of the aging process, 245
   female, 217-218
   regulation of, 87-88
   response to exercise, 88-89
Sucrose, 168
Summation stimuli, 115
Synapse, 113-115
   definition of, 113
   functional characteristics, 114-115
   structural properties of, 113-114
Systemic (or peripheral) circulatory system, 94-109
   regulation of, 101-102
   resistance responses to exercise, 102-106
   resistance to flow, 100-101
   structural properties of, 94-99
   velocity of blood flow, 100

Telemetry, 40-41
Temperature
  age responses to cold acclimatization, 150-151
  diurnal changes, 138
  effects of extreme heat, 143-144
    dehydration, 143
    heat cramps, 143
    heat exhaustion, 144
    heat stroke, 144
  exercise and temperature regulation in cold climates, 148-151
  exercise and temperature regulation in hot climates, 139-143
    hot-humid climates, 141-142
    hot-dry climates, 142-143
  heat acclimatization, 144-146
  individual differences, 139
  measurement of, 136-138
  methods by which heat is lost from the body and gained by the body, 133-135
    conduction, 135
    convection, 133
    evaporation, 133-135
    radiation, 133
  regulation of, 135-136
  sex responses to, 138
Terminal cisternae, 3
Tobacco smoking, 208
Training
  aerobic and anaerobic methods, 272-278
    acceleration sprinting, 277
    continuous fast running, 276
    continuous slow running, 276
    fast interval training, 276-277
    hollow sprints, 277
    interval sprinting, 277
    jogging, 277-278
    repetition running, 277
    repetitions of springs, 276
    slow interval training, 276
    speed play, 277
  of aged, 246-251
  development of aerobic and anaerobic endurance, 267-282
  development of strength and local endurance, 257-265
    eccentric training methods, 262-263
    isokinetic training methods, 263-265
    isometric training methods, 262
    isotonic weight-training methods, 260
    muscular strength, 280
    oxygen debt, 281-282
    pacing, 280
    skill, 280
  factors affecting strength and local endurance, 265-266
    age and sex, 265
    body build, 265
    circulation (affecting local endurance), 266
    muscle length, 266
    nervous system, 265
    strength (affecting local endurance), 266
  female, 223-224, 226
  general principles of, 254-257
    identifying the major energy system(s) involved, 256-257
    individual differences, 255-256
    motivation, 257
    overload principle, 254
    specificity of training, 254-255
  muscular fatigue, 282-283
  physiological adaptations, 267-272
    aerobic endurance changes, 268-272
      blood, 269
      blood distribution, 269
      blood pressure, 269
      capillaries, 269
      cholesterol, 272
      heart rate and heart size, 268
      increased neuromuscular efficiency, 270
      lactic acid, 270
      lungs, 269
      maximal oxygen uptake, 270
      myoglobin, 271
      oxidation of carbohydrates and fats, 271-272
      slow and fast twitch muscle fibers, 270-271
      triglyceride, 272
    anaerobic endurance changes, 268
      increase activity of phosphofructokinase, 268
      increase capacity of ATP-CP system, 268
      increase glycolytic capacity, 268
      increase level of creatine kinase, 268
  relative contributions of the various energy systems during track events, 257
  retention of strength and local endurance, 266-267
  time needed for developing various energy systems of several sports, 258
  various energy systems predominantly needed for selected sports and recreational activities, 256
Treadmill, 28-31
Triad, 3
Tricarboxylic acid (TCA) cycle (also krebs cycle or the citric acid cycle), 21
Triglycerides, 169, 272
Tropomyosin, 2
Troponin, 2
T-Tubules (transverse tubules), 2-3

Underwater weighing, 188-192
Unsaturated and saturated fats, *see* Fatty acids

Vasoconstriction, 101
Vasodilatation, 101
Vital capacity, 61, 218-219, 244
Vitamins, 171-172, 181-183

Water, 172-174, 208-209

Water density, 191
Water-soluble vitamins, 171-173, 182
Weight
    determining desired weight, 195
    making weight for wrestlers, 146-148
    weight-control and exercise, 183-185
Work
    definition of, 15
    determined by bench-stepping, 28
    determined on a bicycle ergometer, 31-32
    determined on a treadmill, 28-31
    negative, 42
Wrestlers, 146-148

Xanthines, 205

Z-line, 2-3